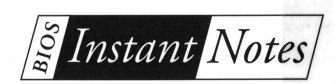

Immunology

Second Edition

BIOS INSTANT NOTES

Series Editor: B. D. Hames, School of Biochemistry and Molecular Biology, University of Leeds, Leeds, UK

Biology

Animal Biology, Second Edition	9781859963258
Biochemistry, Third Edition	9780415367783
Bioinformatics	9781859962725
Chemistry for Biologists, Second Edition	9781859963555
Developmental Biology	9781859961537
Ecology, Second Edition	9781859962572
Genetics, Third Edition	9780415376198
Human Physiology	9780415355469
Immunology, Second Edition	9781859960394
Mathematics & Statistics for Life Scientists	9781859962923
Medical Microbiology	9781859962541
Microbiology, Third Edition	9780415390880
Molecular Biology, Third Edition	9780415351676
Motor Control and Development	9780415391399
Neuroscience, Second Edition	9780415351881
Plant Biology, Second Edition	9780415356435
Sport & Exercise Biomechanics	9781859962848
Sport & Exercise Physiology	9781859962497

Chemistry

Analytical Chemistry	9781859961896
Inorganic Chemistry, Second Edition	9781859962893
Medicinal Chemistry	9781859962077
Organic Chemistry, Second Edition	9781859962640
Physical Chemistry	9781859961940

Psychology
Sub-series Editor: Hugh Wagner, Dept of Psychology, University of Central Lancashire, Preston, UK

Cognitive Psychology	9781859962237
Physiological Psychology	9781859962039
Psychology	9781859960974
Sport & Exercise Psychology	9781859962947

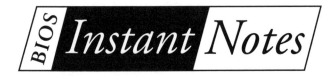

Immunology

Second Edition

Peter M Lydyard

Department of Immunology and Molecular Pathology,
Royal Free and University College Medical School,
University College London, London, UK

Alex Whelan

Department of Immunology, Trinity College and
St James' Hospital, Dublin, Ireland

and

Michael W Fanger

Department of Microbiology and Immunology,
Dartmouth Medical School,
Lebanon, New Hampshire, USA

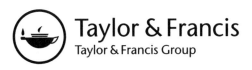
Taylor & Francis
Taylor & Francis Group

Published by:
Taylor & Francis Group
In US: 270 Madison Avenue
           New York, NY 10016
In UK: 2 Park Square, Milton Park
           Abingdon, OX14 4RN

© 2004 by Taylor & Francis Group

Reprinted in 2005, 2007

10-digit ISBN: 1-8599-6039-1
13-digit ISBN: 978-1-85996-039-4

This book contains information obtained from authentic and highly regarded sources. Reprinted material is quoted with permission, and sources are indicated. A wide variety of references are listed. Reasonable efforts have been made to publish reliable data and information, but the author and the publisher cannot assume responsibility for the validity of all materials or for the consequences of their use.

A catalog record for this book is available from the British Library.

Editor: Elizabeth Owen
Production Editor: Andrew Watts
Typeset by: Phoenix Photosetting, Chatham, Kent, UK
Printed by: Cromwell Press

Front cover: Confocal images of human dendritic cells stained by immunofluorescence for mannose receptors (green), HLA Class 1 (red) and colocalisation (yellow). Image kindly supplied by John Connolly, PhD.

Printed on acid-free paper

10 9 8 7 6 5 4 3

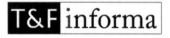

Taylor & Francis Group
is the Academic Division of T&F Informa plc.   Visit our web site at http://www.garlandscience.com

CONTENTS

Abbreviations		viii
Preface		x
Key to cell symbols		xi

Section A – Overview of the immune system
A1	The need	1
A2	External defenses	2
A3	Immune defense	5
A4	Antigens	9
A5	Hemopoiesis – development of blood cells	12

Section B – Cells and molecules of the innate immune system
B1	Cells of the innate immune system	15
B2	Molecules of the innate immune system	23
B3	Recognition of microbes by the innate immune system	33
B4	Innate immunity and inflammation	36

Section C – The adaptive immune system
C1	Lymphocytes	41
C2	Lymphoid organs and tissues	48
C3	Mucosa-associated lymphoid tissues	53
C4	Lymphocyte traffic and recirculation	56
C5	Adaptive immunity at birth	59

Section D – Antibodies
D1	Antibody structure	61
D2	Antibody classes	65
D3	Generation of diversity	68
D4	Allotypes and idiotypes	78
D5	Monoclonal antibodies	80
D6	Antigen/antibody complexes (immune complexes)	83
D7	Immunoassay	87
D8	Antibody functions	93

Section E – The antibody response
E1	The B cell receptor complex, co-receptors and signaling	99
E2	B cell activation	102
E3	The cellular basis of the antibody response	108
E4	Antibody responses in different tissues	112

Section F – The T cell response – cell-mediated immunity
F1	The role of T cells in immune responses	115
F2	T cell recognition of antigen	117
F3	Shaping the T cell repertoire	124
F4	T cell activation	127

F5   Clonal expansion and development of effector function   132
F6   Cell-mediated immunity in context   138

Section G – Regulation of the immune response
G1   Overview   141
G2   Central and peripheral tolerance   145
G3   Acquired tolerance   149
G4   Regulation by antigen and antibody   152
G5   Genes, T helper cells, cytokines and the neuroendocrine
      system   155

Section H – Immunity to infection
H1   The microbial cosmos   159
H2   Immunity to different organisms   162
H3   Pathogen defense strategies   167

Section I – Vaccination
I1   Principles of vaccination   171
I2   Immunization   174
I3   Antigen preparations   177
I4   Vaccines to pathogens and tumors   181

Section J – Immunodeficiency – when the immune system fails
J1   Deficiencies in the immune system   183
J2   Primary/congenital (inherited) immunodeficiency   185
J3   Secondary (acquired) immunodeficiency   189
J4   Diagnosis and treatment of immunodeficiency   192

Section K – Hypersensitivity – when the immune system overreacts
K1   Definition and classification   197
K2   IgE-mediated (type I) hypersensitivity: allergy   199
K3   IgG and IgM-mediated (type II) hypersensitivity   204
K4   Immune-complex-mediated (type III) hypersensitivity   208
K5   Delayed (type IV) hypersensitivity   210

Section L – Autoimmunity and autoimmune diseases
L1   The spectrum and prevalence of autoimmunity   215
L2   Factors contributing to the development of autoimmune
      disease   217
L3   Autoimmune diseases – mechanisms of development   222
L4   Disease pathogenesis – effector mechanisms   227
L5   Diagnosis and treatment of autoimmune disease   231

Section M – Transplantation
M1   The transplantation problem   235
M2   Transplantation antigens   237
M3   Rejection mechanisms   240
M4   Prevention of graft rejection   243

Section N – Tumor immunology

N1	Origin and host defense against tumors	249
N2	Tumor antigens	250
N3	Immune responses to tumors	253
N4	Immunodiagnosis	256
N5	Cytokine and cellular immunotherapy of tumors	259
N6	Immunotherapy of tumors with antibodies	262
N7	Tumor vaccines	266

Section O – Gender and the immune system

O1	Overview	269
O2	Immune cells and molecules associated with the reproductive tracts	271
O3	Functional effects of sex hormones on the immune system	279

Section P – Aging and the immune system (immunosenescence)

P1	Overview	283
P2	Developmental changes in primary lymphoid tissue and lymphocytes with age	285
P3	Effects of aging on innate immunity	288
P4	The effects of aging on T cell immunity	290
P5	The effects of aging on humoral immunity	292
P6	Immunosenescence and morbidity, mortality and longevity	294

Further reading	297
Multiple Choice Questions	299
Appendix I – Selected CD molecules	315
Appendix II – The principal cytokines	317
Glossary	319
Index	325

ABBREVIATIONS

5HT	5'hydroxytryptamine
ADA	adenosine deaminase
ADCC	antibody-dependent cell/cellular cytotoxicity
AFP	alpha-fetoprotein
AICD	activation-induced cell death
AIDS	acquired immune deficiency syndrome
AIHA	autoimmune hemolytic anemia
BALT	bronchus-associated lymphoid tissue
BCR	B cell receptor
CEA	carcinoembryonic antigen
CGD	chronic granulomatous disease
CMV	cytomegalovirus
CRD	carbohydrate recognition domain
CRH	corticotrophin-releasing hormone
CRP	C-reactive protein
CTL	cytolytic/cytotoxic T lymphocyte
CVID	common variable immunodeficiency
DAF	decay-accelerating factor
DAG	diacyl glycerol
DC	dendritic cell
DHEA	dehydroepiandrosterone
DHEAS	dehydroepiandrosterone sulfate
DTH	delayed-type hypersensitivity
EAE	experimental allergic encephalomyelitis
EBV	Epstein–Barr virus
ELISA	enzyme-linked immunosorbent assay
ER	endoplasmic reticulum
FDC	follicular dendritic cell
FRT	female reproductive tract
GALT	gut-associated lymphoid tissue
GC	germinal center
G-CSF	granulocyte colony-stimulating factor
GI	gastrointestinal
GOD	generation of diversity
HAMA	human anti-mouse antibody
HBV	hepatitis B virus
HEV	high endothelial venules
HHV8	human herpes virus 8
HIV	human immunodeficiency virus
HLA	human leukocyte antigen
HPA	hypothalamus/pituitary/adrenal
HPV	human papilloma virus
HSC	hemopoietic stem cell
HTLV	human T cell leukemia virus
IDC	interdigitating cell
IEL	intraepithelial lymphocyte
IF	immunofluorescence
IFN	interferon
IL	interleukin
ITAM	immunoreceptor tyrosine-based activation motif
ITIM	immunoreceptor tyrosine-based inhibitory motif
ITP	immune thrombocytopenic purpura
KAR	killer activation receptor
KIR	killer inhibitory receptor
LAK	lymphokine-activated killer
LCMV	lymphocytic choriomeningitis virus
LFA	leukocyte function antigen
LGL	large granular lymphocyte
LH	Langerhans cell
LP	late proliferative
LPS	lipopolysaccharide
LRR	leucine-rich repeat
LS	late secretory
LSC	lymphoid stem cells
MAC	membrane attack complex
MALT	mucosa-associated lymphoid tissue
MBP	mannose-binding protein
MCP	membrane co-factor protein
M-CSF	monocyte/macrophage colony-stimulating factor
MDP	muramyl dipeptide
MHC	major histocompatibility complex
MØ	macrophage
MS	multiple sclerosis
MZ	marginal zone
NALT	nasal-associated lymphoid tissue
NBT	nitroblue tetrazolium test
NK	natural killer
NO	nitric oxide
NSAID	nonsteroidal anti-inflammatory drugs
PAF	platelet-activating factor
PALS	periarteriolar lymphoid sheath
PCR	polymerase chain reaction
PMN	polymorphonuclear cell

PRR	pattern recognition receptor	SV	splenic vein
PS	phosphatidyl serine	TAA	tumor-associated antigens
PSA	prostate-specific antigen	TBII	thyrotropin-binding inhibitory
RAST	radioallergosorbent test		immunoglobulin
RFLP	restriction fragment length	TCR	T cell antigen receptor
	polymorphism	TGF	transforming growth factor
RIA	radioimmunoassay	TGSI	thyroid growth-stimulating
RP	red pulp		immunoglobulin
SAA	serum amyloid protein A	TIL	tumor-infiltrating lymphocyte
SCF	stem cell factor	TLR	Toll-like receptor
SCID	severe combined immunodeficiency	TNF	tumor necrosis factor
SDS-PAGE	sodium dodecyl sulfate-	TSA	tumor-specific antigen
	polyacrylamide gel electrophoresis	TSH	thyroid-stimulating hormone
SE	staphylococcal enterotoxins	TSST	toxic shock syndrome toxin
SLE	systemic lupus erythematosus	VIP	vasoactive intestinal peptide
SR	scavenger receptor		

PREFACE

Immunology as a science probably began with the observations by Metchnikoff in 1882 that starfish when pierced by a foreign object (a rose thorn) responded by coating it with cells (later identified as phagocytes). Immunology – the study of the way in which the body defends itself against invading organisms or internal invaders (tumors) – has developed rapidly over the last 40 years, and particularly during the last 10 years with the advent of molecular techniques. It is now a rapidly moving field that is contributing critical tools for research and diagnosis, and therapeutics for treatment of a wide range of human diseases. Thus, it is an integral part of college life science courses and medical studies.

In this second edition, we have: (i) updated all of the material presented, including more figures and tables; (ii) modified the presentation of the material to enhance its continuity; and (iii) added additional sections on Aging and Gender, topics that are essential to a comprehensive understanding of immune defense. Of particular note, these changes have significantly enhanced the continuity of presentation of the material, creating a flow of information optimal for original presentation and teaching of Immunology. In so doing, we have not only maintained but increased the value of this book in revision.

For ease of understanding, we have divided the subject matter in this book into six main areas:

1. Cellular and molecular components of the Immune System (Sections A–D).
2. Mechanisms involved in the development of Immunity (Sections E–G) – antibody and cellular responses and their regulation.
3. The Immune System in action (Section H–I) – immunity to infection and vaccination.
4. Diseases and deficiencies of the Immune System (Sections J–L) – allergy, autoimmunity and congenital and acquired immune deficiency.
5. The Immune Response to tumors and transplants (Sections M, N).
6. The influence of Gender and Aging on the Immune Response (Sections O, P).

Finally, we have added Appendices for **CD molecules** and for **Cytokines** and have included a **Glossary**. These should provide resources for rapidly identifying important molecules and concepts in Immunology.

In order to test your understanding of the subject, we have included 125 multiple choice questions with answers at the back of the book. These questions are in the format used in the US National Boards (USMLE) Step 1, and in degree courses in the UK.

We would like to acknowledge the help of Dr Michael Cole and Dr Peter Delves for looking at sections of the manuscript, and in particular, Professor Paul Guyre who helped enormously with advice and support on the whole manuscript. We also thank Professor Randy Noelle who allowed us to use diagrams and tables he currently uses in teaching and Professor Eamon Sweeney for his helpful suggestions. Finally, we would like to thank our wives, Meriel, Annette and Sharon for support and understanding during preparation of the book.

KEY TO CELL SYMBOLS

Lymphocyte

Monocyte

Polymorphonuclear phagocyte (PMN)

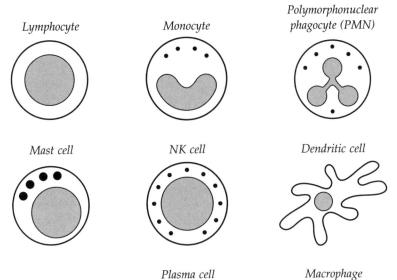

Mast cell

NK cell

Dendritic cell

Plasma cell

Macrophage

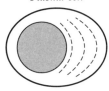

A1 THE NEED

Key Note

The ubiquitous enemy	Infectious microbes and larger organisms such as worms are present in our environment. They range from being helpful (e.g. *E. coli*) to being major pathogens which can be fatal (e.g. HIV).
Related topic	The microbial cosmos (H1)

The ubiquitous enemy

Microbes are able to survive on animal and plant products by releasing digestive enzymes directly and absorbing the nutrients, and/or by growth on living tissues (extracellular), in which case they are simply bathed in nutrients. Other microbes infect (invade and live within) animal/human cells (intracellular), where they not only survive, but also replicate utilizing host-cell energy sources. Both extracellular and intracellular microbes can grow, reproduce and infect other individuals. There are many different species of microbes and larger organisms (such as worms) that invade humans, some of which are relatively harmless and some even helpful (e.g. *E. coli* in the intestines). Many others cause disease (human pathogens). There is a constant battle between invading microbes and the immune system (Topic H2). Some microbes can even cause the death of their hosts, although most successful microbes do not have this property. Table 1 shows the range of organisms that can infect humans.

Table 1.   Range of infectious organisms

Worms (helminths)	e.g. tapeworms, filaria
Protozoans	e.g. trypanosomes, leishmania, malaria
Fungi	e.g. Candida, aspergillus
Bacteria	e.g. *Bacteroides, Staphylococcus, Streptococcus*, mycobacteria
Viruses	e.g. polio, pox viruses, influenza, hepatitis B, HIV

A2 EXTERNAL DEFENSES

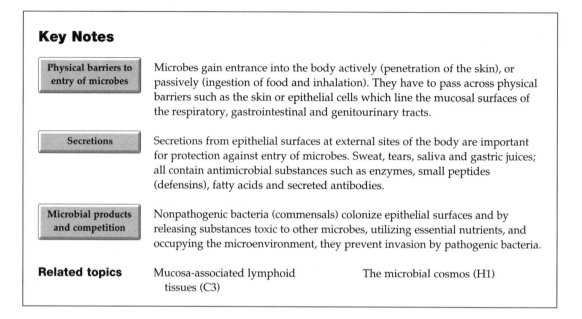

Key Notes

Physical barriers to entry of microbes	Microbes gain entrance into the body actively (penetration of the skin), or passively (ingestion of food and inhalation). They have to pass across physical barriers such as the skin or epithelial cells which line the mucosal surfaces of the respiratory, gastrointestinal and genitourinary tracts.
Secretions	Secretions from epithelial surfaces at external sites of the body are important for protection against entry of microbes. Sweat, tears, saliva and gastric juices; all contain antimicrobial substances such as enzymes, small peptides (defensins), fatty acids and secreted antibodies.
Microbial products and competition	Nonpathogenic bacteria (commensals) colonize epithelial surfaces and by releasing substances toxic to other microbes, utilizing essential nutrients, and occupying the microenvironment, they prevent invasion by pathogenic bacteria.
Related topics	Mucosa-associated lymphoid tissues (C3) The microbial cosmos (H1)

Physical barriers to entry of microbes

Before a microbe or parasite can invade the host and cause infection, it must first attach to and penetrate the surface epithelial layers of the body. Organisms gain entrance into the body by active or passive means. For example, they might burrow through the skin, or be ingested in food, inhaled into the respiratory tract or penetrate through an open wound. In practice, most microbes take advantage of the fact that we have to breathe and eat, and therefore enter the body through the respiratory and gastrointestinal tracts. Whatever their point of entry, they have to pass across physical barriers such as the dead layers of the skin or living epithelial cell layers which line the cavities in contact with the exterior such as the respiratory, genitourinary or gastrointestinal tracts. In fact, the main entry of microbes into the body is via these tracts.

Many of the cells at the interface with the outside world are mucosal epithelial cells which secrete mucus. In addition to providing a physical barrier, these cells have other properties useful in minimizing infection. For example, epithelial cells of the nasal passages and bronchi of the respiratory system have **cilia** (small hair-like structures) that beat in an upward direction to help remove microorganisms that enter during breathing. This is the **mucociliary escalator** (*Fig. 1*).

Secretions

A variety of secretions at epithelial surfaces are important in defense (*Table 1*), as they help to create a hostile environment for microbial habitation. Some substances are known to directly kill microbes, e.g. lysozyme digests proteoglycans in bacterial cell walls; others compete for nutrients (e.g. transferrin, Fe), and others interfere with ion transport (e.g. NaCl). Mucus (containing mucin)

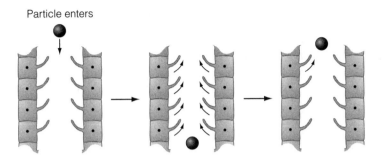

Fig.1. *The mucociliary escalator. When a particle is inhaled, it comes into contact with cilia of the bronchial or nasal epithelia which beat in an upwards direction to a position where the particle can be coughed up or sneezed out.*

Table 1. *Secretions at epithelial surfaces*

Site	Source	Specific substances secreted
Eyes	Lacrimal glands (tears)	Lysozyme, IgA and IgG
Ears	Sebaceous glands	Oily, waxy secretion, fatty acids
Mouth	Salivary glands (saliva)	Digestive enzymes, lysozyme, IgA, IgG, lactoferrin
Skin	Sweat glands (sweat) Sebaceous glands	Lysozyme, high NaCl, short chain fatty acids Oily secretion and fatty acids (sebum)
Stomach	Gastric juices	Digestive enzymes (pepsin, rennin), acid (low pH, 1–2)

secreted by the mucosal epithelial cells coats their surfaces and makes it difficult for microbes to contact and bind to these cells – a prerequisite for entry into the body.

The washing action of tears, saliva and urine also helps to prevent attachment of microbes to the epithelial surfaces. In addition, IgA **antibodies** in tears and saliva prevent the attachment of microbes. These antibodies are also secreted across epithelial cells in the respiratory, gastrointestinal and genitourinary tracts.

Gastrointestinal, respiratory epithelia and phagocytes throughout the body are also known to produce a number of small peptides which have potent antibacterial properties (**peptide antibiotics**). These peptides have molecular weights of 3–5 kDa and include cecropins, magainins and defensins. They are part of the body's innate defense mechanisms and are highly conserved throughout species, probably representing one of the most primitive defense mechanisms against microbes. Although their mechanisms of action are different, these peptides are effective against both Gram-positive and Gram-negative bacteria. Whereas **cecropins** and **magainins** cause lysis, others interfere with ion transport. Secretion of these peptides is upregulated as a result of bacterial infection.

Microbial products and competition

Normal commensals (**nonpathogenic bacteria**) are also important in protection from infection. These nonpathogenic microorganisms are found on the skin, in the mouth and in the reproductive and gastrointestinal tract. The gastrointestinal tract contains many billions of bacteria that have a symbiotic relationship with the host. These bacteria help to prevent pathogens from colonizing the site, by preventing attachment, by competing for essential nutrients and by releasing antibacterial substances such as **colicins** (antibacterial proteins) and short-chain fatty acids. Gut flora also perform such house-keeping duties as further degrading waste matter and helping gut motility. Normal microbial flora occupying the site of entry (e.g. throat and nasal passages) of other microbes probably function in a similar manner. Some bacteria such as lactobacilli, which inhabit the vagina, cause their environment to become acidic (pH 4.0–4.5) which probably discourages the growth of many microbes.

A3 IMMUNE DEFENSE

Key Notes

The immune system

The immune system protects us from attack by microbes and worms. It uses specialized organs designed to filter out and respond to microbes entering the body's tissues and a mobile force of molecules and cells in the bloodstream to respond rapidly to attack. The system can fail, giving rise to immunodeficiency, or 'over-react' against foreign microbes giving rise to tissue damage (immunopathology). It has complex and sophisticated mechanisms to regulate it.

Innate versus adaptive immunity

The innate immune system is the first line of defense against infection. It works rapidly, gives rise to the acute inflammatory response, and has some specificity for microbes, but no memory. In contrast, the adaptive immune system takes longer to develop, is very highly specific, and remembers that it has encountered a microbe previously (i.e. shows memory).

Interaction between innate and adaptive immunity

The innate and adaptive immune systems work together through direct cell contact and through interactions involving chemical mediators, cytokines and chemokines. Moreover, many of the cells and molecules of the innate immune system are also used by the adaptive immune system.

Adaptive immunity and clonal selection

All immunocompetent individuals have many distinct lymphocytes, each of which is specific for a different foreign substance (antigen). When an antigen is introduced into an individual, lymphocytes with receptors for this antigen seek out and bind it and are triggered to proliferate and differentiate, giving rise to clones of cells specific for the antigen. These cells or their products specifically react with the antigen to neutralize or eliminate it. The much larger number of antigen-specific cells late in the immune response is responsible for the 'memory' involved in adaptive immunity.

T and B cells and cell cooperation

There are two major types of lymphocytes, B cells and T cells. T cells mature under the influence of the thymus and, on stimulation by antigen, give rise to cellular immunity. B cells mature mainly under the influence of bone marrow and give rise to humoral immunity, immunity that involves production of soluble molecules – immunoglobulins. Interactions between T and B cells, as well as between T cells and antigen-presenting cells, are critical to the development of specific immunity.

Related topics

The adaptive immune system (C)
Antibodies (D)
The cellular basis of the antibody response (E3)
The T cell response – cell-mediated immunity (F)

Regulation of the immune response (G)
Immunity to infection (H)

The immune system

The immune system is composed of a number of different cell types, tissues and organs. Many of these cells are organized into separate lymphoid organs or glands (Topic C2). Since attack from microbes can come at many different sites of the body, the immune system has a mobile force of cells in the bloodstream that are ready to attack the invading microbe wherever it enters the body. Although many of the cells of the immune system are separate from each other, they maintain communication through cell contact and molecules secreted by them. For this reason the immune system has been likened to the nervous system. Again like the other body systems, the immune system is only apparent when it goes wrong. This can lead to severe, sometimes overwhelming infections and even death. One form of dysfunction is **immunodeficiency** which can result from infection with the human immunodeficiency virus (HIV) causing AIDS. On the other hand, the immune system can be 'hypersensitive' to a microbe (or even to a substance such as pollen) and this itself can cause severe tissue damage sometimes leading to death. Thus, the immune system must strike a balance between producing a life-saving response and a response that causes severe tissue damage. This regulation is maintained by cells and molecules of the immune system and from without by nonimmune cells, tissues and their products (Section G).

Innate versus adaptive immunity

Having penetrated the external defenses, microbes come into contact with cells and products of the immune system and the battle commences. A number of cell types and defense molecules are usually present at the site of invasion or migrate (**home**) to the site. This 'first line of defense' is the '**innate immune system**'. It is present at birth and changes little throughout the life of the individual. The cells and molecules of this innate system are mainly responsible for the first stages of expulsion of the microbe and may give rise to inflammation (Topic B4). Some of the most important cells in the innate immune system are phagocytes, since they are able to ingest and kill microbes.

The second line of defense is the '**adaptive immune system**', which is brought into action even as the innate immune system is dealing with the microbe, and especially if it is unable to remove the invading microbe. The key difference between the two systems is that the adaptive system shows far more specificity and remembers that a particular microbe has previously invaded the body. This leads to a more rapid expulsion of the microbe on its second and third time of entry. The cells, molecules and characteristics of innate and adaptive immune systems are shown in *Table 1*.

Table 1. The innate and adaptive immune systems

Characteristics	Cells	Molecules
Innate immunity		
Responds rapidly	Phagocytes (PMNs and macrophages)	Cytokines
Has some specificity	Natural killer cells	Complement
No memory	Mast cells	Acute phase proteins
	Dendritic cells	
Adaptive immunity		
Slow to start		
Highly specific	T and B cells	Antibodies
Memory		Cytokines

Interaction between innate and adaptive immunity

Although innate and adaptive immunity are often considered separately for convenience and to facilitate their understanding, it is important to recognize that they frequently work together. For example, macrophages are phagocytic but produce important **cytokines** (Topic B2) that help to induce the adaptive immune response. Complement components of the innate immune system can be activated directly by microbes, but can also be activated by antibodies, molecules of the adaptive system. The various cells of both systems work together through direct contact with each other, and through interactions with chemical mediators, the cytokines and chemokines (Topic B2). These chemical mediators can either be cell bound or released as localized **hormones**, acting over short distances. Cells of both systems have a large number of surface receptors: some are involved in adhesion of the cells to blood endothelial walls (e.g. leukocyte function antigen – LFA-1), some recognize chemicals released by cells (e.g. complement, cytokine and chemokine receptors) and others trigger the function of the cell such as activation of the phagocytic process.

Adaptive immunity and clonal selection

All immunocompetent individuals have many distinct lymphocytes. Each of these cells is specific for a different foreign substance (**antigen**). This specificity results from the fact that each lymphocyte possesses cell surface receptors all of which are specific for a particular antigen. When this antigen is introduced into an individual, lymphocytes with appropriate receptors seek out and bind the antigen and are triggered to proliferate and differentiate into the effector cells of immunity (i.e., they give rise through division to large numbers of cells). All members of this **clone** of cells are specific for the antigen initially triggering the response and they, or their products, are capable of specifically reacting with the antigen or the cells that produce it and to mediate its elimination. In addition, there are a much larger number of cells specific for the immunizing antigen late in the immune response. These cells are able to respond faster to antigen challenge giving rise to the '**memory**' involved in immunity. That is, individuals do not usually get infected by the same organism twice, as their immune system remembers the first encounter and protects against a second infection by the same organism. Of particular importance, all immunocompetent individuals have developed enough different specific lymphocytes to react with virtually every antigen with which an individual may potentially come in contact. How this diversity is developed is considered in Topic D3.

Clonal selection as it applies to the B cell system is shown in *Fig. 1* and is presented in more detail in Topic E3. In particular, when antigen is introduced into an individual, B cells with receptors for that antigen bind and internalize it and receive help from T cells (Topic F5). These B cells are triggered to proliferate, giving rise to clones of daughter cells. Some of these cells serve as memory cells, others differentiate and become **plasma cells** (Topic C1) which make and secrete large quantities of specific antibody.

T and B cells and cell cooperation

The lymphocytes selected for clonal expansion are of two major types, B cells and T cells, each giving rise to a different form of immunity. T lymphocytes mature under the influence of the thymus and, on stimulation by antigen, give rise to cellular immunity. B lymphocytes mature mainly under the influence of bone marrow and give rise to lymphoid populations which, on contact with antigen, proliferate and differentiate into **plasma cells**. These plasma cells make a humoral factor (**antibody = immunoglobulin**) which is specific for the antigen and able to neutralize and/or eliminate it.

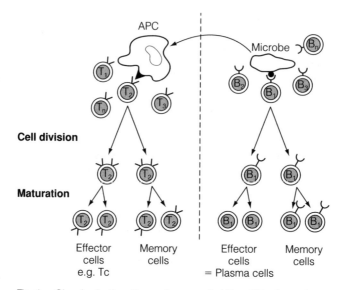

Fig. 1. Clonal selection. From a large pool of B and T cells, antigen selects those which have receptors for it (e.g. T2 and B1) and stimulates their expansion and differentiation into memory and effector cells. Although B cells can recognize and bind native antigen, T cells only see antigen associated with MHC molecules on antigen presenting cells (APC).

The development of the immune response to an antigen also requires cell co-operation. T and B cell populations, as well as antigen-presenting cells, interact in the development of specific immunity. In particular, subpopulations of T cells regulate (e.g. help) humoral and cellular immune responses. Although immune responses to most antigens (especially proteins) require cell cooperation, some antigens (**T-independent**) are able to initiate an immune response in the absence of T lymphocytes.

A4 ANTIGENS

Key Notes

Range of antigens	Antigens are defined as substances which induce an immune response. They include proteins, carbohydrates, lipids and nucleic acids. Microbes have many different antigens which can be recognized by the immune system.
Antigen structure	Antigens may contain a number of different antigenic determinants to which individual antibodies or T cell responses are made. The smallest unit (antigenic determinant) to which an antibody can be made is about three to six amino acids or about five to six sugar residues. All large molecules are multideterminant. Antibodies bind to conformational antigenic determinants (dependent on folding of the molecule) while T cell receptors recognize linear amino acid sequences. Molecules which can stimulate an immune response ('immunogens') can be distinguished from those that react with antibodies but cannot initiate an immune response (haptens or individual antigenic determinants).
Related topics	The B cell receptor complex, co-receptors and signaling (E1) T cell recognition of antigen (F2) Transplantation antigens (M2)

Range of antigens The first stage of removing an invading organism is to recognize it as being foreign, i.e. not 'self' (Sections E and F). The immune system sees the invader as having a number of antigens. An antigen is any substance which induces an immune response resulting in proliferation of lymphocytes and production of antibodies specific for the antigen introduced. This usually includes proteins, carbohydrates, lipids and nucleic acids. Responses can be made to virtually anything. Even self molecules or cells can act as antigens under appropriate conditions, although this is quite well regulated in normal healthy individuals (Section G).

Antigen structure On the structural level, an antigen must be sufficiently unique for the immune system to make an immune response to it. It is usual that an antigen, a molecule which is antigenic, possesses several unique molecular structures, each of which can elicit an immune response. Thus, antibodies or cells produced against an antigen are not directed against the whole molecule but against different parts of the molecule. These 'antigenic determinants' or 'epitopes' (*Fig. 1*) are the smallest unit of an antigen to which an antibody or cell can bind. For a protein, an antibody binds to a unit which is about three to six amino acids whilst for a carbohydrate it is about five to six sugar residues. Therefore, most large molecules possess many antigenic determinants per molecule, i.e. they are 'multideterminant'. However, these determinants may be identical or different from each other on the same molecule. For example, a carbohydrate with repeating sugar units will have several identical determinants, while a large

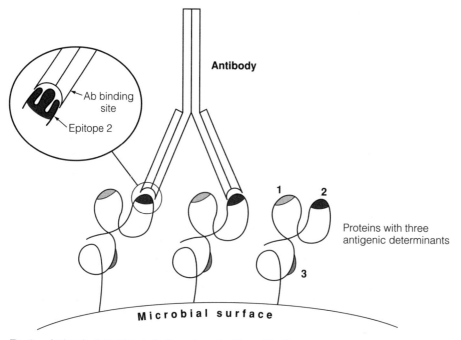

Fig. 1.   Antigenic determinants (epitopes) required by antibodies.

single chain protein will usually not have repeating 3–5 amino acid sequences, and will thus have many different antigenic determinants.

Although the linear sequence of the residues in a molecule has been equated with an antigenic determinant, the physical structures to which antibodies bind are primarily the result of the conformation of the molecule. As a result of folding, residues at different parts of the molecule may be close together and may be recognized by a B cell receptor or an antibody as part of the same determinant (*Fig. 1*). Thus, antibodies made against the native (natural) conformation of a molecule will not, in most instances, react with the denatured molecule even though the primary sequence has not changed. This is in contrast to the way in which T cell receptors recognize antigenic determinants – in the form of linear amino acid sequences (Topic F2) which have to be presented by MHC molecules (*Fig. 2*).

In practical terms, microbes have a large number of different molecules and therefore potentially many different antigenic determinants all of which could stimulate an immune response. However, all antigenic determinants are not

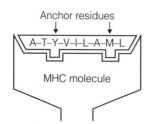

Fig. 2.   Linear sequence of peptides recognized by T cells.

equal, some may elicit strong and others weak responses. This is determined by the health, age and genetics of the individual (Topics G4 and G5).

Very small molecules which can be viewed as single antigenic determinants are incapable of eliciting an antibody response. These **haptens**, as they are called, can be attached covalently to larger molecules (**carriers**) and in this physical form can, with the help of T cells, induce the formation of antibodies. Therefore, one can distinguish between molecules which can stimulate an immune response (**immunogens**) and those which react with antibodies but cannot initiate an immune response (haptens or individual antigenic determinants).

A5   HEMOPOIESIS – DEVELOPMENT OF BLOOD CELLS

Key Notes

A common stem cell	The majority of the cell types involved in the immune system are produced from a common hemopoietic stem cell (HSC). HSC are found in the fetal liver, fetal spleen and neonate and adult bone marrow. They differentiate into functionally mature cells of all blood lineages.
Stromal cells	Direct contact with stromal cells (including epithelial cells, fibroblasts and macrophages) is required for the differentiation of a particular lineage. Adhesion molecules and cytokines are involved in this process.
Role of cytokines	Stromal cells produce many cytokines, including stem cell factor (SCF), monocyte colony-stimulating factor (M-CSF) and granulocyte-colony stimulating factor (G-CSF). Interaction of stem cells with stromal cells and M-CSF or G-CSF results in the development of monocytes and granulocytes, respectively.
Related topic	Molecules of the innate immune system (B2)

A common stem cell

The majority of the cell types involved in the immune system are produced from a common hemopoietic stem cell (HSC) and develop through the process of differentiation into functionally mature blood cells of different lineages, e.g. monocytes, platelets, lymphocytes, etc. (hemopoiesis: *Fig. 1*). These stem cells are replicating self-renewing cells, which in early embryonic life are found in the yolk sac and then in the fetal liver, spleen and bone marrow. After birth the bone marrow contains the HSCs.

The lineage of cells differentiating from the HSC is determined by the microenvironment of the HSC and requires contact with stromal cells and inter-action with particular cytokines. These interactions are responsible for switching on specific genes coding for molecules required for the function of the different cell types, e.g. those used for phagocytosis in macrophages and neutrophils, and the receptors on lymphocytes which determine specificity for antigens. This is, broadly speaking, the process of differentiation.

Stromal cells

Stromal cells, including epithelial cells and macrophages, are necessary for the differentiation of stem cells to cells of a particular lineage, e.g. lymphocytes. Direct contact of the stromal cell with the stem cell is required. Within the fetal liver, and in the thymus and bone marrow, different stromal cells (including macrophages, endothelial cells, epithelial cells, fibroblasts and adipocytes) create discrete foci where different cell types develop. Thus, different foci will

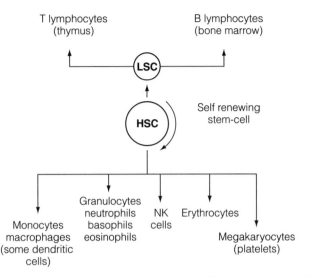

Fig. 1.   Origin of blood cells (hemopoiesis); LSC, lymphoid stem cell; HSC, hemopoietic stem cell.

contain developing granulocytes, monocytes or B cells. Cytokines are essential for this process, and it is thought that adhesion molecules also play an important role (*Fig. 2*).

Role of cytokines   Different cytokines are important for renewal of HSC and their differentiation into the different functionally mature blood cell types. Although an oversimplification, the processes related to HSC regeneration depend largely on SCF, IL-1 and IL-3. The development of granulocytes and monocytes require, among other cytokines, monocyte colony-stimulating factor (M-CSF) and granulocyte colony-stimulating factor (G-CSF), both of which are produced by stromal cells. Thus, interaction of stem cells with stromal cells and with M-CSF or G-CSF results in the development of monocytes and granulocytes, respectively (*Fig. 3*). Other cytokines are important for the early differentiation of T cells in the thymus and B cells in particular locations within the bone marrow.

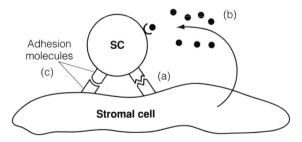

Fig. 2.   Role of stromal cells in hemopoiesis. (a) Stromal cell bound cytokine (e.g. stem cell factor) and (b) released cytokines (e.g. IL-7) determine the differentiation pathway of the stem cell (SC) attached through (c) specific adhesion molecules (e.g. CD44) on the SC attached to hyaluronic acid molecules on the stromal cell.

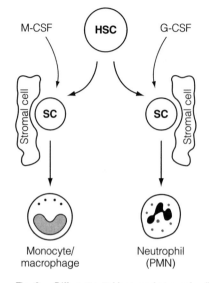

Fig. 3.   Different cytokines and stromal cells induce different pathways of differentiation.

B1 CELLS OF THE INNATE IMMUNE SYSTEM

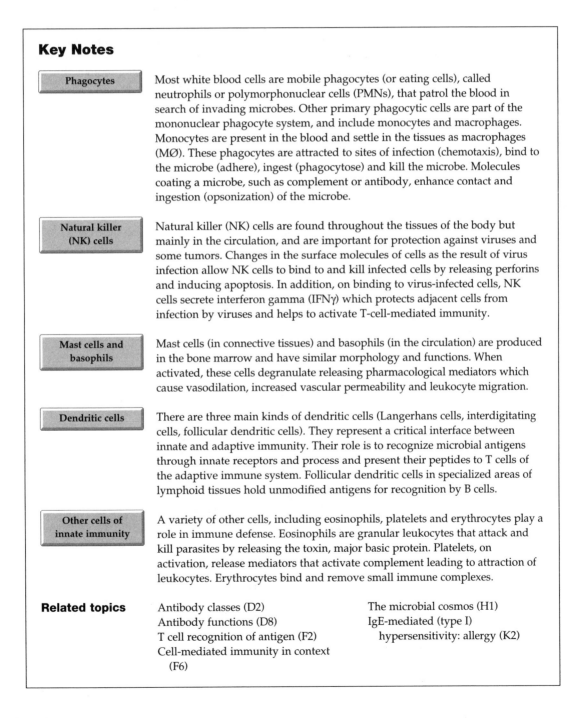

Key Notes

Phagocytes	Most white blood cells are mobile phagocytes (or eating cells), called neutrophils or polymorphonuclear cells (PMNs), that patrol the blood in search of invading microbes. Other primary phagocytic cells are part of the mononuclear phagocyte system, and include monocytes and macrophages. Monocytes are present in the blood and settle in the tissues as macrophages (MØ). These phagocytes are attracted to sites of infection (chemotaxis), bind to the microbe (adhere), ingest (phagocytose) and kill the microbe. Molecules coating a microbe, such as complement or antibody, enhance contact and ingestion (opsonization) of the microbe.
Natural killer (NK) cells	Natural killer (NK) cells are found throughout the tissues of the body but mainly in the circulation, and are important for protection against viruses and some tumors. Changes in the surface molecules of cells as the result of virus infection allow NK cells to bind to and kill infected cells by releasing perforins and inducing apoptosis. In addition, on binding to virus-infected cells, NK cells secrete interferon gamma (IFNγ) which protects adjacent cells from infection by viruses and helps to activate T-cell-mediated immunity.
Mast cells and basophils	Mast cells (in connective tissues) and basophils (in the circulation) are produced in the bone marrow and have similar morphology and functions. When activated, these cells degranulate releasing pharmacological mediators which cause vasodilation, increased vascular permeability and leukocyte migration.
Dendritic cells	There are three main kinds of dendritic cells (Langerhans cells, interdigitating cells, follicular dendritic cells). They represent a critical interface between innate and adaptive immunity. Their role is to recognize microbial antigens through innate receptors and process and present their peptides to T cells of the adaptive immune system. Follicular dendritic cells in specialized areas of lymphoid tissues hold unmodified antigens for recognition by B cells.
Other cells of innate immunity	A variety of other cells, including eosinophils, platelets and erythrocytes play a role in immune defense. Eosinophils are granular leukocytes that attack and kill parasites by releasing the toxin, major basic protein. Platelets, on activation, release mediators that activate complement leading to attraction of leukocytes. Erythrocytes bind and remove small immune complexes.

Related topics	Antibody classes (D2)	The microbial cosmos (H1)
	Antibody functions (D8)	IgE-mediated (type I)
	T cell recognition of antigen (F2)	hypersensitivity: allergy (K2)
	Cell-mediated immunity in context (F6)	

Phagocytes   Phagocytes are specialized 'eating' cells (phagein – to eat, *Greek*) of which there are two main types, neutrophils and macrophages. Neutrophils, often called polymorphonuclear cells (PMNs) because of the multilobed nature of their nuclei (*Fig. 1*), are mobile phagocytes that comprise the majority of blood leukocytes (about 8×10^6/ml of blood). They have a very short half-life (days) and die in the bloodstream by apoptosis (programmed cell death). They have granules that contain peroxidase, alkaline and acid phosphatases, and defensins (small antibiotic peptides) which are involved in microbial killing. These granulocytes stain with neutral dyes and have a different function from granulocytes that stain with eosin (eosinophils), or basic dyes (basophils). PMNs have receptors for chemotactic factors released from microbes, e.g. muramyl dipeptide (MDP), and for complement components activated by microbes (*Table 1*). Their

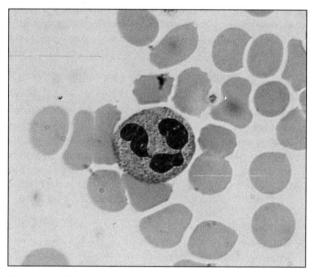

Fig. 1.   A polymorphonuclear cell (neutrophil) in the blood. Reproduced from Immunology 5th edn., 1998, Roitt, Brostoff and Male, with permission from Mosby.

Table 1.   Surface receptors on polymorphonuclear cells (PMNs)

Surface molecules	Function
Fc Receptors	
CD16 (FcγRIII), Fc receptor for IgG	Binds to IgG-antigen complexes (opsonization)
CD32 (FcγRII), Fc receptor for IgG	Binds to IgG-antigen complexes (opsonization)
Complement receptors	
C5aR	Binds to C5a for attraction towards microbe having activated C
CR1 (CD35)	Binds to C3b, iC3b, C4b and mannose binding ligand (opsonization)
CR3 (CDIIb/CD18)	Binds to C3b, iC3b; permits removal of complement coated antigens and microbes (opsonization)
Adhesion molecules	
LFA-1	Binds to ICAM-1 on endothelium for extravasation
VLA4	Binds to VCAM-1 on endothelium for extravasation

main function is to patrol the body via the bloodstream in search of invading microbes. As such they are pivotal cells in acute inflammation. Like the majority of cells involved in the immune system, these phagocytes are produced in the bone marrow (Topic A5).

The mononuclear phagocyte system (previously called the reticuloendothelial system) is a widely distributed tissue-bound phagocytic system whose major function is to dispose of microbes and dead body cells through the process of phagocytosis. Monocytes (*Fig.* 2) are bloodborne precursors of the major tissue phagocytes, macrophages. Different organs/tissues each have their versions of monocyte-derived phagocytic cells (*Table 2*).

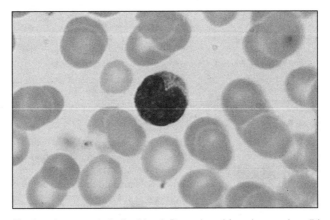

Fig. 2.   A monocyte in the blood. Reproduced from Immunology 5th edn., 1998, Roitt, Brostoff and Male, with permission from Mosby.

Table 2.   Cells of the mononuclear phagocyte system

Cells	Location
Monocytes	Bloodstream
Kupffer cells	Liver
Mesangial cells	Kidney
Alveolar macrophages	Lungs
Microglial cells	Brain
Sinus macrophages	Spleen, lymph nodes
Serosal macrophages	Peritoneal cavity

Phagocytosis is a multistep process (*Table 3*) and the major mechanism by which microbes are removed from the body. It is especially important for defense against extracellular microbes (Topic H2).

Opsonization is the process of making a microbe easier to phagocytose. A number of molecules called 'opsonins' ('to make more tasty' – *Greek*) do this by coating the microbe. They aid attachment of the microbe to the phagocyte and also trigger activation of phagocytosis. Opsonins include the complement component C3b and antibody itself, the latter acting as a bridge between the innate and adaptive immune systems (Topics B2 and D8). Phagocytes use their surface receptors (*Table 4*) which bind to C3b, or to the Fc region of IgG

Table 3.   Stages in phagocytosis

Stage	Mechanism
1 Movement of phagocyte towards the microbe	Chemotactic signals, e.g. MDP, complement (C5a)
2 Attachment of microbe to the phagocyte surface	Binding to mannose, complement and/or Fc receptors
3 Endocytosis of microbe leads to formation of a phagosome	Invagination of surface membrane
4 Fusion of phagosome with lysosome	Microtubules involved
5 Killing of microbe	Oxygen-dependent killing, e.g. O_2-radicals; oxygen independent, e.g. myeloperoxidase, nitric oxide

Table 4.   Surface receptors on monocytes/macrophages

Molecules	Function
Microbial recognition receptors	
Mannose receptors	Mediate both phagocytosis of microbes and induction of adaptive immune responses
Toll-like receptors	Mediate cytokine production and induce adaptive immune responses
Scavenger receptors	Bind bacterial and yeast cell wall carbohydrates or lipids
CD14	Receptor for lipopolysacchardide (LPS) binding protein (associated with toll-like receptor 4)
Fc Receptors	
CD16 (FcγRIII)	Binds to IgG–antigen complexes and IgG-coated target cells, mediating phagocytosis and cytokine production
CD32 (FcγRII)	Binds to IgG–antigen complexes and IgG-coated target cells, mediating phagocytosis and cytokine production
CD64 (FcγRI)	Binds to IgG–antigen complexes and IgG-coated target cells, mediating phagocytosis and cytokine production
CD89 (FcαR)	Binds to IgA–antigen complexes, mediating phagocytosis and cytokine production
Complement receptors	
CD35 (CR1)	Complement receptor involved in enhancing phagocytosis of IgM/IgG-coated microbes on which complement has been activated
Adhesion receptors	
CD18/11a,b,c (LFA-1, CR3, CR4)	Adhesion molecules facilitating interactions with other cells
MHC molecules (HLA)	
MHC Class I (HLA A,B,C)	Presentation of peptides to Tc cells
MHC Class II (HLA D)	Presentation of peptides to Th cells

antibody (Fc receptors, FcR) to attach to C3b or IgG coating the microbes, respectively.

Killing by mononuclear phagocytes is generally very efficient, as there are many cytotoxic mechanisms available to these cells. In particular, these cells contain many different enzymes, cationic proteins and polypeptides (defensins) that in concert can mediate killing and digestion of the microbe. In addition, on activation, these mononuclear phagocytes produce oxygen metabolites, including superoxide, and nitric oxide, both of which are important in killing intracellular pathogens.

Natural killer (NK) cells

Natural killer (NK) cells, also termed 'large granular lymphocytes' (or LGLs), differ from classical lymphocytes in that they are larger, contain more cytoplasm, and have (electron) dense granules (*Fig. 3*). They are produced in the

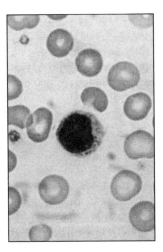

Fig. 3. An NK cell in the blood. Reproduced from Immunology 4th edn, Roitt, Brostoff and Male, with permission from Mosby.

bone marrow and are found throughout the tissues of the body, but mainly in the circulation where they comprise 5–15% of the total lymphocyte fraction (Topic C1). They have a variety of cell surface receptors (*Table 5*), including Fc receptors for IgG (FcγRIII) and receptors for certain cell surface molecules called killer activation receptors (KARs) and killer inhibitory receptors (KIRs).

The main function of NK cells is to kill virus-infected self cells, as well as some tumor cells. When NK cells bind to uninfected self cells, their KIRs provide a negative signal to the NK cell, preventing it from killing the self cell. This is because KIRs recognize MHC class I (Topic F2) leader peptides presented in an MHC-like molecule, HLA-E. However, infection of cells by some viruses reduces the expression of MHC molecules, and therefore decreases the loading of class I peptides in HLA-E, thus allowing the activation through KARs to induce NK cell killing of the infected cell. This is an important

Table 5. Surface receptors on natural killer cells

Molecules	Function
Fc receptors	
CD16 (FcγRIII)	Binds to IgG-coated target cells and mediates ADCC*
Adhesion/accessory molecules	
CD2	Binds to LFA-3
CD56 (NCAM, neural adhesion molecule)	
LFA-1	Binds to ICAM-1
Activation/inhibitory receptors	
KIR (Killer inhibitory receptors)	Contain ITIMs and bind to MHC class I-like molecules associated with self peptide and prevent NK cells from killing
KAR (Killer activation receptors)	Bind to self antigens (e.g. carbohydrate on self cells) and are associated with other molecules which contain ITAMs. On activation by KAR binding (in the absence of simultaneous engagement of KIRs) they initiate release of cytotoxic molecules from the NK cells

*ADCC, antibody-dependent cell cytotoxicity; ITIMs, immunoreceptor tyrosine-based inhibitory motifs; ITAMs, immunoreceptor tyrosine-based activation motifs.

mechanism, allowing NK cells to recognize normal self cells and ignore them, while killing infected or malignant self cells.

The mechanisms by which NK cells mediate killing are identical to those used by cytotoxic T cells (Topic F5) and involve release of granule contents (perforins and granzymes) onto the surface of the infected cell. Perforin has a structure similar to that of C9, a component of complement which can create pores in the cell membrane (Topics B2 and D8), allowing the passage of the granzymes (proteolytic enzymes) into the cell to induce apoptosis. NK cells, like cytotoxic T cells, are also able to induce target cell apoptosis through binding of their surface FasL molecules to Fas molecules on the surface of the virus-infected cell (Topic F5).

IL-2 induces NK cells to become lymphokine-activated killer (LAK) cells which have been used in clinical trials to treat tumors (Topic N5). When NK cells are 'activated' by recognizing a virus-infected cell they secrete IFNγ. This helps to protect surrounding cells from virus infection, although IFNα and IFNβ are probably more important in this role (Topic B2). In addition, IFNγ can also enhance the development of specific T cell responses directed to virus-infected cells (Topics F4 and F5).

Mast cells and basophils

Mast cells (*Fig. 4*) are found throughout the body in connective tissues close to blood vessels and particularly in the subepithelial areas of the respiratory, genitourinary and gastrointestinal tracts. Basophils are granulocytes which stain with basic dyes and are present in very low numbers in the circulation (<0.2% of the granular leukocytes). Basophils and mast cells are very similar in morphology. Both have large characteristic electron-dense granules in their cytoplasm which are very important for their function. Like all the granulocytes, basophils, and probably mast cells as well, are produced from stem cells in the bone marrow.

Mast cells/basophils can be stimulated to release their granules as a result of:

- their binding to C3a and C5a (anaphylatoxins);
- binding of allergens to anti-allergen IgE bound to their cell surface FcεR, and the resulting crosslinking of FcεR; and
- binding to lectins (molecules that bind carbohydrates).

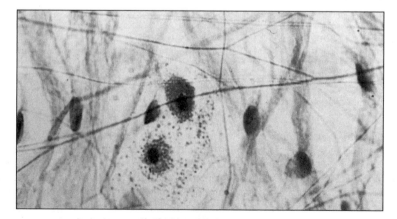

Fig. 4.   Mast cells. Note the large granules in the cytoplasm which contain pharmacological mediators. Reproduced from A Photographic Atlas for the Microbiology Laboratory, 1996, Leboffe and Pierce, with permission from Morton Publishing.

This stimulation results in the fusion of the intracellular granules with the surface membrane and the release of their contents to the exterior by the process of exocytosis. This release is almost instantaneous and is essential in the development of the acute inflammatory response (Topic B4). Granule contents include a variety of pre-formed pharmacological mediators, whereas other pharmacological mediators are produced *de novo* when the cells are stimulated (*Table 6*). When large numbers of mast cells/basophils are stimulated to degranulate, severe anaphylactic responses can occur, which in their mildest form give rise to the allergic symptoms seen in Type I hypersensitivity.

Table 6. *Main mediators released and their effects*

Mediators	Effect
Histamine	Vasodilation, vascular permeability
Cytokines	
*TNFα, IL-8, IL-5	Attracts neutrophils and eosinophils
PAF	Attracts basophils

*TNFα, tumor necrosis factor; PAF, platelet-activating factor.

Dendritic cells

Dendritic cells (DCs) are so called because of their many surface membrane folds that are similar in appearance to dendrites of the nervous system (*Fig. 5*). These folds allow maximum interaction with other cells of the immune system. There are three main kinds of dendritic cells (*Table 7*): Langerhans cells (LH); interdigitating cells (IDC); follicular dendritic cells (FDC).

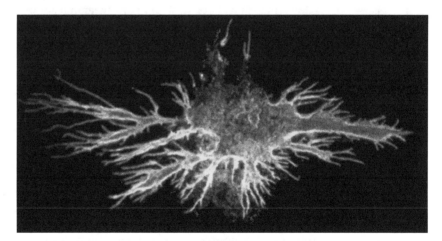

Fig. 5. *Dendritic cell. Note the many membrane processes to allow interactions with lymphocytes. Surface stained with anti CD44 (shown white, see Topic V3). CD44 is an adhesion molecule which allows the dendritic cell to attach to connective tissue and other cells. (Figure courtesy of Dr M. Binks.)*

DCs represent a primary interface between the innate and adaptive immune systems in that they recognize microbial antigens through innate receptors and, through the endogenous processing pathway, are able to initiate adaptive immune responses by presenting peptide antigens to T helper (CD4) cells.

Table 7. Dendritic cells

Dendritic cell type	Localization
Langerhans cells (LH)	Skin
Interdigitating cells (IDC)	Lymph node T cell areas
Follicular dendritic cells (FDC)	B cell follicles of the lymphoid tissues

Since the T cell antigen receptor can only recognize 'pieces' of proteins in association with MHC molecules, proteins first need to be 'processed' (cut up into short peptides). These peptides are then attached to MHC molecules (Topic F2) for display on the surface of the DC. LH and IDC have large amounts of surface MHC class II to present foreign peptides to T cells. Although macrophages can process and present antigen to T cells, the LH and IDC are much more efficient in carrying out this function.

FDC do not express MHC class II molecules, are present within the B cell follicles of lymphoid tissues and function to hold intact antigens on their surface for recognition by B cells. It is thought that this interaction is important not only in B cell stimulation, but also in B cell survival within the primary follicles.

Other cells of innate immunity

Eosinophils are granular leukocytes which stain with eosin. They are present at low levels in the circulation (2–5% of blood leukocytes), have some phagocytic activity, but are primarily responsible for extracellular killing of large parasites (e.g. schistosome worms) which cannot be phagocytosed (Topic H2). They usually bind to an antibody-coated parasite through surface Fc receptors and release the contents of their granules (degranulate) onto the parasite surface. The granules contain peroxides and a toxin, major basic protein, which kill the parasite. Histaminase is also present in the granules. This anti-inflammatory substance dampens the effects of histamine released by mast cells earlier in the response.

As well as having a major role in blood clotting, **platelets** contain important mediators which are released when they are activated at the site of a damaged blood vessel. Parasites coated with IgG and/or IgE antibodies are also thought to activate platelets through surface Fc receptors for these antibody classes. Released mediators activate complement, which in turn attracts leukocytes to the site of tissue damage caused by trauma or infection by a parasite (Section B4).

Erythrocytes have surface complement receptors which bind to complement attached to small circulating immune complexes. They carry these complexes to the liver where they are released to Kupffer cells which phagocytose them. Thus, erythrocytes play an important immunological role in clearing immune complexes from the circulation in persistent infections and in some autoimmune diseases.

B2 MOLECULES OF THE INNATE IMMUNE SYSTEM

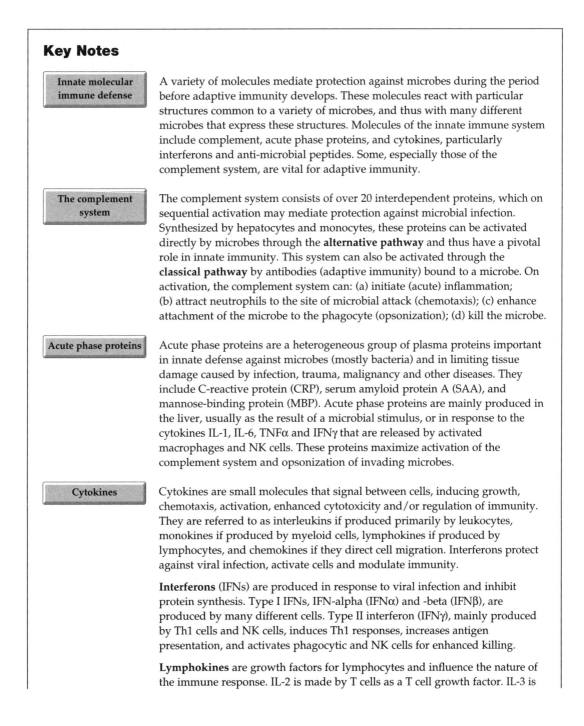

Key Notes

Innate molecular immune defense

A variety of molecules mediate protection against microbes during the period before adaptive immunity develops. These molecules react with particular structures common to a variety of microbes, and thus with many different microbes that express these structures. Molecules of the innate immune system include complement, acute phase proteins, and cytokines, particularly interferons and anti-microbial peptides. Some, especially those of the complement system, are vital for adaptive immunity.

The complement system

The complement system consists of over 20 interdependent proteins, which on sequential activation may mediate protection against microbial infection. Synthesized by hepatocytes and monocytes, these proteins can be activated directly by microbes through the **alternative pathway** and thus have a pivotal role in innate immunity. This system can also be activated through the **classical pathway** by antibodies (adaptive immunity) bound to a microbe. On activation, the complement system can: (a) initiate (acute) inflammation; (b) attract neutrophils to the site of microbial attack (chemotaxis); (c) enhance attachment of the microbe to the phagocyte (opsonization); (d) kill the microbe.

Acute phase proteins

Acute phase proteins are a heterogeneous group of plasma proteins important in innate defense against microbes (mostly bacteria) and in limiting tissue damage caused by infection, trauma, malignancy and other diseases. They include C-reactive protein (CRP), serum amyloid protein A (SAA), and mannose-binding protein (MBP). Acute phase proteins are mainly produced in the liver, usually as the result of a microbial stimulus, or in response to the cytokines IL-1, IL-6, TNFα and IFNγ that are released by activated macrophages and NK cells. These proteins maximize activation of the complement system and opsonization of invading microbes.

Cytokines

Cytokines are small molecules that signal between cells, inducing growth, chemotaxis, activation, enhanced cytotoxicity and/or regulation of immunity. They are referred to as interleukins if produced primarily by leukocytes, monokines if produced by myeloid cells, lymphokines if produced by lymphocytes, and chemokines if they direct cell migration. Interferons protect against viral infection, activate cells and modulate immunity.

Interferons (IFNs) are produced in response to viral infection and inhibit protein synthesis. Type I IFNs, IFN-alpha (IFNα) and -beta (IFNβ), are produced by many different cells. Type II interferon (IFNγ), mainly produced by Th1 cells and NK cells, induces Th1 responses, increases antigen presentation, and activates phagocytic and NK cells for enhanced killing.

Lymphokines are growth factors for lymphocytes and influence the nature of the immune response. IL-2 is made by T cells as a T cell growth factor. IL-3 is important in hematopoiesis. IL-4 is produced by Th2 cells and mast cells and is a growth and differentiation factor for Th2 cells and B cells. IL-5, also produced by Th2 cells and mast cells, is important to B cell activation and production of IgA. IL-10, which is produced by Th2 cells and MØ, induces Th2 responses.

Monokines have activities critical to immune defense and inflammation. IL-1, tumor necrosis factor α (TNFα), and IL-6 activate lymphocytes, increase body temperature, activate and mobilize phagocytes and activate vascular endothelium. TNFα also activates MØ. IL-8 is chemotactic for PMNs. IL-12 activates NK cells to produce IFNγ.

Chemokines are small cytokines produced by many cell types in response to infection or physical damage. They activate and direct effector cells expressing appropriate chemokine receptors to sites of tissue damage and regulate leukocyte migration into tissues. CC chemokines are chemotactic for monocytes, CXC chemokines are chemotactic for PMNs.

Other cytokines include colony-stimulating factors (CSFs) that drive development, differentiation and expansion of cells of the myeloid series. GM-CSF induces commitment of progenitor cells to the monocyte/granulocyte lineage, G-CSF and M-CSF commitment to the granulocyte or monocyte lineage, respectively. Transforming growth factor β (TGFβ) inhibits activation of MØ and growth of B and T cells. Tumor necrosis factor β (TNFβ) is cytotoxic.

Other molecules	Collectins, a group of carbohydrate-binding proteins, act as opsonins to facilitate the removal and destruction of microbes. Peptide antibiotics, produced by a variety of cells, are able to eradicate bacterial infections.
Related topics	External defenses (A2) T cell recognition of antigen (F2)

Related topics

External defenses (A2)
Hemopoiesis – development of
   blood cells (A5)
Cells of the innate immune system
   (B1)
Innate immunity and inflammation
   (B4)
Lymphocytes (C1)
B cell activation (E2)

T cell recognition of antigen (F2)
T cell activation (F4)
Clonal expansion and development
   of effector function (F5)
Genes, T helper cells, cytokines and
   the neuroendocrine system (G5)
Immunity to different organisms
   (H2)

Innate molecular immune defense

There are many molecules of the innate immune system which are important in mediating protection against microbes during the period before the development of adaptive immunity. Although these molecules react with particular structures associated with microbes, they are nonspecific in that they can react with many different microbes that express these structures. The major molecules are those of the complement system, acute phase proteins and cytokines, especially the interferons. Most of the molecules which play a role in the innate immune system are also associated with adaptive immunity. Thus, the complement system can be activated by antibodies, and cytokines are involved in activation of antigen-presenting cells critical to triggering T lymphocyte responses. Cytokines released by macrophages also play a role in acute inflammation. Thus, the immune response to microbes is continuous with both systems being intimately involved and synergistic. A variety of other molecules are also important to the innate immune system, including the antibiotic peptides.

The complement system

The complement system is a protective system common to all vertebrates (Topic D8). In man it consists of 20 soluble glycoproteins (usually designated as C1, C2, etc., or as factors, e.g. factor B), many of which are produced by hepatocytes and monocytes. They are constitutively present in blood and other body fluids. On appropriate triggering, these components interact sequentially with each other (i.e. in a domino-like fashion). This 'cascade' of molecular events involves cleavage of some complement components into active fragments (e.g. C3 is cleaved to C3a and C3b) which contribute to activation of the next component, ultimately leading to lysis of, and/or protection against, a variety of microbes. This system can be 'activated' (*Fig. 1*) directly through the **alternative pathway** by certain molecules associated with microbes, or through the **classical pathway** by antibodies bound to a microbe or other antigen (Topic D8).

The alternative pathway is activated by interaction of C3 with certain types of molecules on microbes or by self-molecules (e.g. CRP, see below) which react with these microbes. Complement component C3 is critical to this interaction and its cleavage into C3a and C3b is the single most important event in the activation of the complement system. More specifically, the alternative pathway depends on the normal continuous low-level breakdown of C3 (*Table 1*). One of the fragments of C3, C3b, is very reactive and can covalently bind to virtually any molecule or cell. If C3b binds to a self cell, regulatory molecules associated with this cell (Topic D8) inactivate it, protecting the cell from complement-mediated damage. However, if C3b binds to a microbe, Factor B is activated and its cleavage product Bb binds to C3b on the microbe. This C3bBb complex (C3 convertase) is enzymatically active and amplifies the breakdown of addi-

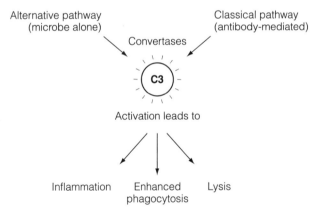

Fig. 1.   The complement system.

Table 1.   Sequence of complement activation by the alternative pathway leading to cell lysis

Microbe (M) + C3b	M-C3b
MC3b + factor B	M-C3b-Bb
M-C3b-Bb + C3b	M-C3b-Bb-C3b
M-C3b-Bb-C3b + C5	M-C3b-Bb-C3b-C5b + C5a
M-C3b-Bb-C3b-C5b + C6 + C7	M-C3b-Bb-C3b-C5b-C6-C7
M-C3b-Bb-C3b-C5b-C6-C7 + C8	M-C3b-Bb-C3b-C5b-C6-C7-C8
M-C3b-Bb-C3b-C5b-C6-C7-C8 + C9	M-C3b-Bb-C3b-C5b-C6-C7-C8-C9 Lysis of M

tional C3 to C3b. Equally important, the resulting enzyme cleaves C5 into C5a and C5b, both of which have critical protective functions. C5b is crucial to formation of the 'membrane attack complex' (MAC), C5b-C6-C7-C8-C9 which mediates lysis of the microbe. This alternative pathway is important for control of infection in the absence of specific immunity. Thus, many different organisms are handled and eliminated as a result of their activation of the alternative pathway.

The major functions of the complement system are:

- Initiation of (acute) inflammation by direct activation of mast cells (C3a, C5a).
- Attraction of neutrophils (chemotaxis) to the site of microbial attack (C5a).
- Enhancement of the attachment of the microbe to the phagocyte (opsonization) (C3b).
- Killing of the microbe activating the membrane attack complex (lysis) (C9).

Acute phase proteins

Acute phase proteins are important in innate defense against microbes (mostly bacteria and protozoa) and in limiting tissue damage caused by microbial infection, trauma, malignancy and other diseases, e.g. rheumatoid arthritis. They are also important in tissue repair. These molecules include C-reactive protein (CRP), complement components, opsonic proteins such as mannose-binding protein (MBP), metal-binding proteins and protease inhibitors. The major acute phase proteins, CRP and serum amyloid protein A (SAA), have similar structures and are termed pentraxins, based on the pentagonal association of their subunits. CRP, which was named based on its ability to react with the C-protein of pneumococcus, is composed of five identical polypeptides associated by noncovalent interactions. MBP binds residues of mannose on glycoproteins or glycolipids expressed by microbes in a form different from that on mammalian cells. Its binding properties permit it to interact with a variety of pathogens.

These proteins, mainly produced by the liver, can either be produced *de novo* (e.g. CRP is increased by as much as 1000-fold within a few hours), or are present at low levels and rapidly increase following infection (fibrinogen). They are produced by hepatocytes in response to the cytokines IL-1, IL-6, TNFα and IFNγ released by activated macrophages and NK cells. IL-6 is important in enhancing production of acute phase proteins.

Acute phase proteins have several functions (*Table 2*), the most important being to maximize activation of the complement system and opsonization of invading microbes, and to limit tissue damage caused by these microbes. CRP

Table 2.   Acute phase proteins and their functions

Protein	Function
C-reactive protein (CRP)	Binds to bacterial phosphoryl choline, activates complement through C1q, acts as an opsonin
Serum amyloid A (SAA)	Activates complement (through C1q), acts as an opsonin
Mannose binding protein (MBP)	Binds to mannose on bacteria, attaches to phagocyte MBP receptors (opsonization), activates complement via classical pathway (Topic D8)
Complement components	Chemotaxis, opsonization and lysis (Topic D8)
Metal binding proteins	Removal of essential metal ions required for bacterial growth
Fibrinogen	Coagulation factor
α1 anti trypsin, α1 anti chymotrypsin	Protease inhibitors

binds to a wide variety of microbes and on binding activates complement through the alternative pathway, causing C3b deposition on the microbe (opsonization) and thus ultimately its phagocytosis by phagocytes expressing receptors for C3b. MBP binding to microbes also initiates complement activation and subsequent opsonization mediated by C3b, but in addition it directly opsonizes these organisms for phagocytosis. In addition, metal-binding proteins inhibit microbial growth, and protease inhibitors limit tissue damage by neutralizing lysosomal enzymes released from phagocytes.

Both CRP and SAA, as well as having complement activation properties, bind to DNA and other nuclear material from cells, helping in their clearance from the host. Quantitation of CRP in the serum of patients with inflammatory diseases (e.g. rheumatoid arthritis) is used as a way to assess the inflammatory activity of the disease. High levels of CRP signify a high level of disease activity.

Cytokines

Cytokines are small molecules, secreted by cells in response to a stimulus. They may have an effect on the cell that produces them and are critical to signaling between cells, with each cytokine often inducing several different biological effects. Many different cells release cytokines, but each cell type releases only certain of these molecules. Cytokines may induce growth, differentiation, chemotaxis, activation, and/or enhanced cytotoxicity. Moreover, it is not uncommon for different cytokines to have similar activities and for many cytokines, some with opposing activities, to be released by a particular stimulus. Thus, the resulting biological effect is a factor of the sum of all of these activities.

To some extent cytokines can be grouped by the cell populations that secrete them. **Monokines** are cytokines secreted by cells of the myeloid series (monocytes, macrophages) and **lymphokines** are cytokines secreted primarily by lymphocytes, although some cytokines are produced by both lymphocytes and myeloid cells. The term **interleukin** (IL) is often used to describe cytokines produced by leukocytes, although some interleukins are also produced by other cell populations. A group of small heparin-binding cytokines, **chemokines**, direct cell migration, and may also activate cells in response to infectious agents or tissue damage. **Interferons** are produced by a variety of cells in response to viral infection.

It is important to note that the same cytokine can be made by several different cell populations. For example, IFNα is made by most if not all nucleated cells in response to viral infection. IFNγ is produced both by Th1 cells and by NK cells. IL-1 is produced by macrophages, B cells and nonimmune keratinocytes. Many different cell types make IL-6, several make IL-4, etc. Moreover, the same cytokine can induce different functions in different cell types. For example, TNFα can promote the proliferation of B cells but activate killing mechanisms in other cell populations. IFNγ activates macrophages to kill intracellular microbes, induces B cells to switch their antibody class to IgG and induces endothelial cells to increase expression of MHC class II molecules.

Interferons

Interferons are pro-inflammatory molecules which can mediate protection against virus infection, and are thus particularly important in limiting infection during the period when specific humoral and cellular immunity is developing. They can be divided into two groups, type I IFN (IFNα and IFNβ) and type II IFN (IFNγ) also called immune IFN (*Table 3*).

Table 3. The interferons

	Type I (IFN-α/β)	Type II (IFNγ)
Chromosomal location	9	12
Origin	All nucleated cells, especially fibroblasts, macrophages and dendritic cells	NK cells and Th1, γδ and CD8 T cells
Induced by	Viruses, other cytokines, some intracellular bacteria and protozoans	Antigen-stimulated T cells
Functions	Antiviral, increases MHC class I expression, inhibits cell proliferation	Antiviral, increases MHC I and II expression, activates macrophages

IFNα and IFNβ are produced by many different cells in response to viral or bacterial infections, especially by intracellular microbes. At least 12 different, highly homologous species of IFNα are produced, primarily by infected leukocytes as well as by epithelial cells and fibroblasts. In contrast, a single species of IFNβ is produced, normally by fibroblasts and epithelial cells. The proinflammatory cytokines IL-1 and TNFα are potent inducers of IFN-α/β secretion, as are endotoxins derived from the cell wall of Gram-negative bacteria.

The receptor for both IFNα and IFNβ is the same and found on most nucleated cells. Binding of IFNα and IFNβ to this receptor inhibits protein synthesis and thus viral replication as a result of the induction of the synthesis of inhibitory proteins and of preventing mRNA translation and DNA replication. In addition, these interferons inhibit cell proliferation, increase the lytic activity of NK cells and induce increased expression of MHC class I and other components of the class I processing and presentation pathway leading to induction of antigen-specific cytolytic T lymphocyte (CTL) responses against virally infected cells. Induction of MHC class I is also important for protection of uninfected cells from killing by NK cells (Topic B1). The importance of IFN-α/β in innate defense against viral infections is indicated by animal studies in which treatment of virus-infected mice with antibodies to IFN-α/β resulted in death.

In contrast to the broad and rather nonspecific antiviral activity of IFN-α/β, IFNγ is primarily a cytokine of the adaptive immune system, as it is important not only for antiviral activity but also plays a major role in regulation of the development of specific immunity and in activation of cells of the immune system. Produced primarily by Th1 cells and NK cells, IFNγ plays a critical role in induction of Th1 immune responses. That is, early in the development of a specific immune response, IFNγ is involved in inducing Th0 cells to differentiate to Th1 cells which make more IFNγ and provide help for development of CTL responses and for IgG antibody production. In addition, Th1 cells or CTLs responding to peptides presented in MHC molecules produce IFNγ which acts both locally and systemically to activate monocytes, MØ, and PMNs which are then better able to kill intracellular pathogens. In particular, IFNγ increases the expression of Fc receptors for IgG on macrophages and PMNs (Topic D8) as well as MHC Class II expression on a wide variety of cells. This enhances the phagocytic function of these cells as well as the antigen-presenting capabilities of professional antigen-presenting cells. IFNγ, which is crucial for macrophage function, enhances macrophage killing of intracellular bacteria and parasites probably as a result of its stimulation of their production of reactive oxygen and reactive nitrogen intermediates.

Lymphokines

A variety of cytokines are produced by lymphocytes and lymphocyte subsets (*Table 4*), many of which are growth factors for lymphocytes and/or influence the nature of the immune response. As an example, IL-2 is made by T cells as a critical autocrine growth factor that is required for proliferation of T cells, especially Th0 and Th1 cells and CTL. On activation (as a result of the interaction of their antigen receptor complexes with antigenic peptide in MHC molecules on APCs) these T cells make IL-2 for secretion and at the same time IL-2 receptors with which to bind and be stimulated by the secreted IL-2. In the absence of IL-2 and/or its receptor, many antigen-specific T cells do not expand, severely compromising immune responses.

IL-3 is involved in the growth and differentiation of a variety of cell types as a result of its synergistic activity with other cytokines in hematopoiesis. IL-4 is produced by Th2 cells and mast cells and is a growth and differentiation factor for Th2 cells and B cells, and can induce B cell class switch to IgE antibodies. IL-4 is important in influencing the nature of the immune response, as it can induce the development of Th2 cells from Th0 cells and can inhibit the development of Th1 responses (*Table 4*). Thus, IL-4 is not only involved in B cell growth, but it can also influence the B cell and its subsequent plasma cells to produce IgE antibody (Topic D3). IL-5 is also produced by Th2 cells and mast cells and is important to B cell activation and in induction of B cell class switch to IgA antibody. It also has a role in eosinophil growth and differentiation. IL-10, which is produced by Th2 cells and MØ, induces B cell activation and Th2 responses and inhibits Th1 responses, perhaps by enhancing IL-4 production and/or by suppressing MØ activity and production of IL-12, a Th1-stimulatory cytokine.

Monokines

This group of cytokines (*Table 4*) has many different local and systemic activities that are critical to immune defense. In addition, these pro-inflammatory

Table 4. *Representative lymphokines and monokines*

Cytokine	Produced by	Activity
IL-1	MØ, epithelial cells	Activates vascular endothelium; tissue destruction; increased effector cell access; fever; lymphocyte activation; mobilization of PMNs; induction of acute phase proteins (CRP, MBP)
IL-2	T cells	Proliferation of T and NK cells
IL-3	T cells, thymic cells	Proliferation and differentiation of hematopoietic cells
IL-4	Th2 cells, mast cells	B cell activation and proliferation; induces Th2 IgE responses and inhibits Th1 responses
IL-5	Th2 cells, mast cells	Eosinophil growth, differentiation; B cell activation, induces IgA responses
IL-6	T cells, MØ	Lymphocyte activation; fever; induction of acute phase proteins
IL-8	Mo, MØ, Fb, Kr	Increases tissue access for, and chemotaxis of PMNs
IL-10	Th2 cells, MØ	B cell activation; suppression of MØ activity; induces Th2 and inhibits Th1 responses
IL-12	B cells, MØ	Induces Th1 and inhibits Th2 responses; activates NK cells
IFNγ	T cells, NK cells	MØ and PMN activation; induces Th1 and inhibits Th2 responses
TNFα	MØ, T cells	Activates vascular endothelium; fever; shock; increases vascular permeability; induces mobilization of metabolites

Monocytes (Mo), macrophages (MØ), endothelial cells (En), fibroblasts (Fb), keratinocytes (Kr), neutrophils (PMNs), chondrocytes (Co).

cytokines are important mediators of inflammation. In particular, as a result of an appropriate stimulus, including ingestion of Gram-negative bacteria and subsequent activation by LPS, MØ secrete IL-1, IL-6, IL-8, IL-12 and TNFα. IL-1, TNFα and IL-6 have activities which include: (a) increasing body temperature and lymphocyte activation, which decrease pathogen replication and increase specific immune responses; (b) mobilization of neutrophils for phagocytosis; (c) induction of release of acute phase proteins (CRP, MBP) and thus complement activation and opsonization.

IL-1 also activates vascular endothelium (in preparation for neutrophil chemotaxis) and induces systemic production of IL-6. IL-8 increases access for, and chemotaxis of, neutrophils. It also activates binding by integrins, which facilitates neutrophil binding to endothelial cells and migration into tissues. Like IL-1, TNFα also activates vascular endothelium and is able to increase vascular permeability. It activates MØ and induces their production of nitric oxide (NO). Although produced by monocytes and MØ, TNFα is also produced by some T cells. Finally, IL-12, which is also produced by B cells, activates NK cells which then produce IFNγ, a cytokine important to inducing differentiation of Th0 cells to Th1 cells (*Table 4*).

Chemokines

This group of more than 50 small, closely related cytokines (MW 8–10 kDa) are primarily involved in chemoattraction of lymphocytes, monocytes and neutrophils (*Table 5*). They are made by monocytes/macrophages, but also by other cells including endothelial cells, platelets, neutrophils, T cells, keratinocytes and fibroblasts. Chemokines can be divided into four different groups based on unique aspects of their amino acid sequence, and in particular the position of conserved cysteine residues. One group has two adjacent cysteines (CC), a second has two cysteines separated by another amino acid (CXC), another has one cysteine, and the last has two cysteines separated by three other amino acids. For the most part, CC chemokines such as monocyte chemotactic protein (MCP-1) are chemotactic for monocytes, inducing them to migrate into tissues and become macrophages, whereas CXC chemokines such as IL-8 are chemotactic for neutrophils inducing them to leave the blood and migrate into tissues. Some of these chemokines are also chemotactic for T cells. Chemokines are produced in response to an infectious process or to physical damage and not only direct cells to the source of infection/damage, but may also enhance their ability to deal with tissue damage.

Receptors for chemokines are all integral membrane proteins with the characteristic feature that they span the membrane seven times. These molecules are coupled to G (guanine nucleoside binding) proteins which act as the signaling moiety of the receptor. Although most of these receptors can bind more than one type of chemokine, they are usually distributed only on particular cell populations, permitting different chemokines to have selective activity.

Some chemokines, for example IL-8 and MCP-1, have been shown to work by first binding to proteoglycan molecules on endothelial cells or on the extracellular matrix. On this solid surface they then bind blood neutrophils or monocytes, slowing their passage and directing them to migrate down a chemokine concentration gradient toward the source of the chemokine. Although the role that each plays in immune defense and pathology is still being clarified, it is evident

Table 5. *Representative chemokines**

Class	Name	Source	Chemoattractant for activation of
CXC (α)	IL-8	Mo, MØ, Fb, Kr	Naive T cells, PMNs
	NAP-2	Platelets	Neutrophils
	MIP-1b	Mo, MØ, En, PMNs	CD8 T cells
CC (β)	MCP-1	Mo, MØ, Fb, Kr	Memory T cells, Mo
	Rantes	T cells	Memory Th cells
C (γ)	Lymphotactin		Lymphocytes
CX$_3$C (δ)	Fractalkine		Lymphocytes, monocytes, NK cells

*See footnote *Table 4.*

that these molecules are potent agents for activating and directing effector cell populations to the site of infection and/or tissue damage as well as for controlling leukocyte migration in tissues.

Other cytokines
Of the many other cytokines which are important to immune defense, several are particularly noteworthy (*Table 6*). A group of CSFs, including granulocyte-monocyte CSF (GM-CSF), granulocyte CSF (G-CSF) and monocyte CSF (M-CSF) drive the development, differentiation and expansion of cells of the myeloid series (Topic A5). GM-CSF induces expansion of myeloid progenitor cells and their commitment to the monocyte/MØ and granulocyte lineage, after which G-CSF and M-CSF induce specific commitment to the granulocyte or monocyte lineage, respectively, and then their subsequent expansion. These factors, and especially G-CSF, are important clinical tools in a number of disease situations as they can be used to expand myeloid effector cell populations critical to defense against pathogens.

TGFβ is produced by a variety of cells including monocytes, MØ, T cells and chondrocytes, and plays an important role in suppressing immune responses, as it can inhibit activation of MØ and growth of B and T cells. TNFβ (lymphotoxin) is a molecule which is cytotoxic to a variety of cell types, including ineffectual chronically infected MØ.

Other molecules   Collectins are a group of carbohydrate-binding proteins structurally related to the complement component C1q. These molecules act as opsonins and are important in the innate immune response to infections. They include mannose-

Table 6. *Other cytokines**

Cytokine	Produced by	Activity
GM-CSF	MØ, T cells	Stimulates growth, differentiation and activation of granulocytes, Mo, MØ
G-CSF	Mo, Fb, En	Stimulates PMN development
M-CSF	Fb	Stimulates Mo, MØ development
TGFβ	Mo, T cells, Co	Inhibits cell growth and inflammation
TNFβ (lymphotoxin)	T cells	Cytotoxic to T, B and other cells

*See footnote *Table 4.*

binding protein, an acute phase protein, and conglutinin. Receptors for collectins are present on macrophages, thus facilitating the removal and destruction of the microbe, and on epithelial cells in the lung and gastrointestinal tract. Mannose-binding protein is also able to activate complement via the classical pathway (Topic D8) and therefore to engage host inflammatory, lytic and phagocytic responses.

Peptide antibiotics, including cecropins, magainins and defensins are part of the body's innate defense mechanisms against microbial infection and have potent antibacterial activities (Topic A2).

B3 RECOGNITION OF MICROBES BY THE INNATE IMMUNE SYSTEM

Key Notes

Pattern recognition receptors	Receptors of the innate immune system interact with, and facilitate removal of, groups of organisms with similar structures. These pattern recognition receptors (PRR) recognize molecular patterns associated with certain groups of microbes, and act not only as a first line of defense against microbes, but also to prime the adaptive immune system.
Mannose receptor	This receptor is expressed on macrophages, dendritic cells and endothelial cells and recognizes a Ca^{2+}-dependent, mannosyl/fucosyl pattern. It mediates phagocytosis of microbes and processing and presentation of microbial peptides on MHC Class II molecules, thus permitting induction of specific anti-microbial T and B cell responses.
Toll-like receptors	Toll proteins or toll-like receptors (TLRs) are a family of germline encoded cell surface proteins that recognize and distinguish between molecular patterns of different groups of pathogens. They not only signal the presence of a pathogen, but trigger the expression of co-stimulatory molecules and effector cytokines important in the development of adaptive immune responses.
CD14	This molecule is expressed on macrophages, binds LPS on Gram-negative bacteria, and facilitates destruction of the microbe and induction of secretion of cytokines involved in triggering adaptive immune responses.
Scavenger receptors	Scavenger receptors on macrophages recognize carbohydrates or lipids in bacterial and yeast cell walls, as well as damaged, modified or apoptotic self cells, and mediate their removal.
Related topics	Cells of the innate immune system (B1) The microbial cosmos (H1)

Pattern recognition receptors

In addition to the soluble molecules of the innate immune system, an increasing number of cell surface receptors have been identified that not only act as a first line of defense against many infectious organisms, but also are important to the development of an adaptive immune response. These pattern recognition receptors (PRR) do not have the remarkable specificity of the T and B cell systems, but have developed over evolutionary time to recognize molecular patterns associated with certain kinds of microbes and to facilitate removal of groups of organisms with similar structures. Moreover, the receptors involved are expressed on a variety of cells some of which are critical to adaptive immunity. These molecules include mannose receptors, CD14 and scavenger receptors, all expressed on macrophages (*Fig. 1*), as well as a recently identified family of

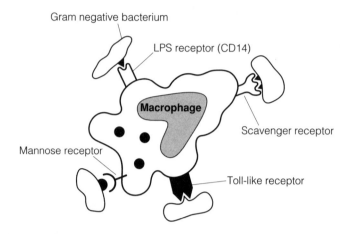

Fig. 1.   Macrophage expression of receptors involved in nonself recognition.

molecules, the Toll-like receptors (*Table 1*). It seems very likely that additional cell surface receptors important to innate immunity will also be found.

Mannose receptor

The mannose receptor is a 180 kDa transmembrane receptor expressed on macrophages, dendritic cells and subsets of endothelial cells. This receptor has eight carbohydrate recognition domains (CRDs), at least some of which have different pattern recognition motifs, making this one receptor fairly broad in the number and range of ligands it can recognize. Its Ca^{2+}-dependent, mannosyl/fucosyl recognition pattern permits it to interact with a variety of pathogens that enter through mucosal surfaces (*Table 2*). Because the mannose receptor is expressed on macrophages throughout the body, it is likely to be one of the first of the innate receptors to interact with microbes (*Fig. 1*). Furthermore, this receptor mediates phagocytosis and destruction of microbes even before the adaptive immune response is induced.

Table 1.   Cell surface receptors recognizing nonself

Name	Specificity	Cellular location
Mannose receptors	Mannosyl/fucosyl structures	Macrophages, endothelial cells, dendritic cells
Toll-like receptors	LPS, peptidoglycan, glucans, teichoic acids, arabinomannans	APCs, B cells, macrophages, other
CD14	LPS	Macrophages
Scavenger receptors	Carbohydrates or lipids	Macrophages, dendritic cells, endothelial cells

Table 2.   Microorganisms that express ligands to which the mannose receptor binds

Pseudomonas aeruginosa	*Mycobacterium tuberculosis*
Candida albicans	*Pneumocystis carinii*
Klebsiella pneumoniae	*Leishmania donovani*

In addition to its role as a front-line receptor mediating destruction of a wide range of organisms, the mannose receptor represents an important direct link to the adaptive immune system. Thus, microbes bound by mannose receptor are internalized and degraded in endosomes. Peptides from the microbe are loaded on MHC class II molecules for display on the surface of these APCs so that T cells of the adaptive immune system can now recognize microbe determinants, thus permitting induction of microbe-specific T and B cell responses.

Toll-like receptors Toll proteins or Toll-like receptors (TLRs) are a family of closely related proteins that all have an extracellular leucine-rich repeat (LRR) domain and a cytoplasmic domain that mediates signal transduction of a variety of effector genes. One of these TLRs (TLR4) has been found to induce cytokine and co-stimulatory molecule expression on APCs. This also binds LPS and induces intracellular signaling. Furthermore, a molecule very similar to the TLRs, RP105, has been found on human B cells and dendritic cells. Cross-linking of this molecule on B cells induces expression of co-stimulatory molecules and proliferation.

Thus, different Toll proteins are able to recognize molecular patterns of different pathogens and to distinguish between different groups of pathogens. In fact, it is now thought that different TLRs discriminate between the major molecular signatures of pathogens, including: peptidoglycan, teichoic acids (Gram-positive bacteria), LPS (Gram-negative bacteria), arabinomannans, and glucans. Of particular importance, these germline-encoded molecules of the innate immune system are not only able to signal the presence of a pathogen, but trigger expression of co-stimulatory molecules and effector cytokines, and in so doing prepare the cell for its involvement in the development of the adaptive immune response.

CD14 CD14 is a phosphoinositolglycan-linked cell surface receptor on macrophages (*Table 1*) that binds to lipopolysaccharide (LPS), a unique bacterial surface structure found only in the cell walls of Gram-negative bacteria, e.g. *E. coli*, *Neisseria*, *Salmonella*. The core carbohydrate and lipid A of LPS are virtually the same for these microbes and are the target for binding by CD14. Binding of LPS on a Gram-negative bacteria to macrophage CD14 and TLR4 facilitates destruction of the microbe as well as induction of secretion of various cytokines involved in triggering a wide array of immune responses.

Scavenger receptors (SR) SR are a group of transmembrane cell surface molecules that mediate binding and internalization (endocytosis) of microbes (both Gram-negative and Gram-positive) as well as certain modified, damaged or apoptotic self cells. These molecules are expressed on macrophages and dendritic cells as well as on some endothelial cells and have specificity for polyanionic molecules and the cells with which they are associated. At least seven different SR that may interact with microbes have been identified, including SR-A I and II, MARCO, SR-CL I and II, dSR-C1 and LOX-1. Of note, SR-A has apparent specificity for the lipid A component of lipopolysaccharide and of lipoteichoic acid which are associated with bacteria. Another SR, LOX-1 not only binds oxidized LDL and therefore appears to play a role in atherogenesis, but can also recognize certain microbes (e.g. *S. aureus* and *E. coli*) and may be important in innate immunity.

B4 INNATE IMMUNITY AND INFLAMMATION

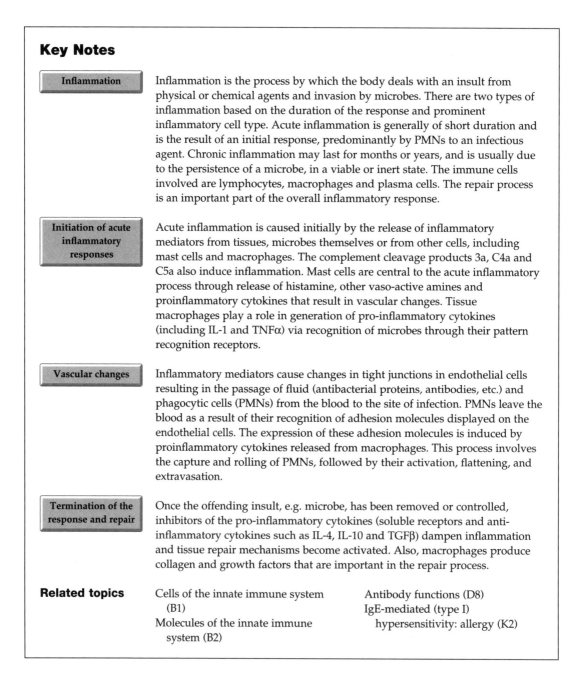

Key Notes

Inflammation

Inflammation is the process by which the body deals with an insult from physical or chemical agents and invasion by microbes. There are two types of inflammation based on the duration of the response and prominent inflammatory cell type. Acute inflammation is generally of short duration and is the result of an initial response, predominantly by PMNs to an infectious agent. Chronic inflammation may last for months or years, and is usually due to the persistence of a microbe, in a viable or inert state. The immune cells involved are lymphocytes, macrophages and plasma cells. The repair process is an important part of the overall inflammatory response.

Initiation of acute inflammatory responses

Acute inflammation is caused initially by the release of inflammatory mediators from tissues, microbes themselves or from other cells, including mast cells and macrophages. The complement cleavage products 3a, C4a and C5a also induce inflammation. Mast cells are central to the acute inflammatory process through release of histamine, other vaso-active amines and proinflammatory cytokines that result in vascular changes. Tissue macrophages play a role in generation of pro-inflammatory cytokines (including IL-1 and TNFα) via recognition of microbes through their pattern recognition receptors.

Vascular changes

Inflammatory mediators cause changes in tight junctions in endothelial cells resulting in the passage of fluid (antibacterial proteins, antibodies, etc.) and phagocytic cells (PMNs) from the blood to the site of infection. PMNs leave the blood as a result of their recognition of adhesion molecules displayed on the endothelial cells. The expression of these adhesion molecules is induced by proinflammatory cytokines released from macrophages. This process involves the capture and rolling of PMNs, followed by their activation, flattening, and extravasation.

Termination of the response and repair

Once the offending insult, e.g. microbe, has been removed or controlled, inhibitors of the pro-inflammatory cytokines (soluble receptors and anti-inflammatory cytokines such as IL-4, IL-10 and TGFβ) dampen inflammation and tissue repair mechanisms become activated. Also, macrophages produce collagen and growth factors that are important in the repair process.

Related topics

Cells of the innate immune system (B1)
Molecules of the innate immune system (B2)

Antibody functions (D8)
IgE-mediated (type I) hypersensitivity: allergy (K2)

Inflammation

Inflammation is the process by which the body deals with an insult from physical or chemical agents and invasion by microbes. It is recognized by its cardinal signs, including redness, heat, swelling and pain. The cells of the immune system contribute to the inflammatory response.

There are two types of inflammation based on the duration of the response and the prominent inflammatory cell type. **Acute inflammation** is generally of short duration, lasting from minutes to a few days, and is the result of an initial response by immune cells (primarily PMNs) to an infectious agent (mainly bacteria). **Chronic inflammation** may last months to years, usually results from the persistence of a microbe in a viable or inert state, and involves lymphocytes, macrophages and plasma cells of the immune system.

An inflammatory response always results in some tissue damage. Moreover, cells of the immune system are important in the repair process that follows successful elimination of a microbe.

Apart from physical and chemical agents and microbes, immune mechanisms themselves can lead to inflammatory responses (hypersensitivity reactions), e.g. allergies and granulomatous lesions (Section K). A summary of the main causes of acute inflammation is shown in *Fig 1*.

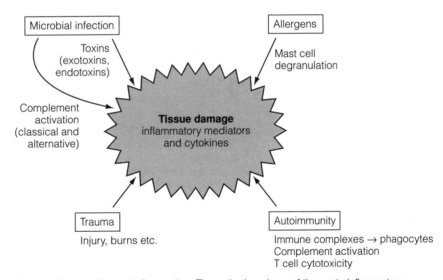

Fig. 1.   *Causes of acute inflammation. The activation phase of the acute inflammatory response may be initiated by trauma, infection, allergy and autoimmune reactions, although the latter is more often associated with the chronic form of inflammation. While the initiating events may be different, the overall inflammatory response is similar, with the exception of inflammation caused by IgE/mast cell interactions where the response may be immediate and more systemic.*

Initiation of acute inflammatory responses

Acute inflammation is caused initially by the release of inflammatory mediators from microbes, damaged tissues, or other cells including mast cells and macrophages (*Table 1*). Complement cleavage products C3a, C4a and C5a may also be involved, as they trigger release of histamine from mast cells, which induces vascular changes leading to edema. Moreover, C5a is chemotactic for PMNs, and C3a, C4a and C5a increase neutrophil and monocyte adherence to endothelial cells. Tissue macrophages also play a role in generation of

Table 1.   Source of inflammatory mediators resulting from microbial infection

Source of initiating factors	Mechanism of induction
Exotoxins	**Via damage to tissues:** Prostaglandins and leukotrienes have a direct effect on vascular endothelium
Endotoxins (from Gram-positive bacteria)	**Via pattern recognition receptors:** Direct effects on macrophages to release proinflammatory cytokines (via toll receptors) eg. IL-1, IL-6, IL-12, IL-18, TNFα and IFNγ
Lipopeptides, etc. (from Gram-positive bacteria)	Direct effects of macrophages to release proinflammatory cytokines (via toll receptors).
C3a derived by alternative or classical pathways	Causes mast cell degranulation

pro-inflammatory cytokines (including IL-1 and TNFα) via recognition, through their pattern recognition receptors (Topic B3), of structures associated with microbes.

Mast cells, which are distributed throughout the body (Topic B1), are central to the acute inflammatory process in that, on stimulation, they release histamine and other vasoactive amines that result in the vascular changes seen in acute inflammation. Other pro-inflammatory substances released by mast cells include IL-1, TNFα, leukotrienes, PAF and nitric oxide, some of which cause blood vessel dilation and edema and increase adhesion of neutrophils and monocytes to endothelium (see below). Vasoactive amines such as histamine can also have an effect on smooth muscle contraction, which is important in defense against worms in the intestine (Topic H2). Thus, while the inflammatory mediators associated with the initiating events of acute inflammation may be different, they share common pathways in the inflammatory process as a result of the intimate involvement of mast cells in this process.

Vascular changes   The inflammatory mediators released by tissues, mast cells and macrophages cause dilation of the blood vessels (vasodilation), which increases blood flow and smooth muscle contraction. These inflammatory mediators also cause rapid alterations in the blood vessel endothelium and induce increased expression of cellular adhesion molecules, which assist in the transfer of blood leukocytes. Overall, changes in tight junctions in endothelial cells occur that permit the passage of fluid (containing antibacterial proteins, clotting factors, and antibodies, etc.) and PMNs from the bloodstream to the site of release of these inflammatory mediators (Fig. 2), so as to combat the microbe and/or repair the damage. Vasodilation and increased blood flow result in the redness and heat, and the edema (fluid accumulation) results in swelling. Fluid accumulation together with tissue damage gives rise to the pain through specialized receptors. Overall, the mast cell plays a major role in acute inflammation initiated by injury or infection by microbes (Fig. 2).

PMNs leave the bloodstream as a result of their recognition of adhesion molecules displayed on the endothelial cells. The expression of these adhesion molecules is induced by pro-inflammatory cytokines released from macrophages. In particular, IL-1 and TNFα cause increased expression of ICAM-1 and VCAM-1, adhesion molecules central to the progression of acute

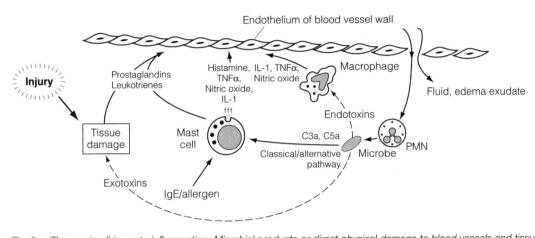

Fig. 2. The mast cell in acute inflammation. Microbial products or direct physical damage to blood vessels and tissues leads to release of mediators, e.g. prostaglandins and leukotrienes, which like mast cell mediators (e.g. histamine) increase vascular permeability and vasodilation. Mast cells release their mediators following microbial activation of complement (classical and alternative pathways) and via IgE/allergen complexes. Microbial endotoxins also activate macrophages to release TNFα and IL-1, which have vasodilatory properties. The outcome of this barrage of mediators is the loosening of the endothelial tight junctions, increased adhesion of intravascular neutrophils (and monocytes) and their passage from blood vessels into the surrounding tissues where they can phagocytose the microbes. Serum proteins (fibrinogen, antibodies, etc.) also pass into the tissues and the accumulating fluid (edema) protects the damaged area during repair.

inflammation. Adhesion molecules expressed on the surface of endothelial cells interact with their counter-receptor (ligand) on PMNs (e.g. ICAM-1 binds to LFA-1, VCAM-1 binds to VLA-4). This process involves the capture and rolling of PMNs, followed by their activation, flattening and extravasation (*Fig. 3*).

Termination of the response and repair

Once the offending insult, e.g. microbe, has been removed or controlled, inhibitors dampen inflammation and tissue repair mechanisms become activated. Inhibitors of the pro-inflammatory cytokines include their soluble recep-

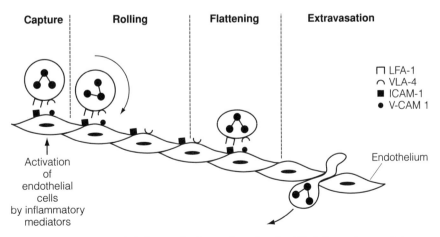

Fig. 3. Adhesion to endothelium and extravasation of neutrophils. Inflammatory mediators activate endothelial cells resulting in expression of adhesion molecules (e.g. ICAM-1 and VCAM-1). These capture leukocytes expressing LFA-1 and VLA-4 (e.g. PMNs) respectively causing them to roll, flatten and squeeze through tight junctions between the endothelial cells (extravasation) and into the tissues where inflammatory mediators are being released.

tors (e.g. receptors for IL-1, TNFα, IL-6 and IL-12), the anti-inflammatory cytokines (IL-4, IL-10 and TGFβ), components of the hemostasis and thrombosis system, and glucocorticoids.

The Th2 cytokine IL-4 downregulates the production of pro-inflammatory cytokines from Th1 cells and TGFβ is a potent inhibitor of many immune functions. Protein C, a component of the hemostasis and thrombosis system, is an anti-inflammatory agent and functions by inhibiting cytokines such as TNFα. Glucocorticoids are well known anti-inflammatory agents and inhibit production of nearly all pro-inflammatory mediators (Section G). Other hormones such as α-melanocyte-stimulating hormone reduce fever, IL-2 synthesis and prostaglandin production, while corticotrophin inhibits macrophage activation and IFNγ synthesis. The neuropeptides somatostatin and VIP reduce inflammation by inhibiting T cell proliferation and migration.

As the inflammatory phase is neutralized by these anti-inflammatory molecules, repair of the damage begins. Various cells including myofibroblasts and macrophages, both of which make collagen, mend tissues. Macrophage products including epidermal growth factor, platelet-derived growth factor, fibroblast growth factor and transforming growth factor are important in the repair process.

C1 LYMPHOCYTES

Key Notes

Specificity and memory

Lymphocytes provide both the specificity and memory which are characteristic of the adaptive immune response. The two types of lymphocytes involved in the adaptive response are T cells and B cells, both of which have similar morphology. They have specific but different antigen receptors and additional surface molecules necessary for interaction with other cells.

T lymphocytes

Large numbers of antigen-specific T cells are produced in the thymus from circulating T cell precursors derived from stem cells in the bone marrow. Each T cell has receptors specific for only one antigen that are generated by gene rearrangement from multiple, inherited germline genes. T cells then undergo selection to remove those that are highly self-reactive. In the process, two different kinds of T cells develop. T helper (Th) cells, of which there are two types (Th1 and Th2), express CD4 and provide help for B cell growth and differentiation. T cytotoxic (Tc) cells express CD8 and recognize and kill virally infected cells. Functionally mature T cells then migrate to secondary lymphoid tissues to mediate protection.

B lymphocytes and plasma cells

HSC differentiation into B cells occurs within the fetal liver and, after birth, the bone marrow. In the bone marrow, B cell precursors rearrange multiple, inherited, germline genes that encode B cell antigen receptors (antibodies), thus creating many different B cells, each with a unique specificity for antigen. Many B cells with antigen receptors that react with self are eliminated. In addition, two kinds of B cells (B1 and B2) with different properties develop. IgM is the first antibody expressed on B cells followed by co-expression of IgD. Mature B cells migrate into the secondary lymphoid tissues where they respond to foreign antigens. When activated by antigen, in most cases with T cell help, they proliferate in germinal centers and mature into memory cells or into plasma cells that produce and secrete large amounts of antibody.

Related topics

Hemopoiesis – development of blood cells (A5)

The B cell receptor complex, co-receptors and signaling (E1)

The role of T cells in immune responses (F1)

T cell recognition of antigen (F2)

Specificity and memory

Lymphocytes are responsible for the specificity and memory in adaptive immune responses. They are produced in the primary lymphoid organs (Topic C2) and function in the secondary lymphoid organs/tissues where they recognize and respond to foreign antigens. There are three types of lymphocytes – NK cells, T cells and B cells, although only T and B cells have true antigen specificity and memory. NK cells were considered earlier (Topic B1) and function in innate protection against viruses and some tumors.

T cells and B cells mature in the thymus and bone marrow, respectively. In the resting state both T and B lymphocytes have a similar morphology with a small amount of cytoplasm (*Fig. 1*). They have specific but different antigen receptors and a variety of other surface molecules necessary for interaction with other cells (*Table 1*). These include molecules required for their activation and for movement into and out of the tissues of the body. This ability to migrate into the tissues and return via the lymphatic vessels to the bloodstream (recirculation) is a unique feature of lymphocytes.

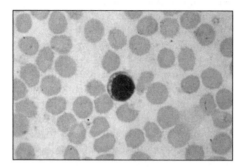

Fig. 1.   A blood lymphocyte. Reproduced from Immunology 4th edn, Roitt, Brostoff and Male, with permission from Mosby.

Table 1.   Characteristics of human B and T cells

	T cells	B cells
Site of maturation	Thymus	Bone marrow
Antigen receptor	TCR	Antibody
Requirement of MHC for recognition	Yes	No
Characteristic 'markers'	All have TCR, CD3 Th – CD4 Tc – CD8	Surface Ig, CD19, CD20, CD21 CD79
Main location in lymph nodes	Paracortical area	Follicles
Memory cells	Yes	Yes
Function	Protect against intracellular microbes Provide help for Ab responses	Protect against extracellular microbes
Products	Th1 – IFNγ, TNFα Th2 – IL-4, IL-5, IL-6 Tc – Perforins	Antibodies (B cells mature into plasma cells)

There are two classes of T lymphocytes, T helper (Th) cells and T cytotoxic (Tc) cells. All T lymphocytes have antigen receptors (TCR) (Topic F2) that determine their specificity and CD3, which is essential for their activation (Topic F4). These molecules also serve as 'markers' to identify T cells. B lymphocytes make and use antibodies as their specific antigen receptor. They have molecules similar to CD3, i.e. CD79, which are important in their activation. B lymphocytes can mature into plasma cells that produce and secrete large amounts of antibody.

T lymphocytes

T cell ontogeny

The thymus is derived from the third and fourth pharyngeal pouches during embryonic life and attracts (with chemoattractive molecules) circulating T cell precursors derived from hemopoietic stem cells (HSC) in the bone marrow. In the thymus, these precursors differentiate into functional T lymphocytes under the influence of thymic stromal cells and cytokines. In particular, in the thymic cortex the precursors (now thymocytes) associate with cortical epithelial nurse cells critical to their development. In this site there is major thymocyte proliferation, with a complete turnover of cells approximately every 72 hours. Thymocytes then move into the medulla, where they undergo further differentiation and selection. Most of the thymocytes generated each day in the thymus die by apoptosis with only 5–10% surviving. Molecules important to T cell function such as CD4, CD8 and the T cell receptor develop at different stages during the differentiation process (*Fig. 2*).

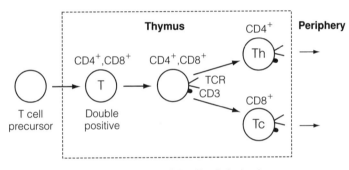

Fig. 2.   Development of CD4$^+$ and CD8$^+$ T cells in the thymus.

Thymus function

The main functions of the thymus as a primary lymphoid organ are to: (a) produce sufficient numbers (millions) of different T cells each expressing unique T cell receptors (generate diversity) such that in every individual there are at least some cells potentially specific for each foreign antigen in our environment; (b) select T cells for survival in such a way that the chance for an auto-immune response is minimized. It is important to note that T cell development within the thymus is *independent* of exogenous (foreign) antigens.

Generation of T cell diversity in the thymus

Millions of T cells, each with receptors specific for different antigens, are generated by gene rearrangement from multiple (inherited) germline genes. Each of the T cells produced in the thymus has only one specificity coded for by its antigen receptor.

Positive and negative selection

Once produced in the thymus, T cells undergo selection using their newly produced receptors. T cells with receptors that bind weakly to MHC molecules are selected whilst those with receptors which bind strongly to MHC and self antigens die through apoptosis (central tolerance to self, Topic G2) and are removed by phagocytic macrophages.

Mature T cells and their subsets

T cells which survive the selection process mature into functionally distinct subsets (*Fig. 3*). These cells migrate to the peripheral lymphoid tissues where they complete their functional maturation and provide protection against invading microbes. Some T cells reside, at least temporarily, in T-cell-dependent areas of tissues. T cells can be identified using monoclonal antibodies specific for characteristic molecules such as the T cell receptor (TCR) or CD3 (*Table 2*). These cells function to control intracellular microbes and to provide help for B cell (antibody) responses. Two different kinds of T cells are involved in these functions, T helper (Th) cells and T cytotoxic (Tc) cells.

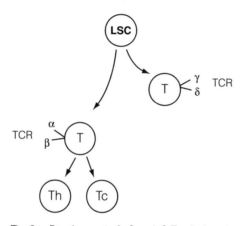

Fig. 3.   Development of αβ and γδ T cells from lymphocyte stem cells (LSC). Two types of T cells are produced in the thymus with different TCRs (αβ and γδ). The classical T cells (Th and Tc) utilize αβ for their TCR.

Th cells provide help for B cells through direct cell surface signaling and by producing cytokines that are critical to B cell growth and differentiation. In addition to TCR and CD3, Th cells also express cell surface CD4 molecules that bind to MHC class II molecules, an interaction required for their activation by antigen (Topic F2). Th cells can be further subdivided into Th1 and Th2 cells based on their ability to help in the development of different immune responses (Topic F5), which is in turn related to their cytokine profiles. The average percentages of these cells in the peripheral blood are shown in *Table 3*. T cytotoxic (Tc) cells mediate killing of infected cells, primarily those infected with virus. These cells express, in addition to TCR and CD3, a cell surface molecule, CD8, that binds to MHC class I and is important for these cells to interact effectively with virally infected cells.

B lymphocytes and plasma cells

The bone marrow and B cell ontogeny

B cells develop from hemopoietic stem cells primarily (perhaps exclusively) in the microenvironment of the fetal liver and, after birth, the bone marrow. The two main functions of the bone marrow as a primary lymphoid organ are to: (a) produce large numbers of B cells, each with unique antigen receptors (antibodies) such that, overall, there is sufficient B cell diversity to recognize all of the antigens in our environment (generate diversity); (b) eliminate B cells with antigen receptors for self molecules. The early stages of B cell development (like that of T cells) is independent of exogenous antigen. Mature B cells leave the bone marrow and migrate via the bloodstream to the secondary lymphoid organs/tissues where they can be found in loose aggregates (primary follicles) in lymphoid tissues or in well-defined proliferating foci (germinal centers).

Two kinds of B cells (B1 and B2) have been identified. The B2 cells are produced in the bone marrow (*conventional B cells*) as described and with the help of Th cells produce IgG, IgA and IgE antibodies. However, B1 cells arise

Table 2. Surface receptors on T cells

Surface molecules	Function
The T cell receptor complex	
TCR	Antigen specific receptor (most T cells utilize $\alpha\beta$ dimers; some use $\gamma\delta$ dimers
CD3 ($\gamma,\delta,\varepsilon$ and ζ (zeta) chains)	Signaling complex associated with the TCR: mediates T cell activation on binding of TCR to MHC–peptide complexes
Subset markers	
CD4 (on helper T cells)	Binds to MHC class II molecules and restricts Th cells to recognizing only peptides presented on MHC class II
CD8 (on cytotoxic T cells)	Binds to MHC class I molecules and restricts Tc cells to recognizing only peptides presented on MHC class I
Co-stimulatory molecules	
CD28	Binds to CD80/CD86 on B cells and APC and positively regulates T cell activation
CTLA4	Binds to CD80/CD86 on B cells and APC and downregulates T cell activation
CD154 (CD40L): on activated Th cells	Binds to CD40 on B cells and APC: triggers activation of APC and activation and antibody class switching of B cells
Adhesion molecules	
LFA-1	Binds to ICAM-1 and facilitates interactions with other cells including B cells, APCs and target cells
CD2 (LFA2)	Binds to LFA-3 and facilitates interactions with other cells including B cells, APCs and target cells
CD45RA (on naïve T cells)	Involved in signal transduction
CD45R0 (on activated/memory T cells)	Involved in signal transduction

Table 3. Human peripheral blood lymphocyte populations

	T cells		B cells	NK cells
	Th	Tc		
Percent of lymphocytes	55	25	10	10
Functional properties	Antigen specific, produce cytokines, memory cells, effector cells		Antigen specific, produce cytokines, memory cells, plasma cells (antibody factories)	Mediate ADCC, tumor surveillance, no memory, lyse virus-infected cells and tumor cells lacking MHC class I

early in ontogeny, express mainly IgM antibodies encoded by germline antibody genes, mature independently of the bone marrow and generally recognize multimeric sugar/lipid antigens of microbes and are thymus independent (Topic E2).

Generation of antigen receptor diversity and negative selection of B cells

Antibodies, like T cell receptors, are encoded by multiple genes. These genes, which are distinct from the T cell antigen receptor genes, rearrange during the pro-B cell stage to create a unique cell surface receptor that defines its specificity for antigen (Topic D3). Since rearrangement occurs in millions of different ways in these developing cells, many B cells, each with a different specificity, are generated. This generation of diversity occurs in the absence of foreign protein and yields large numbers of mature B cells, at least some of which have specificity for each foreign substance or microbe. B cells with specificity for self antigens are induced to die by apoptosis (negative selection) during their immature stage, i.e. when they have expressed IgM on their cell surface, but before expression of IgD. As in the thymus, the majority of the B cells die during development as a result of their production of antigen receptors that cannot be assembled or that are directed against self antigens.

Activated B cells and plasma cells

When activated by antigen and, in most cases, with T cell help, B cells (*Table 4*) proliferate and mature into memory cells or plasma cells. Memory cells only produce antibody for expression on their cell surface and remain able to respond to antigen if it is reintroduced. In contrast, plasma cells do not have cell surface antibody receptors. Rather, these cells function as factories producing and secreting large amounts of antibody of the same specificity as the antigen receptor on the stimulated parent B cell. The morphology of a plasma cell (*Fig. 4*) is consistent with its primary function – high-rate glycoprotein (antibody) synthesis. This includes extensive endoplasmic reticulum, mitochondria and Golgi apparatus. It should be noted that a plasma cell only produces antibodies of one specificity, one class and one subclass.

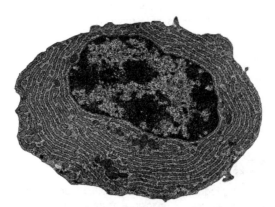

Fig. 4. Ultrastructure of a plasma cell. Note the extensive rough endoplasmic reticulum for antibody production. Reproduced from Immunology 5th edn., 1998, Roitt, Brostoff and Male, with permission from Mosby.

Table 4. Surface receptors on B lymphocytes

Surface molecules	Function
The B cell receptor complex	
Antibody (IgM and IgD on mature B cells)	B cell receptor (BCR) for antigen
CD79a/CD79b (Igα/Igβ) heterodimer	Mediates cellular activation on binding of BCR to antigen
Co-receptors	All these molecules modulate B cell activation
CD19	Influences B cell activation
CD20	Ca^{++} channel
CD21 (complement receptor CR2)	Binds to C3d, C3bi
CD32 (FcγRII: Fc receptor for IgG)	Binds to IgG complexed to antigen
CD40	Signals B cell activation and antibody class switching after engagement with CD40 ligand (CD154) on activated T cells
Molecules required for T cell activation	
MHC class II molecules	Present peptides to Th cells
CD80/86 (B7-1,2)	Binds to CD28 on T cells to trigger their activation
Adhesion molecules	
ICAM-1	Binds to LFA-1 and facilitates interaction with T cells
LFA-3	Binds to CD2 and facilitates interaction with T cells

C2 LYMPHOID ORGANS AND TISSUES

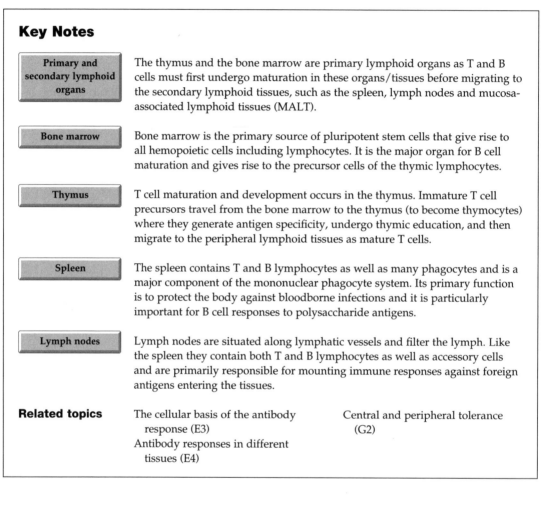

Key Notes

Primary and secondary lymphoid organs

The thymus and the bone marrow are primary lymphoid organs as T and B cells must first undergo maturation in these organs/tissues before migrating to the secondary lymphoid tissues, such as the spleen, lymph nodes and mucosa-associated lymphoid tissues (MALT).

Bone marrow

Bone marrow is the primary source of pluripotent stem cells that give rise to all hemopoietic cells including lymphocytes. It is the major organ for B cell maturation and gives rise to the precursor cells of the thymic lymphocytes.

Thymus

T cell maturation and development occurs in the thymus. Immature T cell precursors travel from the bone marrow to the thymus (to become thymocytes) where they generate antigen specificity, undergo thymic education, and then migrate to the peripheral lymphoid tissues as mature T cells.

Spleen

The spleen contains T and B lymphocytes as well as many phagocytes and is a major component of the mononuclear phagocyte system. Its primary function is to protect the body against bloodborne infections and it is particularly important for B cell responses to polysaccharide antigens.

Lymph nodes

Lymph nodes are situated along lymphatic vessels and filter the lymph. Like the spleen they contain both T and B lymphocytes as well as accessory cells and are primarily responsible for mounting immune responses against foreign antigens entering the tissues.

Related topics

The cellular basis of the antibody
  response (E3)
Antibody responses in different
  tissues (E4)

Central and peripheral tolerance
  (G2)

Primary and secondary lymphoid organs

The thymus and bone marrow are the primary lymphoid organs in mammals. T and B cells with diverse antigen receptors are produced in these organs. Following selection processes (Topics E3, E4 and F3), they migrate to the secondary lymphoid tissues – the lymph nodes, spleen, and the mucosa-associated lymphoid tissues (MALT) (*Fig. 1*).

Bone marrow

During early fetal development blood cells are produced in the mesenchyme of the yolk sac. As the development of the fetus progresses the liver and spleen take over this role. It is only in the last months of fetal development that the bone marrow becomes the dominant site of hemopoiesis (blood cell formation). Bone marrow is composed of hemopoietic cells of various lineages and maturity, packed between fat cells, thin bands of bony tissue (trabeculae), collagen fibers, fibroblasts and dendritic cells. All of the hemopoietic cells are derived

Primary lymphoid organs

Secondary lymphoid organs and tissues

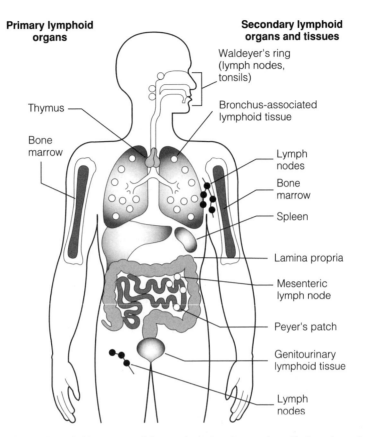

Fig. 1. Lymphoid organs and tissues. Lymphocytes produced in the primary lymphoid organs (thymus and bone marrow) migrate to the secondary organs and tissues where they respond to microbial infections. The mucosa-associated lymphoid tissue (MALT) together with other lymphoid cells in sub-epithelial sites (lamina propria) of the respiratory, gastro-intestinal and genitourinary tracts comprise the majority of lymphoid tissue in the body.

from multipotential stem cells which give rise not only to all of the lymphoid cells found in the lymphoid tissue, but also to all of the cells found in the blood.

Ultrastructural studies show hemopoietic cells cluster around the vascular sinuses where they mature, before they eventually are discharged into the blood. Lymphocytes are found surrounding the small radial arteries, whereas most immature myeloid precursors are found deep in the parenchyma. The bone marrow gives rise to all of the lymphoid cells that migrate to the thymus and mature into T cells, as well as to the major population of conventional B cells. B cells mature in the bone marrow and undergo selection for non-self before making their way to the peripheral lymphoid tissues: there they form primary and secondary follicles and may undergo further selection in germinal centers (Topics E3, E4 and G2).

Thymus

The thymus is a lymphocyte-rich, bilobed, encapsulated organ located behind the sternum, above and in front of the heart. It is essential for the maturation of T cells and the development of cell-mediated immunity. In fact, the term 'T cell' means thymus-derived cell and is used to describe mature T cells. The activity of the thymus is maximal in the fetus and in early childhood and then undergoes atrophy at puberty although never totally disappearing. It is composed of cortical and medullary epithelial cells, stromal cells, interdigitating cells and macrophages. These 'accessory' cells are important in the differentiation of the immigrating T cell precursors and their 'education' (positive and negative selection) prior to their migration into the secondary lymphoid tissues (Topic F3).

The thymus has an interactive role with the endocrine system as thymectomy leads to a reduction in pituitary hormone levels as well as atrophy of the gonads. Conversely, neonatal hypophysectomy (removal of the pituitary gland) results in thymic atrophy. Thymic epithelial cells produce the hormones thymosin and thymopoietin and in concert with cytokines (such as IL-7) are probably important for the development and maturation of thymocytes into mature T cells.

Spleen

The spleen (*Fig. 2*) is a large, encapsulated, bean-shaped organ with a spongy interior (splenic pulp) that is situated on the left side of the body below the diaphragm. The large splenic artery pervades the spleen and branches of this artery are surrounded by highly organized lymphoid tissue (white pulp). The white pulp forms 'islands' within a meshwork of reticular fibers containing red blood cells, macrophages and plasma cells (red pulp). Closely associated with the central arteriole is the 'periarteriolar lymphatic sheath' an area containing mainly T cells and interdigitating cells (IDC). Primary lymphoid follicles, composed mainly of follicular dendritic cells (FDC) and B cells, are contained within the sheath. During an immune response these follicles develop germinal centers (i.e. become secondary follicles). The periarteriolar lymphoid sheath is separated from the 'red pulp' by a marginal zone containing macrophages (MØ) and B cells (*Fig. 2*). The central arterioles in the periarteriolar sheath subdivide like the branches of a tree. The space between the branches is filled with 'red pulp', and vascular channels called splenic sinuses. The spleen is a major component of the mononuclear phagocyte system, containing large

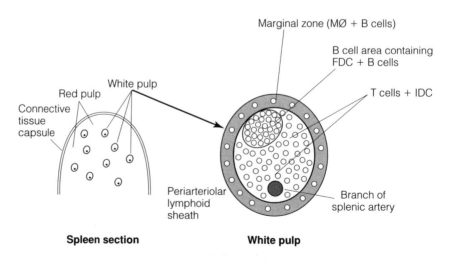

Fig. 2.   Structure of lymphoid tissue in the spleen.

numbers of phagocytes. Unlike lymph nodes, it does not contain either afferent or efferent lymphatics.

The main immunological function of the spleen is to filter the blood by trapping bloodborne microbes and producing an immune response to them. It also removes damaged red blood cells and immune complexes. Those individuals who have had their spleens removed (splenectomized) have a greater susceptibility to infection with encapsulated bacteria, and are at increased risk of severe malarial infections, which indicates its major importance in immunity. In addition, the spleen acts as a reservoir of erythrocytes.

Lymph nodes

Lymph nodes (*Fig. 3*) are small solid structures found at varying points along the lymphatic system, e.g. groin, armpit and mesentery. They range in size from 2 to 10 mm, are spherical in shape and are encapsulated. Beneath the capsule is the subcapsular sinus, the cortex, a paracortical region and a medulla. The cortex contains many follicles and on antigenic stimulation becomes enlarged with germinal centers. The follicles are comprised mainly of B cells and follicular dendritic cells. The paracortical (thymus-dependent) region contains large numbers of T cells interspersed with interdigitating cells.

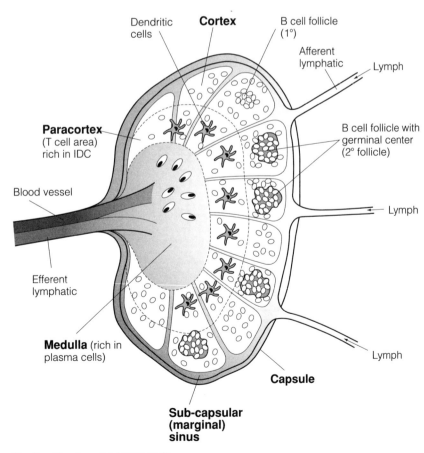

Fig. 3. Structure of a lymph node.

The primary role of the lymph node is to filter the lymph and then produce an immune response against trapped microbes/antigens. Lymph arriving from the tissues or from a preceding lymph node in the chain, passes via the afferent lymphatics into the subcapsular sinus and then into the cortex, around the follicles, into the paracortical area and then into the medulla. Lymph in the medullary sinuses then drains into efferent lymphatics and hence through larger lymphatic vessels back into the bloodstream. Lymphocytes enter the lymph nodes from the tissues via the afferent lymphatics and from the blood-stream through specialized post capillary venules called high endothelial venules that are found in the paracortical region of the node. B cells entering the blood migrate to the cortex where they are found in follicles (B cell areas).

C3 MUCOSA-ASSOCIATED LYMPHOID TISSUES

Key Notes

MALT	The majority (>50%) of lymphoid tissue in the human body is located within the lining of the respiratory, digestive and genitourinary tracts, as they are the main entry sites for microbes into the body; subdivided into NALT, GALT and BALT.
NALT	Nasal-associated lymphoid tissue (NALT) includes immune cells underlying the throat and nasal passages and especially the tonsils. The architecture of these lymphoid tissues, although not encapsulated, is similar to that of the lymph nodes and consists of follicles composed mainly of B cells.
GALT	Gut-associated lymphoid tissue (GALT) is composed of lymphoid complexes (also called Peyer's patches in the ileum) that consist of specialized epithelium, antigen-presenting cells and intraepithelial lymphocytes. These structures occur strategically at specific areas in the digestive tract.
BALT	The lymphoid tissue associated with the bronchus (BALT) is structurally similar to Peyer's patches and other lymphoid tissues of the gut. It consists of lymphoid aggregates and follicles and is found along the main bronchi in the lobes of the lungs.
Related topics	Lymphocyte traffic and recirculation (C4) The microbial cosmos (H1)
	Central and peripheral tolerance (G2) Immune cells and molecules associated with the reproductive tracts (O2)

MALT

The main sites of entry for microbes into the body are through mucosal surfaces. It is therefore not surprising that more than 50% of the total body lymphoid mass is associated with these surfaces. These are collectively called mucosa-associated lymphoid tissues (MALT) and include NALT, BALT, GALT and lymphoid tissue associated with the genitourinary system (see Section O).

NALT

The nasal-associated lymphoid system is composed of the lymphoid tissue at the back of the nose (pharyngeal, tonsil and other tissue) and that associated with the Waldeyer's ring (palatine and lingual tonsils). The strategic location of these lymphoid tissues suggests that they are directly involved in handling airborne microbes. Their composition is similar to that of lymph nodes but they are not encapsulated and are without lymphatics. Antigens and foreign particles are trapped within the deep crypts of their lympho-epithelium from where they are transported to the lymphoid follicles (*Fig. 1*). The follicles are composed mainly of B cells surrounded by T cells and the germinal center within the follicle is the site of antigen-dependent B cell proliferation.

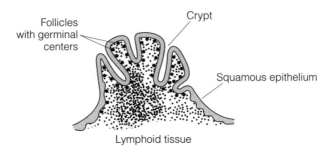

Fig. 1.   *Tonsilar lymphoid tissue: Antigens trapped in the crypts are transported by M cells into the sub-epithelial areas where lymphocytes are stimulated via antigen presenting cells.*

GALT

The primary role of GALT is to protect the body against microbes entering the body via the intestinal tract. It is primarily made up of lymphoid aggregates and lymphoid cells (IELs) between epithelial cells and within the lamina propria. In order to distinguish between harmful invaders or harmless food, the gut has a 'sampling' mechanism that analyzes everything that has been ingested (or in the case of BALT and NALT, inhaled). The analytical, or antigen-sampling machinery of the gut, consists of specialized epithelial cells, M cells, and intimately associated APCs (antigen 'processing and presenting' cells (*Fig. 2*). M cells take up foreign molecules and pass them to underlying APCs, which present them in the context of class I and class II MHC molecules to T cells. The helper T cells help to activate B cells and both T and B cells can migrate to other parts of the GI tract (including salivary glands) and other MALT sites, e.g. lactating mammary glands and respiratory and genitourinary tracts, and protect these surfaces from invasion by the same microbes (Topic E4). Depending on the antigen, the APC and its state, and other factors, toler-

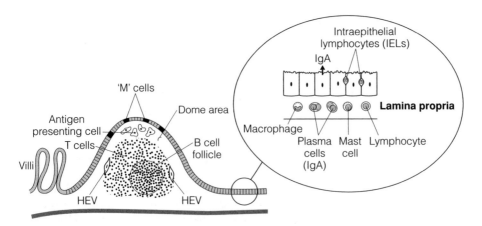

Fig. 2.   *Intestinal lymphoid aggregates: 'M' cells transport luminal antigens into the dome area where they are taken up by antigen-presenting cells, processed and presented to T cells entering the site via the high endothelial venules (HEV). The cells interact with antigen-specific B cells and these migrate via the draining lymph nodes to the sub-epithelial sites (lamina propria) of the intestinal tract but also locations within the other tracts of the body i.e. the respiratory tract and the genitourinary tract.* **Insert:** *Here the B cells develop into IgA-secreting plasma cells and IgA is transported through the epithelium into the lumen of the intestine. CD4 T and, more prominently CD8 T cells are present and the latter are frequently seen between the epithelial cells (IELs). Mast cells and macrophages are also present in the lamina propria.*

ance as well as immunity can be induced to the sampled antigen (Topics G3 and I2).

The combination of specialized epithelium and antigen-processing cells plus lymphocytes constitute what are called lymphoid complexes. These are localized structures that occur regularly at specific areas in the digestive tract and are exemplified by Peyer's patches in the terminal ileum. Lymphoid complexes are not distributed uniformly throughout the gut as one might initially expect, but are congregated in several zones (*Fig. 3*).

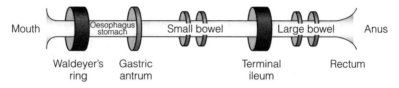

Fig. 3.   *Lymphoid complexes along the gastrointestinal tract; volume of the rings indicates the relative amount of lymphoid tissue.*

BALT

Bronchus-associated lymphoid tissue is similar to Peyers patches. It is composed mainly of aggregates of lymphocytes organized into follicles that are found in all lobes of the lung and are situated under the epithelium mainly along the bronchi. The majority of lymphocytes in the follicles are B cells. Antigen sampling is carried out by epithelial cells lining the surface of the mucosa and by way of M cells which transport antigens to underlying APCs and lymphocytes.

C4 LYMPHOCYTE TRAFFIC AND RECIRCULATION

Key Notes

Lymphocyte traffic and recirculation	T and B cells produced in the thymus and bone marrow, respectively, migrate via the bloodstream to the secondary lymphoid organs/tissues where they carry out their function. They do not stay in one site but continually recirculate through the body in search of antigens.
Trafficking in MALT	Lymphocytes stimulated in one mucosal organ, e.g. the GALT, can migrate to the lamina propria of other sites of the mucosal immune system (e.g. lactating mammary glands and salivary glands), and protect these surfaces from invasion with the same microbes.
Mechanisms of lymphocyte traffic	Lymphocytes have surface 'homing molecules' (adhesion molecules) that they use to attach to endothelial cells of blood vessels to exit the blood system at different anatomical sites.
Related topics	Lymphoid organs and tissues (C2) Mucosa-associated lymphoid tissues (C3)

Lymphocyte traffic and recirculation

Lymphocytes produced in the primary lymphoid organs, thymus (T) and bone marrow (B), migrate via the bloodstream to the secondary lymphoid organs or tissues where they carry out their function. Since these cells have not yet encountered antigen, they are called 'naive cells' and do not remain in one secondary lymphoid organ, but continue to recirculate around the body until they recognize their specific antigen (*Fig. 1*). They enter the lymph nodes via the **high endothelial venules (HEV)** and if they are not activated there, they pass via efferent lymphatic vessels into the thoracic duct and hence back into the bloodstream. Both memory and naive cells recirculate through the lymphoid tissues.

T and B cells migrate to different sites within the lymph nodes. T cells reside in the paracortical region whereas the B cell domain is the lymphoid follicle. B cells must traverse through the T cell area to reach the follicle. In the spleen, lymphocytes enter the periarteriolar lymphoid sheath (PALS) by way of the marginal zone (MZ) and leave through the splenic veins (SV) in the red pulp (RP). The lymphoid tissues are dynamic structures, wherein both T and B lymphocytes are continuously trafficking through each other's territories as well as being challenged by antigen on antigen-presenting cells. Lymphocytes also are able to traffic to specific tissues such as the MALT (see below).

Trafficking in MALT

One of the unique features of MALT is that lymphocytes stimulated in one site can migrate to other sites of the mucosal immune system to protect them

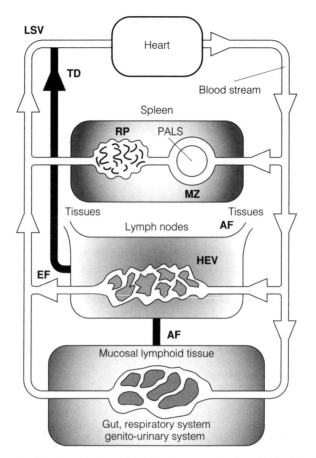

Fig. 1.   Lymphocyte recirculation. Lymphocytes travel in the blood stream to the spleen where they enter the periarteriolar lymphoid sheath (PALS) via the marginal zone (MZ) and re-enter the blood stream via the red pulp (RP). Lymphocytes enter the lymph nodes via high endothelial veins (HEV) in the paracortical regions and pass via the efferent lymphatics (EF) into the lymphatic system and via the thoracic duct (TD) into the left subclavian vein (LSV). Lymphocytes pass into the mucosal tissues through the HEV and return via the afferent lymphatics (AF) of the draining lymph nodes. Lymphocytes stimulated by microbes in the MALT migrate back to the mucosal tissues where they have been stimulated. Thus, lymphocytes stimulated in the intestine will migrate back to sites in the lamina propria along the intestine (as well as to other mucosal sites) to protect the body against the specific microbial attack via this route. Arrows indicate the direction of flow.

against the same antigen or from invasion by the same microbe. Thus for example, lymphocytes that initially encountered and were stimulated by antigen in the GALT can migrate via the blood to distant sites including the salivary glands, lactating mammary glands, the respiratory and reproductive tracts, etc., and mediate protection in these other MALT tissues.

Mechanisms of lymphocyte traffic

Lymphocytes have 'homing' molecules which determine where they exit the bloodstream. These cell surface **adhesion molecules** attach to molecules (**addressins**) on specialized endothelial cells of the HEV. The lymphocytes then migrate between endothelial cells into the tissue (*Fig. 2*). Of note, different

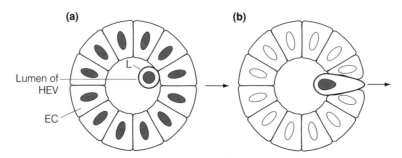

Fig. 2.   *Traffic of lymphocytes from the blood stream via HEV. (a) Lymphocytes (L) attach to the endothelial cells (EC) in the HEV by adhesion molecules. (b) Lymphocytes pass between endothelial cells to exit the HEV into lymph nodes or the MALT.*

lymphocytes express different specific adhesion molecules which attach to specific surface addressins on endothelial cells of blood vessels in particular sites of the body. Thus, some lymphocytes express adhesion molecules that bind to addressins on the HEVs of lymph nodes and home there. Other lymphocytes express adhesion molecules that only bind to addressins on the HEVs of MALT, allowing them to migrate into the MALT areas of the body (*Fig. 3*).

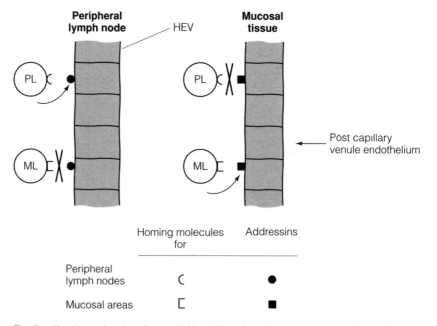

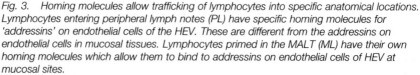

Fig. 3.   *Homing molecules allow trafficking of lymphocytes into specific anatomical locations. Lymphocytes entering peripheral lymph notes (PL) have specific homing molecules for 'addressins' on endothelial cells of the HEV. These are different from the addressins on endothelial cells in mucosal tissues. Lymphocytes primed in the MALT (ML) have their own homing molecules which allow them to bind to addressins on endothelial cells of HEV at mucosal sites.*

C5 ADAPTIVE IMMUNITY AT BIRTH

Colostrum-first breast Milk.

Key Notes

Lymphocytes in the newborn	T and B lymphocytes are present in the blood of newborns in slightly higher numbers than in adults, and many are fully functional. However, their ability to mount an immune response to certain antigens (e.g. polysaccharides) may be deficient, perhaps due to immaturity of some cells, to sequential expression of genes encoding antigen receptors, and/or to maternal antibody.
Antibodies in the newborn	Maternal IgG crosses the placenta (mediated by Fc receptors) and is present at high levels in the newborn. IgG is not synthesized *de novo* by the fetus until birth and IgA not for 1–2 months after birth, whereas IgM is produced late in fetal development. Maternal IgA from colostrum and milk during nursing, coats the infant's gastrointestinal tract and supplies passive mucosal immunity.
Related topics	Antibody classes (D2) Primary/congenital (inherited) immunodeficiency (J2)

---

de novo - latin - from start.

Lymphocytes in the newborn

Slightly higher than normal numbers of apparently mature T and B lymphocyte populations (as well as NK cells) are present in the blood of newborn individuals. Even so, the ability to mount an immune response to certain antigens may be lacking at birth. Thus, children under 2 years do not usually make antibody to the polysaccharides of pneumococcus or *H. influenzae*. In general, the ability to respond to a specific antigen depends on the age at which the individual is exposed to the antigen. There are a variety of explanations for this sequential appearance of specific immunity, including: (a) sequential expression of genes encoding receptors for each antigen; (b) immaturity of some B or helper T cell populations or of antigen-presenting cells (e.g. macrophages and dendritic cells); (c) passive maternal antibody that binds antigen and removes it, thereby interfering with the development of active immunity.

Since hemophilus polysaccharide conjugated to tetanus toxoid evokes protective anti-polysaccharide antibodies during the first year of life, this neonatal deficiency is likely to be in the Th cell population. Delayed maturation of the CD4$^+$ Th population may contribute to the generally low levels of IgG leading to immunodeficiency in transient hypogammaglobulinemia (Topic J2).

Antibodies in the newborn

IgM is produced late during fetal development but IgG is not synthesized *de novo*, until after birth (*Fig. 1*). IgA begins to appear in the blood at 1–2 months of age. However, **maternal IgG** crosses the placenta into the fetus (mediated by Fc receptor, FcRn) and is present at high levels in the newborn. This passive immunity partly compensates for the deficiencies in the ability of the infant to initially synthesize antibody through an immune system some components of which may not be totally mature. Furthermore, maternal IgA obtained by the infant from colostrum and milk during nursing coats the infant's

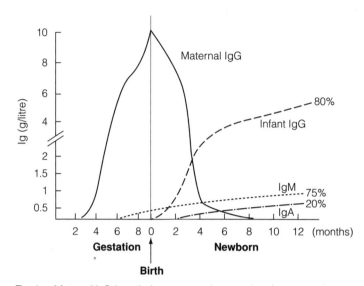

Fig. 1.   Maternal IgG is actively transported across the placenta and accumulates in the
baby's blood until birth. This protective IgG then decreases due to catabolism and disappears
completely by about 6–8 months of age. De novo synthesis of IgM by the baby occurs first at
6–8 months of gestation and this is followed around birth by IgG and later IgA. At one year of
age, the levels of the baby's IgG, IgM and IgA are about 80, 75 and 20% of adult levels,
respectively.

gastrointestinal tract and supplies passive mucosal immunity. As suggested
above, this passive immunity may contribute to the infant's unresponsiveness
to certain antigens until maternal antibodies are degraded or used up, and are
no longer interfering with the development of active immunity.

D1 ANTIBODY STRUCTURE

Key Notes

Molecular components

Antibodies, often termed 'immunoglobulins', are glycoproteins that bind antigens with high specificity and affinity. In humans there are five chemically and physically distinct classes of antibodies (IgG, IgA, IgM, IgD, IgE).

Antibody units

Antibodies have a basic unit of four polypeptide chains – two identical pairs of light (L) chains and heavy (H) chains – bound together by covalent disulfide bridges as well as by noncovalent interactions. These molecules can be proteolytically cleaved to yield two Fab fragments (the antigen-binding part of the molecules) and an Fc fragment (the part of the molecule responsible for effector functions, e.g. complement activation). Both H- and L-chains are divided into V and C regions – the V regions containing the antigen-binding site and the C region determining the fate of the antigen.

Affinity

The tightness of binding of an antibody-binding site to an antigenic determinant is called its affinity. The tighter the binding, the less likely the antibody is to dissociate from antigen. Different antibodies to an antigenic determinant vary considerably in their affinity for that determinant. Antibodies produced by a memory response have higher affinity than those in a primary response.

Antibody valence and avidity

The valence of an antibody is the number of antigenic determinants with which it can react. Having multiple binding sites for an antigen dramatically increases its binding (avidity) to antigens on particles such as bacteria or viruses. For example, two binding sites on IgG are 100 times more effective at neutralizing virus than two unlinked binding sites.

Related topics

Antibody classes (D2)
Generation of diversity (D3)

The B cell receptor complex, co-receptors and signaling (E1)

Molecular components

Antibodies are glycoproteins that bind antigens with high specificity and affinity (they hold on tightly). They are molecules, originally identified in the serum, which are also referred to as 'immunoglobulins,' a term often used interchangeably with antibodies. In humans there are five chemically and physically distinct classes of antibodies (IgG, IgA, IgM, IgD, IgE).

Antibody units

All antibodies have the same basic four polypeptide chain unit: two light (L) chains and two heavy (H) chains (*Fig. 1*). In this basic unit, one L-chain is bound, by a disulfide bridge and noncovalent interactions, to one H-chain. Similarly, the two H-chains are bound together by covalent disulfide bridges as well as by noncovalent hydrophilic and hydrophobic interactions. There are five different kinds of H-chains (referred to as μ, δ, γ, ε and α chains), which determine the class of antibody (IgM, IgD, IgG, IgE and IgA, respectively). There are also two different kinds of L-chains – κ and λ, each with a MW of 23 kDa. Each antibody unit can have only κ or λ L-chains but not both. The properties of the different antibody classes are shown in *Table 1*.

Both H- and L-chains have intrachain disulfide bridges every 90 amino acid residues, which create polypeptide loops, domains, of 110 amino acids. These domains are referred to as VH, VL, CH1, CH2, etc. (*Fig. 1*) and have particular functional properties (e.g. VH and VL together form the binding site for antigen). This type of structure is characteristic of many other molecules, which are thus said to belong to the *immunoglobulin gene superfamily*.

The N terminal half of the H-chain and all of the L-chain together make up what is called a Fab fragment (*Fig. 1*) and contains the antigen-binding site. The actual binding site of the antibody is composed of the N-terminal quarter of the H-chain combined with the N terminal half of the L-chain. The amino acid sequences of these regions differ from one antibody to another and are thus called variable (V) regions and contain the amino acid residues involved in binding an antigenic determinant. Most of the antibody molecule (the C terminal three-quarters of the H-chain and the C terminal half of the L-chain) are

Table 1.   Properties of the human immunoglobulins

	IgG	IgA	IgM	IgD	IgE
Physical properties					
Molecular weight, kDa	150	170–420	900	180	190
H-chain MW, kDa	50–55	62	65	70	75
Physiologic properties					
Normal adult serum (mg/ml)	8–16	1.4–4.0	0.4–2.0	0.03	ngs
Half-life in days	23	6	5	3	<3
Biologic properties					
Complement-fixing capacity	+	–	++++	–	–
Anaphylactic (Type I) hypersensitivity	–	–	–	–	++++
Placental transport to fetus	+	–	–	–	–

There are four IgG (IgG1, IgG2, IgG3, IgG4), two IgA subclasses (IgA1, IgA2) and two L chain types (κ and λ).

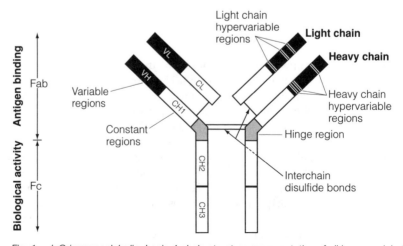

Fig. 1.   IgG immunoglobulin: basic 4 chain structure representative of all immunoglobulins.

constant (C) regions of the antibody molecule and are the same for all antibodies of the same class and subclass. These C regions do not bind antigen, but
rather determine the 'biological' properties of the molecule and thus the fate of
antigen bound by the antigen-binding site. In particular, the C terminal half of
the H-chain, the Fc region (Fragment that crystallized), serves others functions,
i.e., combines with complement, is cytophilic (binds to certain types of cells,
such as macrophages), etc. Carbohydrates are also present on antibodies, primarily on the Fc portion of H-chains.

Affinity

Different antibody molecules produced in response to a particular antigenic
determinant may vary considerably in their tightness of binding to that determinant (i.e., in their **affinity** for the antigenic determinant). The higher the
binding constant the less likely the antibody is to dissociate from the antigen.
Clearly, the affinity of an antibody population is critical when the antigen is a
toxin or virus and must be neutralized by rapid and firm combination with
antibody. Antibodies formed soon after the injection of an antigen are generally
of lower affinity for that antigen whereas antibodies produced later have
dramatically greater affinities (association constants 1000 times higher).

**Antibody
valence and
avidity**

The valence of an antibody is the maximum number of antigenic determinants
with which it can react. For example, IgG antibodies contain two Fab regions
and can bind two molecules of antigen or two identical sites on the same particle, and thus have a valence of two. Valence is important for binding affinity, as
having two or more binding sites for an antigen can dramatically increase the
tightness of binding of the antibody to antigens on a bacteria or virus. This
combined effect, avidity, results from synergy of the binding strengths of each
binding site. Avidity is the firmness of association between a multideterminant
antigen and the antibodies produced against it.

Determining the avidity of an antibody population is very difficult, since it
involves evaluating some function of the group interactions of a large number
of different antibodies with a large number of different antigenic determinants.
Even so, the importance of avidity can be demonstrated both mathematically
and biologically. For example, as a result of working together (being on the
same molecule) two IgG binding sites are 10–100 fold more effective at neutralizing a virus than two unassociated binding sites, and if the antibody has more
binding sites, as in the case of IgM (Topic D2), it may be a million times more
effective (*Fig. 2*). This can be visualized by considering antibodies with one or
two binding sites for a particular antigenic determinant on a microorganism.
The antibody with one site can bind to, but can also dissociate from, a determinant on the organism. When it comes off, it can diffuse away. However, the
antibody with two sites can bind two identical determinants on the organism
(each organism has many copies of each protein or carbohydrate). If one binding site dissociates, the other is probably still attached and permits the first site
to reform its association with the organism. It therefore follows that the larger
the number of binding sites per antibody molecule, the larger the number of
bonds formed with an organism, and the less likely it will be to dissociate.
Thus, an antibody with a poor intrinsic affinity for an antigenic determinant
can, as a result of a large number of combining sites per molecule, be extremely
effective in neutralizing a virus or complexing with a microorganism.

	Fab	IgG	IgM
Binding sites	1	2	10
Relative binding avidity	1	100	1 000 000

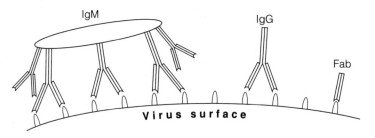

Fig. 2.   Avidity and antibody valence in viral neutralization.

D2 ANTIBODY CLASSES

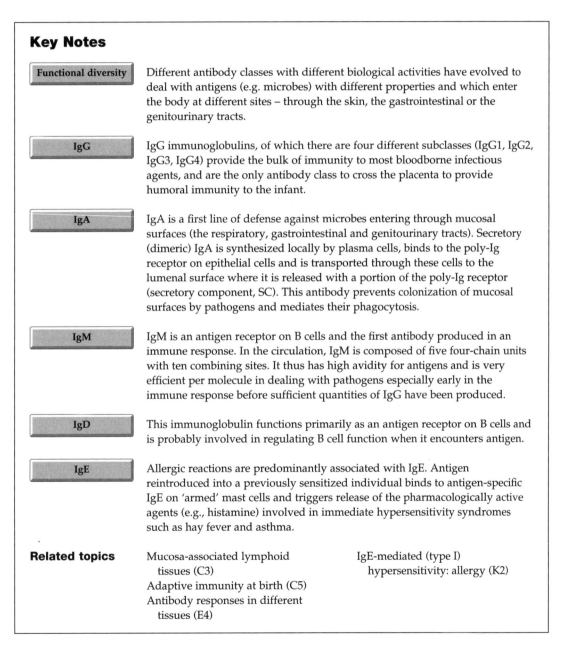

Key Notes

Functional diversity

Different antibody classes with different biological activities have evolved to deal with antigens (e.g. microbes) with different properties and which enter the body at different sites – through the skin, the gastrointestinal or the genitourinary tracts.

IgG

IgG immunoglobulins, of which there are four different subclasses (IgG1, IgG2, IgG3, IgG4) provide the bulk of immunity to most bloodborne infectious agents, and are the only antibody class to cross the placenta to provide humoral immunity to the infant.

IgA

IgA is a first line of defense against microbes entering through mucosal surfaces (the respiratory, gastrointestinal and genitourinary tracts). Secretory (dimeric) IgA is synthesized locally by plasma cells, binds to the poly-Ig receptor on epithelial cells and is transported through these cells to the lumenal surface where it is released with a portion of the poly-Ig receptor (secretory component, SC). This antibody prevents colonization of mucosal surfaces by pathogens and mediates their phagocytosis.

IgM

IgM is an antigen receptor on B cells and the first antibody produced in an immune response. In the circulation, IgM is composed of five four-chain units with ten combining sites. It thus has high avidity for antigens and is very efficient per molecule in dealing with pathogens especially early in the immune response before sufficient quantities of IgG have been produced.

IgD

This immunoglobulin functions primarily as an antigen receptor on B cells and is probably involved in regulating B cell function when it encounters antigen.

IgE

Allergic reactions are predominantly associated with IgE. Antigen reintroduced into a previously sensitized individual binds to antigen-specific IgE on 'armed' mast cells and triggers release of the pharmacologically active agents (e.g., histamine) involved in immediate hypersensitivity syndromes such as hay fever and asthma.

Related topics

Mucosa-associated lymphoid tissues (C3)
Adaptive immunity at birth (C5)
Antibody responses in different tissues (E4)

IgE-mediated (type I) hypersensitivity: allergy (K2)

Functional diversity

Different microbes have different biological properties and can enter the body through different routes (the skin, the gastrointestinal tract, the respiratory tract or the genitourinary tract). It is likely that the five different antibody classes (IgM, IgD, IgG, IgE and IgA; *Fig. 1*) and their subclasses have evolved at least

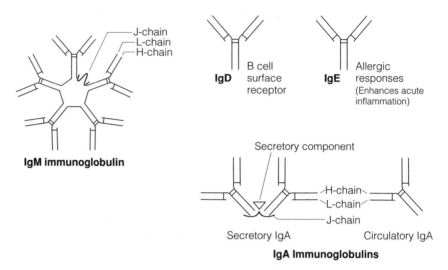

Fig. 1. Chain structures of different classes of immunoglobulins.

partly to facilitate protection against microbes entering at the different sites and with different properties. There is some overlap in their function and in where they are produced, but generally there is a division of labor among the different antibody classes, e.g. IgA is the most common antibody in mucosal secretions while IgM is mainly found in the plasma, and both are most effective at those locations.

IgG

Immunoglobulins of the IgG class have a MW of 150 kDa and are found both in vascular and extravascular spaces as well as in secretions. IgG is the most abundant immunoglobulin in the blood (see *Table 1* in Topic D1), provides the bulk of immunity to most bloodborne infectious agents and is the only antibody class to cross the placenta to provide passive humoral immunity to the developing fetus and thus to the infant on its birth. IgG has two H-chains (referred to as γ chains) with either two κ or two λ L-chains. Furthermore, there are four different subclasses of IgG (designated IgG1, IgG2, IgG3, IgG4), which have slightly different sequences in their H-chains and corresponding differences in their functional activities.

IgA

This immunoglobulin is present in the serum as a 170 kDa, four polypeptide (two L and two H) chain protein. More important, it is the major immunoglobulin present in external secretions such as colostrum, milk, and saliva where it exists as a 420 kDa dimer (*Fig. 1*). In addition to the κ or λ L-chains and the IgA heavy chain (designated α), which distinguishes it from IgG or other antibody classes, secreted IgA also contains two other polypeptide chains – secretory component (SC) and J-chain (Joining chain). SC is part of the poly-Ig receptor involved in the transepithelial transport of exocrine IgA and stabilizes IgA against proteolytic degradation. The two four-chain units composing secretory IgA are held together by the J-chain through disulfide bridges. Most IgA is synthesized locally by plasma cells in mammary and salivary glands, and along the respiratory, gastrointestinal and genitourinary tracts (Topic E4). It is then transported through epithelial cells to the lumen. This antibody is a first line of defense against microbial invaders at mucosal surfaces. Of the two subclasses of IgA, IgA2 rather than IgA1 is primarily found in mucosal secretions.

IgM

IgM is the first antibody produced by, and expressed on the surface of, a B cell. It acts as an antigen receptor for these cells, and is also present as a soluble molecule in the blood. On the B cell surface this molecule is expressed as a four-chain unit – two μ H-chains and two L-chains. In the blood, IgM is composed of five four-chain units held together by disulfide bridges at the carboxy-terminal end of the μ chains (*Fig. 1*). J-chain is also associated with IgM in the blood and initiates the polymerization of its subunits at the time of its secretion from a plasma cell. Because of its size (900 kDa), IgM is found primarily in the intravascular space (i.e. in the bloodstream). As IgM is the first antibody produced in an immune response, its efficiency in combining with antigen is of particular importance until sufficient quantities of IgG antibody have been synthesized. Although IgM antibodies usually have low-affinity binding sites for antigen, they have ten combining sites per molecule which can synergize with each other on the same molecule when it binds to a microbe. Thus, the overall tightness of binding of an IgM molecule (avidity) to a microbe is quite high, making antibodies of this class very effective in removal of the microbe.

IgD

IgD is present in low quantities in the circulation (0.3 mg/ml in adult serum). Its primary function is that of an antigen receptor on B lymphocytes (*Fig. 1*), but it is probably also involved in regulating B cell function when it encounters antigen. B cells thus can express both IgM and IgD and both are specific for the same antigen. When IgM and IgD expressed on a B cell interact with an antigen for which they are specific, the antigen is internalized, and processed and presented to helper T cells which trigger the B cells to proliferate and differentiate into plasma cells, thus initiating the development of a humoral immune response.

IgE

IgE is present in the serum at very low levels (nanograms per milliliter), but plays a significant role in enhancing acute inflammation, in protection from infection by worms, and in allergic reactions (Topics B4, H2, K2). Antibody-mediated allergy is predominantly associated with IgE. After stimulation of the development of IgE-producing plasma cells by an antigen, the IgE produced binds to receptors on mast cells which are specific for the Fc region of IgE. When antigen is *reintroduced* into an individual with such 'armed' mast cells, it binds to the antigen-binding site of the IgE molecule on the mast cell, and as a result of this interaction, the mast cell is triggered to release pharmacologically active agents (e.g., histamine). IgE antibodies are thus important components of immediate hypersensitivity syndromes such as hay fever and asthma (Topic K2, *Fig. 1*).

D3 GENERATION OF DIVERSITY

Key Notes

Antibody genes

The DNA encoding immunoglobulins is found in three unlinked gene groups – one group encodes κ L-chains, one λ L-chains, and one H-chains. Each L-chain gene group has multiple different copies of V gene segments and J gene segments. In addition, in the κ chain group there is one gene segment encoding the constant region of κ chains, while in the λ group there are four λ chain C region gene segments. The H-chain gene group has multiple different copies of V, D and J gene segments and one gene segment for each of the constant regions for the different antibody classes and subclasses.

Gene rearrangement

During its development, a single B cell randomly selects from its H-chain gene group, one V, one D and one J gene segment for rearrangement (translocation). It then selects from the κ or λ gene group one V and one J gene segment for translocation. These gene segments then recombine to create a gene (VJ) encoding a binding site for an L chain and a gene (VDJ) encoding a binding site for an H-chain.

Allelic exclusion

After successful rearrangement of the Ig DNA segments, the cell is committed to the expression of a particular V region for its H-chain and a particular V region for its L-chain and there is active suppression, allelic exclusion, of other H- and L-chain V region rearrangements. Each B cell and all of its progeny will therefore express and produce antibodies, all of which have exactly the same specificity.

Synthesis and assembly of H- and L-chains

After successful rearrangement of L- and H-chain DNA, primary L- and H-chain mRNAs are transcribed and the RNA between the newly constructed V region gene and the constant region gene spliced out. After translation, the L and H polypeptide chains combine in the endoplasmic reticulum (ER) to form an antibody molecule, which then becomes the antigen-specific receptor for that B cell. In plasma cells, the part of the mRNA encoding the H-chain transmembrane domain, which is important for its membrane expression on B cells, is spliced out and the antibody produced is secreted.

Differential splicing and class switching

A mature B cell expresses both IgM and IgD with the same specificity. This results from differential cleavage and splicing of the primary transcript to yield two mRNAs – one for an IgM H-chain and the other for an IgD H-chain – both of which are translated and expressed on the B cell surface with L-chain. B cell class switch to IgG, IgA or IgE requires interaction of CD154 on T cells with CD40 on B cells and cytokines produced by the T helper cell (IL-4 induces switch to IgE; IL-5 to IgA; IFNγ to IgG1). These interactions induce translocation of the VDJ gene segment next to another C region gene with the loss of intervening DNA. The primary transcript is then spliced to give an mRNA for the new H-chain.

Ways of creating diversity

Antibody diversity, i.e. the generation of antibodies with different specificities, is created at the DNA level by multiple germline V, D and J gene segments for heavy, and V and J gene segments for light chains, by their random combination, by imprecise joining, and by subsequent somatic mutations in the resulting V regions. At the protein level, diversity is created as a result of random selection and pairing of L- and H-chains.

B cell development and selection

Gene segments encoding the different parts of the V regions of antibodies rearrange during the pro-B cell stage. The first genes to rearrange encode the variable part of the H chain. This V region is transcribed with the μ constant region gene and an IgM H chain appears in the cytoplasm. At this pre-B cell stage, gene segments that encode the variable region of the L chains rearrange. H and L chains combine and are expressed on the surface of the immature B cell. At this stage, B cells with high affinity for self antigens are induced to die by apoptosis (**negative selection**). Surviving B cells traffic to secondary lymphoid organs and are selected to expand by contact with their specific antigen. During the immune response, the overall affinity of antibodies for an antigen increases with time, partly because B cells expressing higher-affinity antibody compete most successfully for antigen and contribute a higher proportion to the antibody pool.

Affinity maturation

Mutations in VH and VL genes of activated B cells may generate higher affinity antibodies allowing these cells to compete most successfully for antigen. These cells clonally expand and differentiate into plasma cells that contribute to the overall antibody pool.

Related topics

Lymphocytes (C1)
The B cell receptor complex, co-receptors and signaling (E1)

The cellular basis of the antibody response (E3)

Antibody genes

Three unlinked gene groups encode immunoglobulins – one for κ chains, one for λ chains and one for H-chains, each on a different chromosome (*Table 1*). Within each of these gene groups on the chromosome there are multiple coding regions (**exons**) which recombine at the level of DNA to yield a binding site. In a mature B cell or plasma cell, the DNA encoding the V region for the H-chain of a specific antibody consists of a continuous uninterrupted nucleotide sequence. In contrast, the DNA in a germline cell (or non B cell) for this V region exists in distinct DNA segments, exons, separated from each other by regions of noncoding DNA (*Fig. 1*). The exons encoding the V region of the H-chain are: V segment (encoding approximately the first 102 amino acids), D segment (encoding 2–4 amino acids), and J segment (encoding the remaining 14 or so amino acids in the V region). For L-chains there are only V (encoding the first approximately 95 amino acids) and J segment (encoding the remaining 13 or so amino acids) exons. In each gene group, there are from 30–65 functional

Table 1.   Genes for human immunoglobulins

Ig polypeptide	Chromosome
H-chain	14
κ-chain	2
λ-chain	22

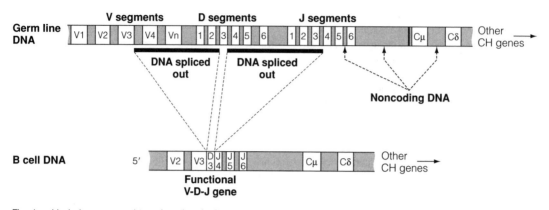

Fig. 1.   H-chain genes and translocation. In the germ line, and therefore in a cell destined to become a B cell, the H-chain gene loci contains many V segment genes. In a developing B cell, one of these V segments recombines with one of many D segments, which has already recombined with one of several J segments, to produce a functional VDJ gene. In each B cell, the rearranged gene is transcribed, spliced and translated into a H-chain protein.

V segment genes. The D and J regions are between the V and C regions on the chromosome and there are multiple different genes for each but fewer in number than those encoding the V segment. Thus, DNA segments that ultimately encode the binding site of antibodies have to be moved over distances (translocated) on the chromosome to form a DNA sequence encoding the V region (**gene 'rearrangement'**).

The DNA sequences encoding the C region of the L- and H-chains are 3' to the V genes, but separated from them by unused J segment genes and noncoding DNA. Furthermore, each gene group usually has one functional C gene segment for each class and subclass. Thus, the H-chain gene group has nine functional C region genes, one each encoding μ, δ, $\gamma1$, $\gamma2$, $\gamma3$, $\gamma4$, ϵ, $\alpha1$, $\alpha2$. For the L-chain gene groups, there is one gene segment encoding the C region of κ L-chains, but four encoding λ L-chain C regions.

Gene rearrangement

During its development, a single B cell randomly selects one V, one D and one J (for H-chains), and one V and one J (for L-chains) for rearrangement (translocation). Gene segments encoding a portion of the V region are moved adjacent to other gene segments encoding the rest of the V region to create a gene segment encoding the entire V region, with the intervening DNA removed. Gene rearrangement in B cells requires the products of two recombination-activating genes, RAG-1 and RAG-2, which appear to be only expressed together in developing lymphocytes. These enzymes break and rejoin the DNA during translocation and are thus critical to the generation of diversity.

The H-chain gene group is the first to rearrange, initially moving one of several D segment genes adjacent to one of several J segment genes. This creates a DJ combination, which encodes the C terminal part of the H-chain V region.

A V segment gene then rearranges to become contiguous with the DJ segment, creating a DNA sequence (VDJ) encoding a complete H-chain V region (*Fig. 1*). This VDJ combination is 5' to the group of H-chain C region genes, of which the closest one encodes the μ chain. A primary mRNA transcript is then made from VDJ through the μ C region gene, after which the intervening message between VDJ and the μ C region gene is spliced out to create an mRNA for a complete μ H-chain.

After the H-chain has successfully completed its rearrangement, one of the V region gene segments in either the λ or κ gene groups (but not both) translocates next to a J segment gene to create a gene (VJ) encoding a complete L-chain V region (*Fig. 2*). For κ chains, the DNA sequences encoding the C region of the

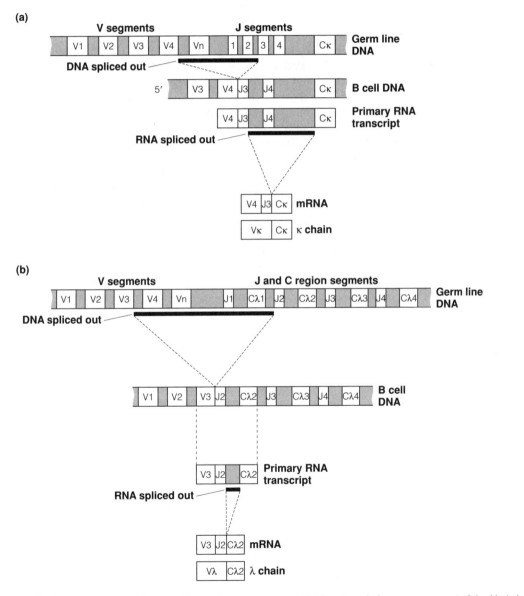

Fig. 2.   L-chain genes and translocation. During differentiation of a B cell, and after rearrangement of the H-chain genes, one of the two L-chain groups rearrange. In particular, either (a) a germ line Vκ gene combines with a J segment gene to form a VJ combination; or (b) a germ line Vλ gene combines with one of the J segment Cλ gene combinations to form a VJ Cλ combination. The rearranged gene is then transcribed into a primary RNA transcript which then has the intervening noncoding sequences spliced out to form mRNA. This is then translated into light chain protein.

L-chains are 3′ to the V genes, but separated from them by unused J segment genes and noncoding DNA (*Fig. 2(a)*). For λ chains, since the J segment genes are each associated with a different Cλ gene, translocation of a V gene segment to a J gene segment results in a V region next to a particular Cλ gene (e.g. Cλ2 as shown in *Fig. 2(b)*). It is important to emphasize that in each B cell, only one of two L-chain gene groups will be used. A primary mRNA transcript is then made from VJ through the L-chain C region gene, after which the intervening message between VJ and the C region gene is spliced out to create an mRNA for a complete L-chain.

Allelic exclusion

After successful rearrangement of the Ig DNA segments, the cell is committed to the expression of a particular V region for its H-chain and a particular V region for its L-chain and *excludes* other H- and L-chain V region rearrangements. This process is referred to as **allelic exclusion** and is unique to B and T cell antigen receptors. If an aberrant rearrangement occurs on the first chromosome the process will continue, i.e., the process does not stop if the cell does not get it right the first time. The process stops, however, if the cell gets it right or runs out of chromosomes to rearrange. In fact, following successful VH gene rearrangement on one chromosome there is active suppression of further rearrangement of the other VH gene segments. Similarly, following successful VL gene rearrangement there is active suppression of further rearrangement of other VL gene segments.

Thus, each B cell makes L-chains all of which contain a V region encoded by the same VJ region sequence and H-chains all of which contain a V region encoded by the same VDJ sequence. Each B cell will therefore express antibodies on its surface, all of which have exactly the same specificity. This cell and all of its progeny are committed to express and produce antibodies with these V regions.

Synthesis and assembly of H- and L-chains

After successful rearrangement of both L- and H-chain DNA, L- and H-chain mRNA is produced and translated into L- and H-polypeptide chains that combine in the endoplasmic reticulum (ER) to form an antibody molecule, which is transported to the plasma membrane as the antigen-specific receptor for that B cell. Since the gene encoding the H-chain also contains coding sequences for a transmembrane domain, the H-chain produced contains a C terminal amino acid sequence which anchors the antibody in the plasma membrane. In plasma cells, the part of the mRNA encoding the H-chain transmembrane domain important for its membrane expression on B cells is spliced out. Thus, the antibody produced by a plasma cell does not become associated with the membrane, but rather is secreted.

Differential splicing and class switching

As indicated above, the first antibody produced by a B cell is of the IgM class. Soon thereafter the B cell produces both an IgM and an IgD antibody, each having the same V regions and thus the same specificity. This is the result of the differential cleavage and splicing of the primary transcript. In particular, a primary transcript is made which includes information from the VDJ region through the Cδ region (*Fig. 3*). This transcript is differentially spliced to yield two mRNAs – one for an IgM H-chain and the other for an IgD H-chain. In a mature B cell both are translated and expressed on the B cell surface with L-chain.

B cells expressing IgM and IgD on their surface are capable of switching to other H-chain classes (IgG, IgA or IgE). This isotype (class) switching requires

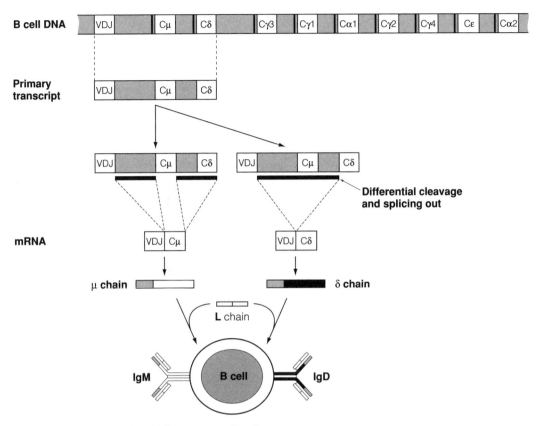

Fig. 3.　Expression of IgM and IgD on a mature B cell.

stimulation of the B cell by T helper cells and in particular requires binding of the CD40 ligand (CD154) on T cells to CD40 on B cells. In addition, the cytokines produced by the T helper cell influence the constant region gene to which class switching occurs. Th2 cells producing IL-4 induce B cells to class switch to IgE; IL-5, which is also produced by Th2 cells, induces B cells to class switch to IgA; IFNγ produced by Th1 cells induces class switching to IgG1 (*Fig. 4*). These signals induce translocation of VDJ and its insertion 5′ to another constant region gene (*Fig. 5*). Class switch is guided by repetitive DNA sequences 5′ to the C region genes and occurs when these **switch regions** recombine. The intervening DNA is cut out and the resulting DNA on the rearranged chromosome in the B cell which has class switched, and in plasma cells derived from this B cell, no longer contains Cμ, Cδ or other intervening H-chain C region genes. A primary transcript is made and the RNA between the VDJ coding region and the new H-chain coding region is spliced out to give an mRNA for the new H-chain.

Ways of creating diversity　　Ig diversity (the generation of antibodies with different specificities) is created by several antigen-independent mechanisms. In addition, in B cells that have been stimulated by antigen and received T cell help, Ig genes undergo increased mutational events that may increase the affinity of the antibody produced by the B cell. Overall, diversity is generated by:

Antigen-independent events

- at the DNA level as a result of multiple germ line V, D and J heavy and V and J light chain genes,
- at the DNA level as a result of random combination of V, D and J segments or V and J segments,
- at the DNA level as a result of imprecise joining of V, D and J segments,
- at the protein level as a result of random selection and pairing of different combinations of L- and H-chain V regions in different B cells.

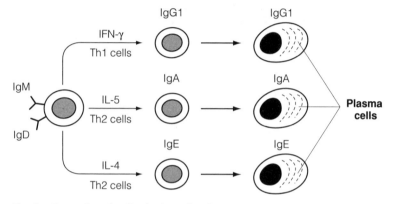

Fig. 4.   Generation of antibody class diversity.

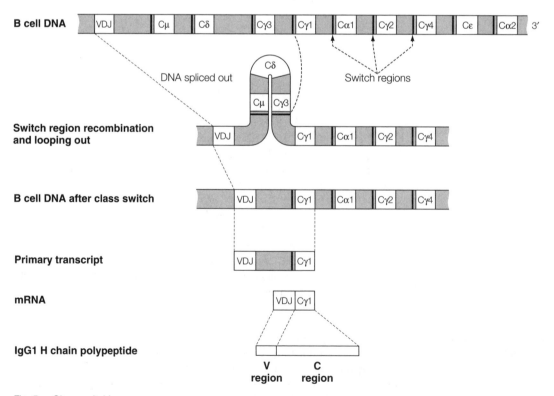

Fig. 5.   Class switching.

Antigen-dependent events
- at the DNA level as a result of somatic mutation in the V region, which may create higher-affinity antibody-binding sites.

Although rearrangement of the gene segments that will make up the V region genes occurs in an ordered fashion, they are chosen at random in each developing B cell. As these events occur in a vast number of cells, the result is that millions of B cells, each with a different antigen specificity, are generated. Additional diversity is created during recombination of V and J (L-chain) and V, D and J (H-chain) gene segments due to imprecise joining of the different gene segments making up the V region. That is, for example, although translocation of a V gene segment to a J gene segment could occur with all three nucleotides of the last codon of the V segment joining with all three nucleotides of the first codon of the J segment, it is also possible that one or two nucleotides at the 3′ end of the V segment could replace the first one or two nucleotides of the J segment. Such a difference in the position at which recombination occurs can change the amino acid sequence in the antigen-binding area of the resulting V region of the antibody, and thus change its specificity. Furthermore, after antigen stimulation of the B cell, the DNA of its L- and H-chain V regions becomes particularly susceptible to somatic mutation and undergoes affinity maturation (see below).

Diversity is also generated as a result of the fact that any L-chain can interact with any H-chain to create a unique binding site. Thus, for example, an L-chain with a particular VJ combination for its binding site could be produced by many different B cells and interact with the different H-chains (i.e. different in their VH region) generated in each of these B cells to create many different specificities.

In sum, almost unlimited diversity is created from a limited number of V region gene segments. The diversity almost certainly exceeds the amount of diversity needed to bind the immunogens of microbes. However, the vast majority of the different B cells generated will never encounter antigen to which they can bind, and thus will not be stimulated to further development. And yet, such apparent wastefulness is justified by the fact that this mechanism of creation of diversity ensures that there are B cells, and thus antibodies, reactive with virtually all antigens that will be encountered. When an antigen to which this antibody binds is encountered, the B cell is triggered to divide and to give rise to a clone of cells, each one of which makes, at least initially, the originally displayed antibody molecule (clonal selection: Topics A3 and E3).

B cell development and selection

Gene segments encoding the variable parts of the V regions of antibodies rearrange during the pro-B cell stage (*Fig. 6*). Since rearrangement occurs in millions of different ways in these developing cells, many B cells, each with a different specificity, are generated. This generation of diversity occurs in the absence of foreign protein and yields large numbers of mature B cells, of which at least some have specificity for each foreign substance or microbe. The first genes to rearrange encode the variable part of the H chain of the antibody which together with the genes of the constant part of the molecule (and in particular genes which code for the μ H chain) are transcribed first in the differentiation process and appear in the cytoplasm. At this stage the genes in these pre-B cells which code for the variable region of the L chains rearrange. The transcribed H- and L-chains combine, giving rise to a functional IgM antigen receptor which is then expressed on the surface of the cell (immature B cell). It

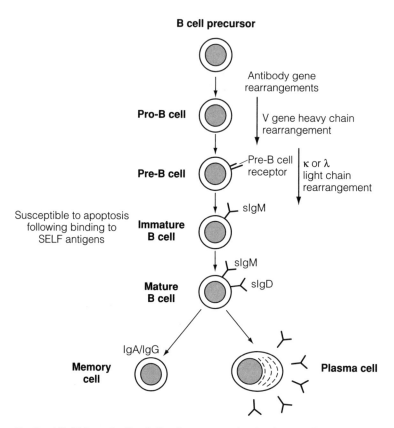

Fig. 6.   Life history of a B cell. B cell precursors develop into pro-B cells which begin to rearrange their H-chain V genes. During the pre-B cell stage the translated heavy chain peptide assembles with surrogate light chain to form the pre-B cell receptor. This is thought to mediate further development of the B cell. During the pre-B cell stage, κ or λ light chain genes rearrange with one class of L-chain being transcribed and translated into protein. The κ or λ light chain then associates with new μ heavy chain to replace the surrogate light chain resulting in expression of surface IgM – the cell's functional antigen receptor. This immature B cell is susceptible to apoptosis/anergy on contact with self-antigen. Mature B cells acquire surface IgD in addition to IgM and migrate to the secondary lymphoid organs and tissues where they respond to foreign antigens by proliferation and development into memory and plasma cells.

is during this stage that B cells with high affinity for self antigens are induced to die by apoptosis (negative selection). As in the thymus, the majority of the B cells die during development from production of antigen receptors which cannot be assembled or those directed against self antigens (Topic G2).

During an antibody response to an antigen, the overall affinity of the antibodies produced increases with time. For example, antibodies produced in the secondary response usually have higher affinity for (tighter binding to) the antigen than those produced in the primary response. This is partly due to clonal selection and the presence of significantly more antigen-binding B cells at the time of the secondary response than during the primary response. If the quantity of antigen is insufficient to stimulate all B cells that could bind the antigen, i.e. when antigen is limited, B cells with the highest affinity antigen receptors will compete most successfully for the antigen. These cell populations are stimulated and give rise to plasma cells making their higher affinity antibody, thus increasing the affinity of the total pool of antibody. These higher-affinity antibodies are also usually more efficient at effector functions than those produced in the primary response.

Affinity maturation

After class switch to IgG, IgA or IgE, the DNA of the L- and H-chain V regions of B cells stimulated by antigen and T cells becomes particularly susceptible to somatic mutation. This results in changes in the nucleotides of the DNA and thus corresponding changes in the amino acid sequence of the V regions of the antibody expressed by the B cell. As a result, the B cell may have a different specificity and not bind to or be stimulated by the original antigen. However, it often happens that at least some mutations result in amino acid changes which increase the tightness of binding of the antibody on the B cell to its antigen. These B cells will compete more efficiently for antigen than the original B cell, and will differentiate into plasma cells producing a higher-affinity antibody (**affinity maturation**), resulting in an overall increase in the affinity of the antibody population to that antigen. Typical antibodies have binding constants of 10^{6-7} M^{-1}. After successive immunization with limiting antigen they are usually 10^{8-9} M^{-1} but may be as high as 10^{12} M^{-1}.

D4 ALLOTYPES AND IDIOTYPES

Key Notes

Allotypes	These are genetic markers on immunoglobulins (Ig) that segregate within the species. If Ig expressing a particular allotype is injected into an individual whose Igs do not express that allotype, an immune response could develop against the allotype. Like blood types, they are inherited in Mendelian fashion but are usually of no functional consequence.
Idiotypes	These are unique antigenic determinants associated with antigen-binding sites of antibodies and are the result of the different amino acid sequences which determine their specificities.
Related topics	Regulation by antigen and antibody (G4) Transplantation antigens (M2)

Allotypes

In addition to class and subclass categories, an immunoglobulin (Ig) can be defined by the presence of genetic markers termed allotypes. These markers are different in different individuals and are thus immunogenic when injected into individuals whose Ig lacks the allotype. Like the blood group antigens (ABO), they are determinants which segregate within a species (the Ig of some members of the species have them, others do not). Allotypes are normally the result of small amino acid differences in Ig L- or H-chain constant regions. For example, the Km (*Inv*) marker is an allotype of human κ L-chains and is the result of a leucine vs valine difference at position 191. The *Gm* markers are allotypes associated with the IgG H-chains. Allotypes are inherited in a strictly Mendelian fashion, and usually have no significance to the function of the antibody molecule.

Idiotypes

Antigenic determinants associated with the binding site of an antibody molecule are called idiotypes and are unique to all antibodies produced by the same clone of B cells. That is, although all antibodies have idiotypic determinants, these determinants are different for all antibodies not derived from the same clone of B cells. Thus, the number of different idiotypes in an individual is at least as numerous as the number of specificities. Antibodies are produced against these idiotypic determinants when they are injected into other animals. In fact, one's own idiotypes may be recognized by one's own immune system. That is, the amino acid sequence associated with the combining site of an antibody (call this idiotype, D) is immunogenic even in the individual in which it is produced. An immune response produced against this idiotype (anti-D) can eliminate the B cells producing the antibody with this idiotype and thus decrease the antibody response to the antigen which initially triggered production of this idiotype. Furthermore, an anti-idiotype immune response (antibody or T-cell-mediated) expresses its own idiotype which in turn can be recognized as foreign and an anti-idiotype immune response made against this idiotype. Jerne (who shared the Nobel prize with Kohler and Milstein in 1984) described a *Network Theory* which proposes that a series of idiotype–anti-idiotype reactions are partially responsible for regulation of the immune response (Topic G4).

D5 MONOCLONAL ANTIBODIES

Key Notes

Monoclonal antibodies	Standardized procedures involving fusion of an immortal cell (a myeloma tumor cell) with a specific predetermined antibody-producing B cell are used to create hybridoma cells producing monospecific and monoclonal antibodies (mAb). These mAb are standard research reagents and many have significant clinical utility.
Humanization and chimerization of mAbs	Most mAbs developed have been mouse, and although useful as research and diagnostic tools, they are not ideal therapeutics because of their immunogenicity in humans. This has been dealt with by humanizing these murine Abs or by making fully human mAbs.
Fv libraries	By randomly fusing heavy (H) and light (L) chain variable (V) region genes from B cells, Fv libraries containing a vast number of binding specificities can be generated and used as a source for creation of specific mAbs.
Related topics	Lymphocytes (C1) Immunotherapy of tumors with Immunodiagnosis (N4) antibodies (N6)

Monoclonal antibodies

In 1975, Kohler and Milstein developed a procedure (for which they received the Nobel Prize) to create cell lines producing predetermined, monospecific and monoclonal antibodies (mAb). This procedure has been standardized and applied on a massive scale to the preparation of antibodies useful to many research and clinical efforts. The basic technology involves fusion of an immortal cell (a myeloma tumor cell) with a specific predetermined antibody-producing B cell from immunized animals or humans (*Fig. 1*). The resulting hybridoma cell is immortal and synthesizes homogeneous, specific mAb, which can be made in large quantities. Thus, MAbs have become standard research reagents and have extensive clinical applications.

Humanization and chimerization of mAbs

The vast majority of mAbs have been developed in mice, and although useful as research and diagnostic tools, they have not been ideal therapeutic reagents at least partly because of their immunogenicity in humans. That is, a murine Ab introduced into a patient will be recognized as foreign by the patient's immune system and a Human Anti-Mouse Ab (HAMA) response will develop that compromises the therapeutic utility of the Ab. This has been dealt with in two basic ways.

Humanized antibodies
Murine mAbs can be genetically modified to be more human (*Fig. 2*). In particular the constant region of the murine IgG heavy (H) and of the murine light (L) chain can be replaced at the DNA level with the constant region genes of

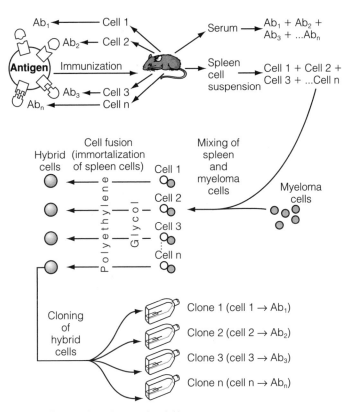

Fig. 1. Preparation of monoclonal Abs.

human IgG1 H and L chains to create a **chimeric Ab** where only the variable (V) regions are murine. This significantly decreases but does not eliminate the immunogenicity of the Ab. Another approach involves sequencing the V regions of the mouse Ab VH and VL regions and then inserting the DNA sequences of the hypervariable regions of these chains into human IgG VH- and VL-chain genes. The resulting Ab is 95% human with only the binding regions being murine.

Fully human mAbs
Human Abs have been made by fusing human B cells with myeloma cells, although this has been very difficult and usually requires immortalizing the B cells using Epstein–Barr virus before fusing. This approach is not ideal as a virus is used, the specificity of the mAbs produced is limited and the yield of the Abs produced is poor. More recently, a human antibody mouse has been created by replacing the genes for mouse immunoglobulins with genes for human immunoglobulins. Thus, when the mouse is immunized it makes fully human Abs against the Ag and the B cells making these Abs can be fused with myeloma cells to generate hybridomas making the human mAb.

Fv libraries   Another way of preparing mAbs involves Fv libraries. This approach initially involves obtaining mRNA for the VH and VL regions from a large number of

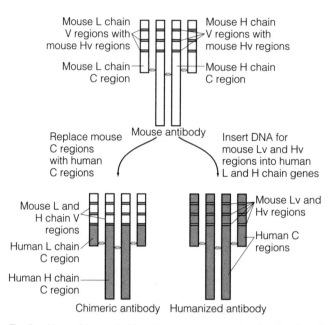

Fig. 2. *Humanizing and chimerizing mouse monoclonal antibodies. Chimeric mAbs are created by replacing the murine genes for the constant region of the light (L) and heavy (H) chain with the corresponding human constant region genes. Humanized mAbs are created by inserting the gene sequences for each of the hypervariable (Hv) regions of the mouse antibody into the corresponding place in the genes for the L and H chains for a human antibody.*

B cells. From this mRNA, cDNA for each H-chain V region is prepared and joined to the cDNA for each L-chain V region (*Fig. 3*) to create all combinations, and thus genes encoding a vast number of different antigen-combining sites (**Fv** regions). These are cloned into cells for production of the antibody-binding site they encode. For example, they can be cloned into bacteriophage (viruses that infect bacteria) and selected for their specificity. Thus, Fvs can be expressed in a replicating bioform and used as a source from which specific mAbs can be created.

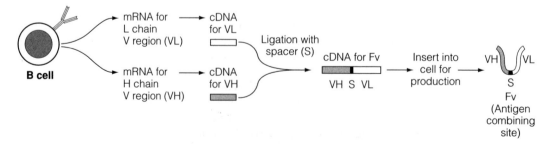

Fig. 3. *Fv preparation. mRNA for the V regions of L- and H-chains is prepared from B cell mRNA using the polymerase chain reaction. From this mRNA, cDNA for each H chain V region is prepared and joined to the cDNA for each L chain V region, with a spacer between. This yields a gene encoding the antigen binding region of the antibody, which is inserted into a cell for production of a protein, Fv, that is the combining site of an antibody.*

D6 ANTIGEN/ANTIBODY COMPLEXES (IMMUNE COMPLEXES)

Key Notes

Immune complexes *in vitro*	Combination of antibody (Ab) with a multideterminant antigen (Ag) results in a lattice of alternating molecules of Ag and Ab, which grows until large precipitating aggregates are formed (equivalence). In Ab excess or in Ag excess, less lattice formation occurs and soluble complexes form.
Immune complexes *in vivo*	Introduction of Ag *in vivo* results in an immune response in which there is initially Ag excess. Within days, as Ab is produced, equivalence is reached and the resulting immune complexes are removed by phagocytic cells. After Ag removal, B cell stimulation stops, and the Ab concentration in the serum decreases as a result of normal catabolism.
Immune complexes and tissue damage	Persistence of Ag (microbial or self) may result in continual formation of immune complexes that with an 'overwhelmed' phagocytic system are deposited in tissues resulting in damage (type III hypersensitivity) mediated mainly by complement and neutrophils.
Precipitation assays	Combination of Ab with Ag results in lattice formation and precipitation if there is sufficient Ag and Ab (equivalence). These reactions are the basis for qualitative and quantitative assays for Ag or Ab, including radial immunodiffusion and immunoelectrophoresis.
Agglutination assays	The interaction of surface Ags on insoluble particles (e.g. cells) with specific Ab to these Ags results in agglutination of the particles. Agglutination can be used to determine blood types; the presence of Ab to bacteria in serum is an indication of previous or current infection; and in the Coomb's test autoantibodies to erythrocytes can be identified.
Related topics	Innate immunity and inflammation (B4) Antibody structure (D1) Antibody classes (D2) IgM and IgG-mediated (type II) hypersensitivity (K3) Immune-complex mediated (type III) hypersensitivity (K4) Transplantation antigens (M2)

Immune complexes *in vitro*

Immunogens have more than one antigenic determinant per molecule (are multideterminant). Immunization with antigen therefore results in many antibody populations, each directed toward different determinants on the protein. Since one molecule of Ab (IgG) can react with two molecules of Ag, and one molecule of Ag can react with many molecules of Ab, a lattice or framework consisting of alternating molecules of Ag and Ab can be produced which precipitates. The extent to which a lattice forms depends on the relative amounts of Ag and Ab present (*Fig. 1*). As the amount of Ag added increases, the amount of precipitate and Ab in the precipitate increases, until a maximum is reached, and then decreases with further addition of Ag. When there is both sufficient Ag and sufficient Ab, the combination of Ag and Ab proceeds until large aggregates are formed, which are insoluble and precipitate (**equivalence**). However, in **Ab excess** or in **Ag excess**, less lattice formation occurs and more soluble complexes are formed.

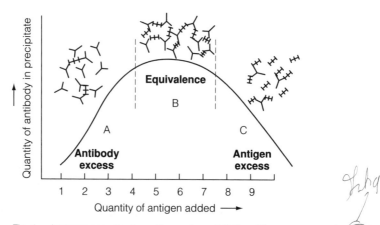

Fig. 1.   *Immune complex formation and precipitation. The same amount of Ab to a protein was added to each of a series of tubes (1–9), followed by the addition of increasing amounts of the protein Ag to each successive tube. (A) The zone of Ab excess; (B) zone of equivalence in which all of the Ag and Ab are incorporated into a precipitate; and (C) the zone of Ag excess.*

Immune complexes in vivo

These reactions occur *in vivo* during an immune response. Initially, there is Ag excess as no Ab to the Ag is present at the time of first contact with the Ag. Within days however, plasma cells develop, producing Ab to the Ag which complex with it (Ag excess). As more Ab is produced, equivalence is reached resulting in large Ag–Ab complexes which are removed by phagocytic cells through interaction with their Fc and complement receptors. Plasma cells continue to produce Ab during their short life, increasing the Ab concentration in the serum (Ab excess). However, once Ag has been removed, no further restimulation of B cells occurs and no more plasma cells develop (Topic G4). Thus, the Ab concentration in the serum begins to decrease as a result of normal catabolism.

Immune complexes and tissue damage

If the Ag persists (e.g. with some infectious organisms such as *Streptococcus*) or is self Ag, immune complexes are continually formed and may not readily be removed due to an 'overwhelmed' phagocytic system. This can lead to the deposition of immune complexes in tissues resulting in damaging reactions (type III hypersensitivity, Topic K4). The complexes activate complement and induce an acute inflammatory response (Topic B4). Direct interaction of the immune complexes with Fc and complement receptors on the neutrophils causes the release of proteolytic enzymes that damage surrounding tissues.

Precipitation assays

As previously described, when there is both sufficient Ag and sufficient Ab, the combination of Ag and Ab proceeds until large aggregates are formed which are insoluble in water and precipitate (equivalence). The extent to which a lattice forms depends on the relative amounts of Ag and Ab present.

Lattice formation and precipitation are the basis for several qualitative and quantitative assays for Ag or Ab. These assays are done in semisolid gels into which holes are cut for Ag and/or for Ab and diffusion occurs until Ag and Ab are at equivalence and precipitate. In **radial immunodiffusion,** Ab (e.g. horse anti-human IgG) is incorporated into the gel and Ag (e.g. human serum) is placed in a hole cut in the gel. Ag diffuses radially out of the well into the gel and interacts with the Ab forming a ring of precipitation, the diameter of which is related to the concentration of the Ag (*Fig. 2*). Similar assays have been developed in which a voltage gradient (electrophoresis) is used to speed up movement of Ag into the Ab containing gel (rocket immunoelectrophoresis).

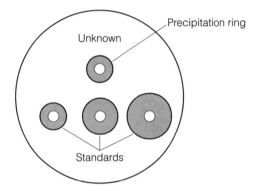

Fig. 2.　*Measurement of Ag by precipitation in gels. Ab-containing gel is placed on a glass or plastic surface. Holes are cut in the gel and filled with Ag which diffuses radially out of the well and interacts with the Ab in the gel. Soluble complexes are initially formed but as more Ag diffuses equivalence is reached resulting in a lattice and precipitation. The diameter of the precipitation ring is related to the concentration of the Ag and, using known standards, can be quantitated and compared with the levels of Ag in other samples.*

In **immunoelectrophoresis**, Ags (e.g. serum) are placed in a well cut in a gel (without Ab) and electrophoresed, after which a trough is cut in the gel into which Abs (e.g. horse anti-human serum) are placed. The Abs diffuse laterally to meet diffusing Ag, and lattice formation and precipitation occur permitting determination of the nature of the Ags (*Fig. 3*).

Agglutination assays

Agglutination involves the interaction of surface Ags on **insoluble particles** (e.g. cells) and specific Ab to these Ags (*Fig. 4*). Ab thus links together (agglutinates) insoluble particles. Much smaller amounts of Ab suffice to produce agglutination than are needed for precipitation. For this reason, agglutination rather than precipitation may be used to determine blood group types or if Ab to bacteria is present in blood as an indication of infection with these bacteria. Since IgM has ten binding sites, whereas IgG has two, IgM is much more efficient at agglutinating particles or cells.

Although Abs are frequently used by themselves to assay for the presence of an Ag, a second Ab is sometimes used in what is known as a **Coomb's test**. In some instances, such as when an autoantibody has been produced against a given cell type, the cells will have human Ab bonded to them, and thus can be identified by a second Ab (an Ab to human immunoglobulin) which will cause agglutination of the cells. In an **indirect Coomb's test**, the presence of circulating Ab to a cell surface Ag is demonstrated by adding the patient's serum to test cells (e.g. erythrocytes) followed by addition of Ab to human Ab.

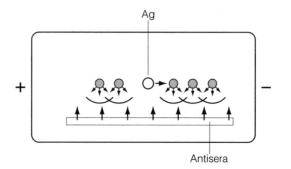

Fig. 3. Identification of antigens using gel electrophoresis. Ag (e.g. serum) is placed in a well cut in a gel and subjected to a voltage gradient which causes the various antigens to migrate different distances through the gel dependent on their charge. After electrophoresis, a trough is cut in the gel into which antibodies (e.g. horse anti-human serum) are placed. The antibodies diffuse laterally from the trough until they meet Ag diffusing from its location after electrophoresis. Again, lattice formation and precipitation occurs and, based on immunoelectrophoresis of defined standards, the identity of the Ag can be determined.

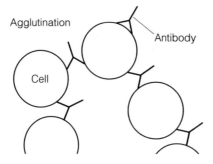

Agglutination: Antigen insoluble before
                    adding antibody

Precipitation: Antigen is initially soluble;
                    antibody binding to it creates
                    a lattice and makes it
                    insoluble

Fig. 4. Agglutination.

D7 IMMUNOASSAY

Key Notes

Ag - Antigen. Ab - Antibody.

Antibodies and assays

A variety of assays have been developed which provide specific qualitative and quantitative measurement of Ag or Ab, both of which are often of considerable research and clinical relevance. Ab to an organism in the serum of a patient demonstrates infection by the organism. Ab with defined specificity is used to determine the presence of disease-associated antigens in a patient. As tools in molecular and cellular research, Abs permit localization and characterization of Ags.

ELISA/RIA

The presence and concentration of a specific Ag or of an Ab to a specific Ag in solution can be determined by radioimmunoassays (RIA) or enzyme-linked immunosorbent assays (ELISA). Ag attached to a solid surface captures the Ab with which it reacts and is quantitated using a labeled second Ab reactive to the first. These assays permit measurement of a wide variety of Ags as well as the concentration and isotype of Abs specific for a given Ag, such as those reactive with an infectious organism.

Immunofluorescence and flow cytometry

Using a fluorescence microscope and Abs labeled with a fluorescent molecule, tissue sections can be examined for cells expressing particular Ags (e.g. those which are tumor associated). Direct or indirect immunofluorescence techniques permit qualitative and quantitative evaluation of several different cell-associated molecules at the same time. Flow cytometers rapidly analyze large numbers of cells in suspension, providing a molecular fingerprint of the cells. Fluorescence-activated cell sorters separate cell subpopulations for more detailed study.

Immunoblotting

Immunoblotting is used to assay for the presence of molecules in a mixture. Western blot analysis involves separating molecules by sodium dedecyl sulfate polyacrylamide gel electrophoresis (SDS-PAGE), transferring them to another matrix and detecting the molecule of interest using ELISA or RIA. This assay is often used to confirm the presence of Abs to infectious agents (e.g. HIV) in patient serum. Immunoblotting can also be used to analyze products of single cells (e.g. cytokines) and the nature of the producing cell.

Affinity purification of Ag and Ab

Ab coupled to an insoluble matrix (e.g. agarose) specifically binds its Ag, which can then be eluted from the Ab yielding relatively pure Ag in one step. Similarly, Ag or protein A coupled to an insoluble matrix permits purification of Ab.

Related topics

Antibody structure (D1)
The cellular basis of the antibody response (E3)
The microbial cosmos (H1)
Immunization (I2)
Diagnosis and treatment of immunodeficiency (J4)

IgE-mediated (type I) hypersensitivity: allergy (K2)
IgM and IgG-mediated (type II) hypersensitivity (K3)
Diagnosis and treatment of autoimmune disease (L5)
Immunodiagnosis (N2)

Antibodies and assays

Methods for measuring antigen–antibody reactions have been well established and include those that have direct biologic relevance (*Table 1*). The combination of Ab with biologically active Ag (virus, toxin, enzyme and hormone) can be detected by neutralization of the virus infection, toxicity, enzymatic and hormonal activity, respectively. Precipitation and agglutination have also been adapted for development of several useful assays.

Table 1.   Effects of combination of antigen and antibody*

Agglutination	Antigenic particle + specific Ab results in aggregation of particles
Precipitation	Soluble Ag + specific Ab results in lattice formation and precipitation
C activation	Ag in solution or on particle + specific Ab results in activation of C
Cytolysis	Cell + anti-cell Ab + C may result in lysis of the cell
Opsonization	Antigenic particle + Ab + C enhances phagocytosis by Mo, MØ, PMNs
Neutralization	Toxins, viruses, enzymes, etc. + specific Abs may result in their inactivation

*C, Complement; Mo, monocytes; MØ, macrophages; Ab, antibody; PMNs, polymorphonuclear cells

A variety of other assays have been developed which provide specific qualitative and quantitative measurement of Ag or Ab for both research and diagnostic purposes. Since the immune system recognizes and remembers virtually all Ags that are introduced into an individual, assays which demonstrate the presence of Ab to an organism in the serum of a patient have become a standard way of determining that the patient has had contact with, was infected by, the organism (e.g. the presence of Ab to HIV in the serum of a patient usually means that the patient has been infected with HIV). Alternatively, Abs with defined specificity (e.g. to Ags associated with cancer cells) can be used to determine the presence of disease-associated Ags in a patient. Abs are also extremely important tools in molecular and cellular research as they permit the localization and characterization of Ags.

ELISA, RIA

The presence of Ab to a particular Ag in the serum of a patient can be determined using very sensitive radioimmunoassays (RIA) or enzyme-linked immunoabsorbent assays (ELISA). Such assays (*Fig. 1*) are of particular value in demonstrating Ab to Ags of infectious agents, e.g. virus, bacteria, etc. The presence of an Ab of a particular isotype can also be determined using a modification of these assays. The radioallergosorbent test (RAST) uses as detecting ligand a radiolabeled Ab to human IgE and permits the measurement of specific IgE Ab to an allergen. ELISA and RIA also provide very specific and sensitive measurement of toxins, drugs, hormones, pesticides, etc., not only in serum, but also in water, foods and other consumer products. Based on these procedures, assays for nearly any Ag or Ab can be readily developed.

Immuno-fluorescence and flow cytometry

Although it is possible to use ELISA and RIA to evaluate the presence of an Ag on a cell, this is usually more conveniently done using Abs to which a fluorescent marker has been covalently attached. Moreover, in most cases a mAb is used and thus is highly specific for a particular molecule and a particular epitope on that molecule. This type of assay can be done using an Ab to the Ag which is directly fluorescent labeled (**direct** immunofluorescence) or by first incubating the unlabeled Ab with the cells (e.g. a mouse mAb to human T cells) and then, after washing away unbound Ab, adding a second fluorescent-labeled Ab that reacts with the first Ab (e.g. a goat Ab to mouse immunoglobulin). This

(a)
Radioimmunoassay (RIA)

(b)
Enzyme-linked immunoabsorbant assay

(c)
Radioallergosorbent test (RAST)

(d)
Sandwich ELISA

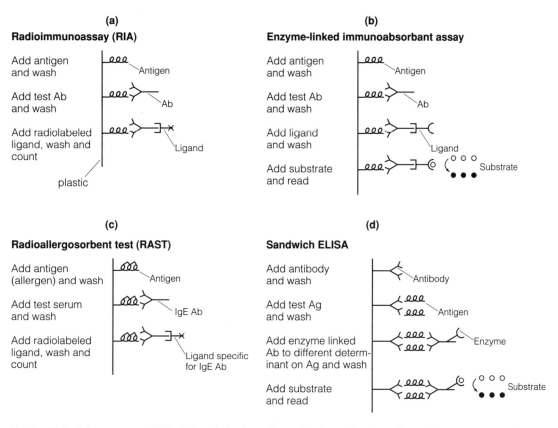

Fig. 1   (a) Radioimmunoassay (RIA). Antigen is incubated in a microtiter well and small quantities are adsorbed. Free antigen is washed away. Test antibody is added, which may bind to the Ag, and unbound Ab washed away. Ab remaining bound to the Ag is detected by a radiolabeled ligand (e.g. an Ab specific for the isotype of the test Ab, or staphylococcal protein A which binds to the Fc region of IgG). (b) Enzyme-linked immunosorbent assay (ELISA). This is similar to RIA except that the ligand (e.g. the Ab that binds the test Ag) is covalently coupled to an enzyme such as peroxidase. This ligand binds the test Ab and after free ligand is washed away the bound ligand is detected by the addition of substrate which is acted on by the enzyme to yield a colored and detectable end product. (c) Radioallergosorbent test (RAST). This measures Ag-specific IgE in an RIA where the ligand is a labeled anti-IgE Ab. (d) The sandwich assay is done as above except that Ab to an antigen is first adsorbed to a micotiter well and unbound Ab washed away. A potential source of Ag is added and what is not bound (captured) by the Ab is washed away. An enzyme-linked Ab to a different determinant on the Ag is then added, followed by washing. The presence of Ag is detected by the change in color of added substrate.

indirect immunofluorescent assay (*Fig. 2*) has two advantages, it has higher sensitivity and requires labeling of only one Ab, the second Ab, because, in the example given, it can detect (react with) mouse Ab to other antigens.

Fluorescent Abs to cell surface molecules (e.g. those which are tumor associated) are very useful in examining tissue sections for cells expressing the Ag. This assay is done by incubating the tissue section with the labeled Ab (for direct immunofluorescence) or unlabeled Ab, followed by labeled second Ab and then examining the tissue section using a fluorescent microscope. These microscopes irradiate the tissue with a wavelength of light that excites the fluorescent label on the Ab to emit light at a different wavelength. This emitted light can be directly visualized, photographed and even quantitated. Moreover, it is possible to analyze a tissue sample using several different Abs at the same

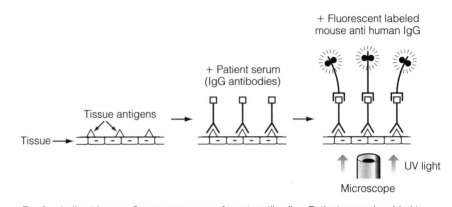

Fig. 2. Indirect immunofluorescence assay for autoantibodies. Patient serum is added to tissue sections and the autoantibodies bind to particular autoantigen(s). After washing, fluorescent antibodies to human IgG are added and viewed under a fluorescence microscope. A green color shows where the human antibodies have bound to the tissue autoantigens.

time, as each Ab could be labeled with a different fluorescent molecule each of which emits light at a wavelength distinct from the others. It is also possible to look for intracellular molecules (e.g. Abs) by first permeabilizing the cells and then doing the staining and fluorescence microscopy. Thus, one can use this approach to develop a molecular fingerprint of the cells associated with a tissue.

Although fluorescence microscopy can be, and is, applied to the analysis of **single cell suspensions**, another rather technologically sophisticated approach, **flow cytometry**, is most often used. This assay uses the same basic staining procedures as described for fluorescence microscopy, followed by automated quantitation of the amount of fluorescence associated with individual cells (*Fig. 3*). In particular, the suspension of stained cells is fed to the flow cytometer which disperses the cells so they then pass single file through a focused laser beam which excites any fluorescent label associated with the cells. Those stained by the fluorescent Ab emit light that is detected and quantitated by optical sensors and the intensity of fluorescence is plotted in histogram form by a computer. This machine can analyze 1000 cells per second and provide quantitative data on the number of molecules of a particular kind on each cell. It can also analyze mixtures of cells and provide data on their size and granularity in addition to their expression of specific molecules. Some versions of this machine (**fluorescence-activated cell sorter**) are also able to separate out cells into microdroplets and sort those expressing a selected amount of a particular Ag into a separate tube for further analysis or culture.

Immunoblotting

It is possible to combine various separation and detection procedures for identification and analysis of Ags and for evaluating the expression of molecules by single cells. Western blot analysis involves separating Ags by polyacrylamide gel electrophoresis (PAGE) in the presence of sodium dodecyl sulfate (SDS) which results in separation of molecules on the basis of size. These molecules are then transferred to another matrix (e.g. nitrocellulose) to form a pattern on the matrix identical to that on the gel. Enzyme-linked Ab to the molecule of

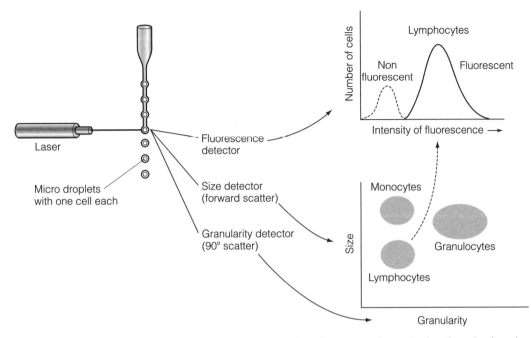

Fig. 3. Flow cytometry. After labeling with fluorescent antibody, cells are passed one at a time through a laser beam. Photodetectors measure the amount of fluorescence which is plotted as a histogram showing the proportion of non-fluorescent (unstained) and fluorescent (stained) cells. Other detectors simultaneously measure scattered laser light, which is used to generate a 'dot blot' in which lymphocytes, monocytes and granulocytes can be discriminated.

interest is then added, the unbound Ab washed off and substrate added (see ELISA) for visualization. This assay permits specific identification of proteins in a mixture and is also often used to confirm the presence of Abs to certain infectious agents (e.g. HIV) in the serum of patients.

Immunoblotting can also be used to assay for the presence of molecules in a mixture as described for the sandwich ELISA. This has now been extended for analysis of products of single cells. For example, to assay for production of a cytokine, Ab to the cytokine is coated onto the nitrocellulose 'floor' of a special culture well (see sandwich ELISA), the unbound Ab is washed off, and cells are then plated on top of this Ab. After incubation, an enzyme-linked Ab to a different determinant on the cytokine is added, followed by washing and substrate addition. Wherever a cell produced the cytokine, it will be captured by the first Ab and will then be detected by the second Ab and its conversion of substrate, forming a colored spot on the nitrocellulose (hence the name ELISPOT assay). The nature of the cell producing the cytokine can also be determined by flow cytometry after staining the cells with a fluorescent-labeled cell-type-specific Ab (e.g. anti-CD4 for T helper cells) and an anti-cytokine Ab labeled with a different fluorochrome.

Affinity purification of Ag and Ab

The specificity of Abs is not only important to the development of many research and diagnostic assays, but can, in some instances, be used to purify, or be purified by, interaction with Ag. This is because Abs do not form covalent bonds when they combine with Ag. Ab coupled to an insoluble matrix (e.g. agarose) specifically binds its Ag, removing it from a mixture of other molecules. After washing to remove all unbound molecules, the Ag can be eluted at low pH and/or at high ionic strength, which breaks the reversible bonds holding it to the Ab. As this can usually be performed without damaging the Ag or Ab, it is possible to obtain relatively pure Ag in one step. Similarly, Ag coupled to an insoluble matrix permits purification of Ab from media or serum. Ab can also be purified based on its binding by proteins (e.g. protein A) isolated from some strains of *Staphylococcus aureus*. Protein A coupled to agarose binds IgG Abs which can be eluted by decreasing the pH and/or by increasing the ionic strength of the eluting buffer, again without damaging the Ab. Using similar techniques, cell subpopulations with characteristic cell surface molecules (e.g. immunoglobulin on B cells) can also be isolated (positive selection) or removed (negative selection) from a mixture of cells.

D8 ANTIBODY FUNCTIONS

Key Notes

Role of antibody alone	Antibody alone can neutralize viruses and toxins if it binds tightly to, and blocks, a part of the toxin or virus critical to its biological activity. Similarly, antibodies can inhibit microbes from colonizing mucosal areas and in some cases may induce programed cell death (apoptosis).
Role of antibody in complement activation	IgG or IgM antibodies can, on binding to antigen, activate the **classical** pathway of complement leading to lysis of the cell on which the antigen is located, and/or to attraction of immune cells (chemotaxis) which phagocytose the antigen-expressing cells.
Role of antibody with effector cells	Phagocytes (PMNs and macrophages) have various receptors including those for complement component C3b, for the Fc region of IgG (FcγR) and for the Fc region of IgA (FcαR). These receptors enhance binding to, and phagocytosis, or ADCC of, antibody and/or complement opsonized microbes. Binding of antigens (e.g. allergens) to IgE already bound to Fc receptors for IgE on mast cells results in degranulation and subsequent enhancement of the acute inflammatory response.
Related topics	Cells of the innate immune system (B1) Innate immunity and inflammation (B4)
	Molecules of the innate immune system (B2) Immunity to different organisms (H2)

Role of antibody alone

Antibody alone can, in some instances, neutralize, and thus protect against, viruses and toxins. However, its effectiveness depends greatly on the specificity and affinity of the antibody. That is, it must react with the part of the toxin or virus critical to its biological activity, and it must bind tightly enough to prevent interaction of the toxin or virus with the cell surface receptor through which it gains entry. Similarly, antibodies, primarily of the IgA class, can bind to bacteria and inhibit their attachment to mucosal epithelial cells. They can also cause their agglutination and thus prevent colonization of mucosal areas (Topic D2). In addition, antibodies specific for certain molecules on the surface of cells can induce programed cell death (apoptosis).

Role of antibody in complement activation

The ability of antibody to protect against infection is, in many instances, greatly enhanced by or dependent on the complement system. As described in Topic B2, the complement system is a protective system common to all vertebrates. In man it consists of a set of over 20 soluble glycoproteins, many of which are produced by hepatocytes and monocytes. These molecules are constitutively present in blood and other body fluids and may be present in large amounts, especially C3, the pivotal molecule of the complement system. The component molecules (C) include C1 (C1q, C1r, C1s), C2, C3, C4, C5, C6, C7, C8, C9 as well as a set of molecules which are primarily associated with the alternative pathway, including Factor B and Factor D (Topic B2). On appropriate triggering, these components interact sequentially with each other. This 'cascade' of molecular events involves cleavage of some complement components into active fragments (e.g. C3 is cleaved to C3a and C3b), which contribute to activation of the next component, ultimately leading to lysis of, and/or protection against, a variety of microbes.

When an antibody of the IgG or IgM class (Topic D1, *Table 1*) attaches to an antigen, **the classical pathway** of complement is activated leading to complement-mediated lysis of the microbe (or other cell) on which the antigen is located. In addition, complement activation can also lead to attraction of immune cells (chemotaxis), and to opsonization and phagocytosis of the cell on which complement is being activated (Topic B2). The classical pathway can also be activated by an Ag–Ab lattice.

Table 1.   Sequence of complement activation by the classical pathway leading to cell lysis

T (target cell) + A (antibody)	TA complex
TA + C1q,r,s	TAC1
TAC1 + C4	TAC1,4b + C4a
TAC1,4b + C2	TAC1,4b,2b + C2a
TAC1,4b,2b + C3	TAC1,4b,2b,3b + C3a
TAC1,4b,2b,3b + C5	TAC1,4b,2b,3b,5b + C5a
TAC1,4b,2b,3b,5b + C6 + C7	TAC1,4b,2b,3b,5b,6,7
TAC1,4b,2b,3b,5b,6,7 + C8	TAC1,4b,2b,3b,5b,6,7,8
TAC1,4b,2b,3b,5b,6,7,8 + C9	TAC1,4b,2b,3b,5b,6,7,8,9 Lysis of T

T refers to target cell, A refers to antibody

Sequence of activation
Formation of a site to which the first component of complement (C1) can bind requires a single bound antibody of IgM, or two IgG molecules bound in close proximity to each other. The Clq component of the C1 complex (C1q, C1r, C1s) then binds to the Fc regions of the cell-bound antibodies (*Fig. 1*). This results in activation of C1 which then catalyzes the cleavage of C4 and C2, pieces of which (C4b and C2b) then bind to the cell surface forming a new cell-bound enzyme, C3 convertase (C4b+C2b). C3 convertase then cleaves C3 into C3a and C3b. C3b binds to the cell surface, forming a C4b, 2b, 3b complex. The cleavage of C3 into C3a and C3b is the single most important event in the activation of the complement system. This may be achieved by two different cleavage enzymes, C3 convertases – one as a component of the alternative pathway (Topic B2), the other a part of the classical pathway. One of the fragments, C3b, is very reactive and can covalently bind to virtually any molecule or cell. If C3b binds to a self cell, regulatory molecules associated with this cell (see below) inactivate it, protecting the cell from complement-mediated damage.

For the classical pathway, the C4b, 2b, 3b complex governs the reaction and binding of the next complement components, C5, C6, C7, C8 and C9 to the cell surface (*Table 1*). More specifically, C5b is crucial to formation of the 'membrane attack complex' (MAC), C5b-C6-C7-C8-C9, which mediates lysis of the microbe. The sequence of activation of the C5–9 components is the same as that described for the alternative pathway (Topic B2), and leads to functional and

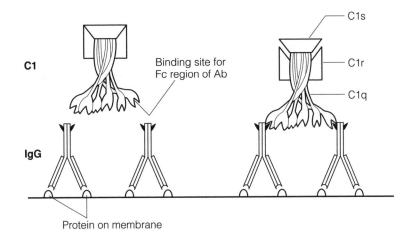

Fig. 1. *Initiation of complement activation by binding of C1 to antibody. The CH2 domains of the Fc regions of adjacent IgG molecules, bound to repeating antigenic determinants on a membrane, interact with the C1q subunit of C1. This results in the activation of C1r and C1s subunits, exposing an enzymatic active site.*

structural damage to the membrane as a result of the formation of pores created by insertion of C9 complexes into the membrane.

The major functions of the complement system
The classical pathway has the same biological activities and major functions as the alternative pathway, including:

- Initiation of (acute) inflammation by direct activation of mast cells.
- Attraction of neutrophils to the site of microbial attack (chemotaxis).
- Enhancement of the attachment of the microbe to the phagocyte (opsonization).
- Killing of the microbe activating the membrane attack complex (lysis).

The components of the complement system most important to these main functions are the inflammatory peptides C3a and C5a (anaphylatoxins), derived from C3 and C5, respectively. C3a and C3b bind to receptors on mast cells causing them to release pharmacological mediators (degranulate) such as histamine, which result in smooth muscle contraction and increased vascular permeability (Topics B2, B4 and K4). C5a is also chemotactic and attracts neutrophils (PMNs) to the site of its generation (e.g. by microbial attack). It also causes PMN adhesion, degranulation and activation of the respiratory burst.

Also important C3b and its split products (and C4b) act as opsonins, marking a target for recognition by receptors on phagocytic cells. These receptors (e.g. complement receptor, CR1 = CD35) are expressed on monocytes/macrophages, PMNs and erythrocytes. PMNs attracted to a site of complement activation by C5a find and bind to C3b through their cell surface complement receptors, an interaction that greatly enhances internalization of the microbe by these cells. Thus, complement can not only lead to lysis of a microbe, but attracts phagocytes and identifies, using C3b, what these cells should phagocytose. Even organisms resistant to direct lysis by complement may be phagocytosed and killed. Binding of C3b-containing complexes to CR1 on erythrocytes shuttles immune complexes to the mononuclear phagocytes of the liver and spleen, facilitating their removal.

Finally, C5b through C9, the MAC, and especially C9 produces 'pores' in the target cell membrane. These pores have diameters of about 10 nm and permit leakage of intracellular components and influx of water that results in disintegration (lysis) of the cell.

Regulation

The complement system is a powerful mediator of inflammation and destruction and could cause extensive damage to host cells if uncontrolled. However, complement components rapidly lose binding capacity after activation, limiting their membrane-damaging ability to the immediate vicinity of the activation site. The complement system is also tightly regulated by inhibitory/regulatory proteins. These regulatory proteins (*Table 2*) include C1 inhibitor, Factor I, C4b binding protein, Factor H, decay-accelerating factor (DAF), membrane co-factor protein (MCP), and CD59 (protectin). They protect host cells from destruction or damage at different stages of the complement cascade. Because regulatory proteins are expressed on the surface of many host cells but not on microbes, they limit damage to the site of activation and usually to the invading microbe which initiated complement activation.

Table 2.   Regulatory proteins of the complement system

Protein	Function
C1 inhibitor	Binds to C1r and C1s and prevents further activation of C4 and C2
Factor I	Enzymatically inactivates C4b and C3b
C4b binding protein	Binds to C4b displacing C2b
Factor H	Displaces C2b and C3b by binding C4b
DAF	Inactivates C3b and C4b
MCP	Promotes C3b and C4b inactivation
CD59	Prevents binding of C5b,6,7 complexes to host cells

Activation equals inactivation

Because the activated complement components are unstable and also readily inactivated by complement regulatory proteins, the activity of complement is short lived. Therefore, activation of complement is equivalent to its inactivation. Thus, depressed complement levels in an individual may indicate that complement is being used up faster than it is being produced, suggesting chronic activation of complement perhaps resulting from continuous *in vivo* formation of antigen–antibody complexes.

Role of antibody with effector cells

A variety of effector cells have receptors for the Fc region of antibodies. Phagocytes (PMNs, macrophages and eosinophils) utilize their Fc receptors (FcR) for IgG (FcγR) or IgA (FcαR) to enhance phagocytosis of antibody opsonized microbes. In addition, these FcR can mediate killing of cells through antibody-dependent cellular cytotoxicity (ADCC). PMNs, monocytes, macrophages, eosinophils and NK cells can kill antibody-coated target cells directly (*Fig. 2*). That is, in ADCC, lysis of the target cell does not require internalization (although that may also happen) and involves release of toxic molecules (e.g. TNFα, Topic B2) at the surface of the target.

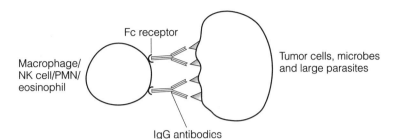

Fig. 2.   Antibody dependent cellular cytotoxicity (ADCC) of an antibody coated target cell. Several effector cell populations have Fc receptors (FcR) for IgG. Antibody coated microbes attach to macrophages or PMNs through these receptors, and their resulting crosslinking leads to release of toxic substances. This extracellular killing probably occurs prior to phagocytosis of opsonized microbes through FcR or complement receptors. This also occurs when the antibody coated target is too large to be phagocytosed, e.g. a worm. Eosinophils are particularly important in killing worms by this mechanism (Topic H2). Macrophages, PMNs, and eosinophils can also use IgA FcR for ADCC. NK cell mediated death of virus-infected cells and tumor cells can be enhanced through ADCC.

Enhanced phagocytosis can also be mediated by phagocyte receptors for the complement component C3b, which is generated by antibody-mediated activation of the complement sequence (classical pathway) or on activation by certain microbes of the alternative pathway of complement. Mast cells and basophils have FcR for IgE (FcεR), which on binding of IgE-coated antigens or cells can trigger degranulation and subsequent enhancement of the acute inflammatory response. Over-stimulation of mast cells/basophils by this mechanism leads to pathology (Topic K2).

E1 THE B CELL RECEPTOR COMPLEX, CO-RECEPTORS AND SIGNALING

Key Notes

The B cell receptor (BCR) complex	The BCR complex consists of the antigen receptor, Ig, in association with two other polypeptides, Igα and Igβ (CD79a and CD79b). Igα and Igβ are signaling molecules for the BCR and are also required for assembly and expression of Ig.
B cell co-receptors	Co-receptors, including CD21, CD32 and CD19 associate with the BCR complex especially when both the BCR and one or more of the co-receptors are linked through an antigen-complement/antibody complex. Depending on which molecules are ligated, signaling by the Ig-Igα/Igβ complex is enhanced or inhibited.
Receptor–ligand interactions	Lymphocytes need to be activated in order to carry out their function. Binding of the lymphocyte to an antigen via its antigen receptor, *signal 1*, is necessary, but not sufficient to stimulate it and may lead to anergy. Accessory and co-stimulatory molecules on the surface of B cells are required for cell–cell interaction and the signal transduction events leading to activation (*signal 2*).
Signaling by co-receptors	B cell signaling is initiated through the Igα/Igβ complex associated with the BCR and results in phosphorylation of tyrosine motifs (ITAMs). This is followed by an ordered series of biochemical events involving kinases and phosphatases. These events are modulated by signals from co-receptors. Second messengers lead to activation of transcription factors and thus to activation of lymphocyte function.
Related topics	Cells of the innate immune system (B1) Lymphocytes (C1) B cell activation (E2)

The B cell receptor (BCR) complex

As described in Topic D2, the receptor for antigen on B cells is immuno-globulin. Initially cells make IgM and then IgD, which are both displayed on the surface of a mature B cell. These Igs are transmembrane molecules although the cytoplasmic domain of each is only three amino acids long, too short to signal the cell when antigen binds to the antibody. However, this membrane-bound Ig is associated with two other polypeptides on the B cell, Igα and Igβ (*Fig. 1*). These small molecular weight (20 kDa) transmembrane molecules are the signaling molecules for the BCR. When IgM, IgD (or other Ig isotypes on the B cell) are cross linked by binding to antigen, Igα and Igβ transduce signals which begin to prepare the cell for a productive interaction with T helper cells. Igα and Igβ are also required for assembly and expression of immunoglobulin, and thus of the B cell receptor complex, in the plasma membrane.

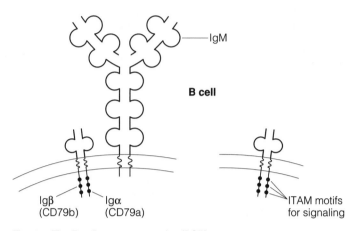

Fig. 1.   The B cell receptor complex (BCR).

B cell co-receptors

Molecules associated with the B cell receptor complex are expressed early in development to enable assembly of a functional antigen receptor on the B cell surface. Other molecules important for B cell functions, including their ability to present antigen, e.g. MHC class II molecules, also develop early in the life of a B cell. Moreover, the co-receptor complex on the surface of B cells can, depending on which molecules are ligated, enhance or inhibit signaling by the Ig-Igα/Igβ complex. This co-receptor complex includes CD21 (complement receptor 2, CR2), CD32 (a receptor for the Fc region of IgG, FcγRIIB), and CD19 (a signaling molecule). These molecules associate with the BCR complex especially when both the BCR and the co-receptor complex interact with the same antigen; i.e., if the BCR binds antigen with which soluble Ab and/or complement have also interacted, CD21 and CD32 will be engaged and, through these signaling molecules, influence signaling by the Igα/Igβ complex (*Fig. 2*).

Receptor–ligand interactions

Lymphocytes need to be activated in order to carry out their function. At the molecular level this means receiving a message from outside the cell via

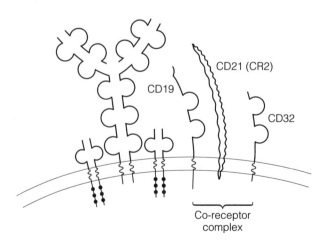

Fig. 2.   The BCR complex and its co-receptor complex.

interaction with a cell surface receptor. This signal is then passed through the cytoplasm to the nucleus (signal transduction) to induce the gene transcription required for cell proliferation and synthesis and release of effector molecules, e.g. cytokines and antibodies. Although binding of the lymphocyte to an antigen via its antigen receptor (*signal 1*) is necessary to stimulate the cell, it is not sufficient and usually results in anergy if signal 2 is not also provided. Certainly, the binding of accessory cell surface molecules (e.g. B7-1 and B7-2 (CD80 and CD86), CD40 and LFA-1, on B cells) with their counter receptors on T cells is important, as these interactions increase the avidity of cell–cell interaction. In addition, co-stimulatory molecules (some of which are also accessory molecules) modulate the signal transduction events leading to activation by providing the critical second signal (*signal 2*). B cells are activated with and without the requirement of T cells. Multimeric antigens can stimulate B cells directly whilst responses to protein antigens require T cell help.

Signaling by co-receptors

The antigen receptors on B cells do not have intracytoplasmic tails of sufficient length and amino acid composition to act as signaling molecules. Thus, B cell signaling is initiated through CD79a/b, which is associated with the BCR. These molecules have immuno-tyrosine activation motifs (ITAMs) that are phosphorylated by kinases to initiate the activation process. Similar to the early events leading to activation of T cells, the molecules of the B cell receptor complex become associated with the enzymes involved in phosphorylation within cholesterol-rich areas of membrane termed 'lipid rafts' (Topic F4). An ordered series of biochemical events then occurs via kinases and phosphatases, which is modulated by signals from other co-receptor cell surface molecules. Second messengers are produced which are eventually responsible for activation of transcription factors inside the nucleus and for production of cell cycle proteins and molecules required for lymphocyte effector functions. Cytokines induce proliferation and further differentiation of activated B cells.

E2 B CELL ACTIVATION

Key Notes

Two kinds of B cells

Two B cell groups can be distinguished based on their requirement for T cell help in order to proliferate and differentiate. *B1 cells* are T cell independent, produce mainly IgM antibodies for secretion, and generally recognize multimeric sugar/lipid (thymus-independent, T-I) antigens of microbes. *B2 cells* (conventional B cells) are dependent on T cell help and are primarily responsible for the development of IgG, IgA and IgE antibody-mediated immunity.

Thymus-independent (T-I) antigens

Although B cell responses to most antigens require T cell help, activation of B cells by certain antigens does not. These T-independent antigens are of two types, both of which generate primarily IgM antibodies of low affinity. Type 1 antigens are bacterial polysaccharide mitogens that activate B cells independently of their antigen receptors. Type 2 antigens are linear, poorly degradable antigens, e.g. pneumococcus polysaccharide. These antigens persist on the surface of macrophages and directly stimulate B cells through cross-linking of their surface receptors.

Thymus-dependent (T-D) antigens

Th cells induce B cells to produce antibodies, to switch the isotype of antibody being produced and to undergo affinity maturation. Binding of most antigens to antigen receptors on B cells provides one signal whilst the cytokines produced by the Th cells, and the engagement of complementary surface molecules on the *cognate* B cell provides the second signal resulting in B cell activation. Th cells recognize antigenic peptides on the surface of antigen-specific B cells because the B cells can capture antigen specifically via membrane Ig and associate its peptidase with class II MHC molecules. Once triggered via the TCR, Th cells express CD40L, which triggers B cell activation via its CD40 surface receptor. Activated B cells reciprocally co-stimulate T cells via CD28, which produce IL-2, IL-4 and IL-5. As a result, both the T cells and B cells clonally expand and differentiate.

Biochemical events leading to B cell activation

Igα/Igβ molecules transmit the first signals following B cell interaction with antigen through ITAMs of their intracytoplasmic tails. Co-receptors of the B cell receptor complex (CD21 and CD19) modulate these initial signals. CD21 binds to C3d if it is bound to the specific antigen and provides an additional positive signal in B cell activation. Cross-linking of membrane receptor antibodies on B cells by T-I antigens induces clustering of co-receptors leading to multiple signals enhancing activation of kinase networks and of IgM-producing B cells. B cells primed by a T-D antigen receive a second signal when the Th cell CD40L binds to CD40 on the B cell. Together with cytokines such as IL-2, IL-4, etc., this signaling induces proliferation and differentiation of the B cells into plasma cells or memory cells.

Related topics

Lymphocytes (C1)
The B cell receptor complex, co-receptors and signaling (E1)
T cell recognition of antigen (F2)
Regulation by antigen and antibody (G4)

Genes, T helper cells, cytokines and the neuroendocrine system (G5)
Primary/congenital (inherited) immunodeficiency (J2)

Two kinds of B cells

Two B cell groups can be distinguished based on their requirement for T cell help in order to proliferate and differentiate. *B1 cells* arise early in ontogeny, produce mainly IgM antibodies for secretion that are encoded by germline antibody genes, and mature independently of the bone marrow. These cells generally recognize multimeric sugar/lipid antigens of microbes and are T-cell-independent (T-I), that is, they do not require T cell help in order to proliferate and differentiate in response to antigen.

B2 cells are the *conventional* B cells primarily responsible for the development of humoral (antibody)-mediated immunity. They are produced in the bone marrow, and are T-cell-dependent (T-D); that is, they require T cell help in order to proliferate and differentiate in response to antigen. B2 cells eventually give rise to plasma cells that produce IgG, IgA and IgE antibodies.

Thymus-independent (T-I) antigens

Although B cell responses to most antigens require T cell help, activation of B cells by certain antigens does not. For the most part, these B1 cells recognize and respond to T-independent (T-I) antigens and produce primarily IgM antibodies of low affinity, whereas T-dependent (T-D) antigens generate much higher-affinity antibodies of the other classes. T-I antigens are of two types.

Type 1 antigens
Bacterial polysaccharides have the ability, at high enough concentration, to activate the majority of B cells independently of their specific antigen receptors. They do this through a mitogenic component that bypasses the early biochemical pathways initiated through the antibody receptor. The B cell focuses the polysaccharide antigen and at sufficiently high concentrations drives its activation (*Fig. 1*).

Type 2 antigens
Some linear antigens that are not easily degraded and have epitopes spaced appropriately on the molecule, e.g. pneumococcus polysaccharide, can directly stimulate B cells in a T-cell-independent fashion. These antigens persist on the

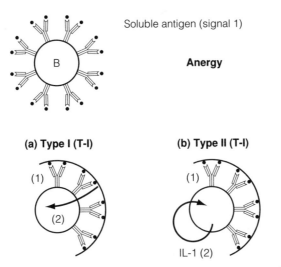

Fig. 1. Activation of B cells through T cell independent antigens. Soluble antigen interaction with the B cell antigen receptor (antibody) results in anergy (signal 1 only). Signal 2 is provided by a mitogenic component (arrow) of the type I antigen (a) and via autocrine activity of IL-1 (arrow) for type II antigen (b).

surface of splenic marginal zone and lymph node subcapsular macrophages and directly stimulate B cells through cross-linking of their surface receptors (*Fig. 1*). Although activation is independent of T cells, cytokines produced by T cells can amplify these responses.

Thymus-dependent (T-D) antigens

The production of antibody to most antigens requires the participation of T cells. In particular, Th cells induce B2 cells to proliferate, differentiate and produce antibodies. In addition, Th cells induce switching of the class of antibody being produced and affinity maturation. To accomplish this, Th cells produce critical cytokines and directly engage the *cognate* B cell and trigger its activation through cell surface receptors. This T cell *collaboration* with B cells is necessary since binding of most (non-multimeric) antigens to antigen receptors on most B cells provides one signal that, in the absence of a second signal, is an anergic signal, i.e. turns off the B cell. The cytokines produced by the Th cells and the engagement of complementary surface molecules provide the essential second signals to the B cell resulting in its activation (*Fig. 2*).

More specifically, Th cells recognize antigenic peptides on the surface of antigen-specific B cells because the B cells are able to capture antigen specifically via membrane (m)IgM and mIgD. This feature of B cells, to capture, process and present specific antigen, makes them unique amongst the antigen-presenting cells which normally take up antigen via scavenger and other receptors (Topic B3). The antigen is then endocytosed, degraded via the exogenous processing pathway and peptides are associated with class II MHC molecules (*Fig. 4*; Topic F2). Th cells whose TCR are specific for that peptide–MHC complex, recognize and bind to B cells via TCR–MHC interactions and through engagement of adhesion molecules.

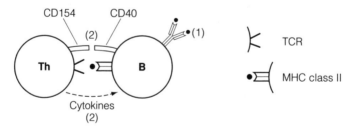

Fig. 2.   *T cell activation of B cells. T cells provide the 2nd signal to B cells via ligation of CD40 by CD 154 (CD40 ligand) but also via cytokines.*

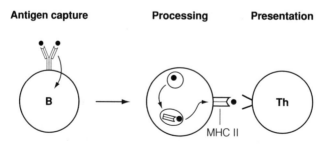

Fig. 3.   *Activation of B cells through T cell help. Captured soluble antigens are processed and presented to Th cells which provide the 2nd signal required for B cell activation.*

Once triggered via the TCR, the Th cell expresses CD40 ligand (CD40L), the ligand for the B cell surface molecule CD40. This Th cell now triggers the activation of the B cell via the CD40 surface receptor (*Fig. 4*). As a result, the activated B cell reciprocally co-stimulates the Th cell via CD28. At this time, both the T cell and B cell are stimulated. T cells then produce cytokines including IL-2 (autocrine growth factor for the Th cells) and IL-4 and IL-5 (growth and differentiation factors for the activated B cells). As a result, both the T cell and B cell clonally expand and differentiate. Ligation of B cell CD40 by CD40L on T cells is also important in that it rescues B cells from death in germinal centers (Topic E3).

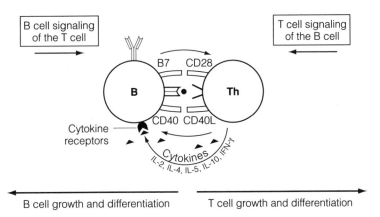

Fig. 4.   Reciprocal activation of T and B cells.

Biochemical events leading to B cell activation

The transmembrane surface immunoglobulin antigen receptors on B cells, like the TCR on T cells have short intracytoplasmic tails unable to transduce signals themselves. Therefore, on engagement of the B cell antigen receptor, other molecules associated with these receptors mediate signaling. In particular, CD79a and b of the B cell receptor complex (Topic E1) contain ITAMs, which are phosphorylated during the early stages of activation and initiate the B cell signaling cascade. Other members of the B cell receptor complex (*Fig. 5*) modulate the initial signals mediated through antigen binding and enhance the strength of cell–cell interaction. For example, CD21, a complement receptor that binds C3d, may provide an additional positive signal in B cell activation as a result of binding to C3d associated with antigen. As with T cell activation, these processes in B cells are mediated through phosphatases and kinases. The importance of one kinase, btk, is indicated by the observation that mutation of the gene encoding it results in the absence of B cells (Bruton's agammaglobulinemia: Topic J2).

B cells like T cells require two signals for their activation. Binding of soluble antigen to the antibody receptor alone (signal 1) results in apoptosis. This is seen experimentally using antibodies to the sIgM on B cells. Proliferation is induced in the presence of a second signal that for B cell activation is provided by interaction of Th cell CD40L with CD40 on the B cell surface. This is also a requirement for class switching. Other cytokines produced by Th cells induce appropriate signals important to differentiation of the B cells into plasma or memory cells (*Fig. 6*). After initial B cell activation and following class switch-

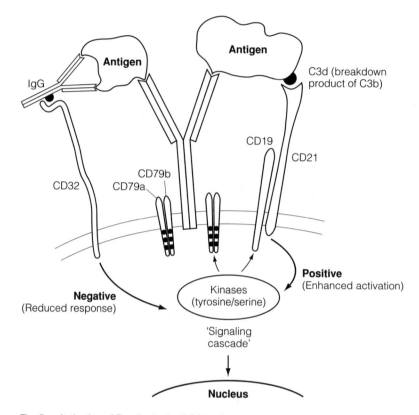

Fig. 5.   *Activation of B cells via the BCR and co-receptor complex. Attachment of antigen results in activation of several kinases and the intracytoplasmic chains of Igα and Igβ are phosphorylated on their ITAMs. Binding of CD21 to antigen bound to complement (C3d) regulates signaling via CD19 in a positive way, whilst interaction of CD32 with IgG antibody bound to antigen and the antigen receptor, provides a negative signal.*

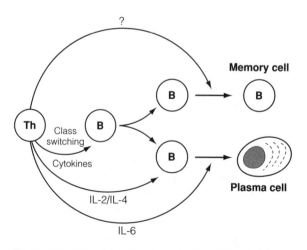

Fig. 6.   *The roles of cytokines in maturation of B cells into memory and plasma cells.*

ing to IgG, B cells are susceptible to regulation by concomitant binding of FcγRII (CD32) and the B cell antigen receptor. In particular, further activation of these cells can be inhibited by their binding of specific antigen attached to IgG. As a result, CD32 transmits a negative signal to the B cell and prevents its activation ('negative feedback': Topic G4).

T-I antigens, which do not induce IgG responses (since their CD40 molecules are not ligated), receive their second signal via the 'mitogenic' component of T-I type I antigens. The second signal via T-I type 2 antigens is through binding of repeating antigenic units by BCR, which leads to clustering of co-receptors. In these cases, the signals transduced are quite different from those resulting in activation of T-D B cells.

E3 THE CELLULAR BASIS OF THE ANTIBODY RESPONSE

Key Notes

Selection and activation of B cells

Antigen introduced into an individual binds specifically to B cells with receptors for that antigen. In the presence of T cell help these B cells clonally expand and some differentiate into plasma cells that make antibody specific for the antigen triggering the response.

Primary and memory responses

On first exposure to antigen, a primary immune response develops resulting in production of IgM antibodies. This is usually followed by an IgG immune response within 4–5 days. This response is self-limiting and will stop when antigen is no longer available to stimulate B cells. When antigen is reintroduced, there are more antigen-specific B cells, which have differentiated to more responsive memory B cells, resulting in a more rapid response and usually in IgG antibody production.

Multiclonal responses

Antibodies produced by a single cell are homogeneous, but the response to a given antigen involves many different specific antibody-producing cells and thus, overall, is very heterogeneous (i.e. multiclonal). Moreover, the effectiveness of an antibody response to a microbe may depend on this heterogeneity.

Cross-reactive responses

Similar or identical antigenic determinants are sometimes found in association with widely different molecules or cells. This cross-reactivity is important: (a) in protection against organisms with cross-reactive antigens; and (b) in autoimmune diseases induced by infectious organisms bearing antigens cross-reactive with normal self antigens (e.g. streptococcal infections which predispose to rheumatic fever).

Related topics

Lymphocytes (C1)
Antibody classes (D2)
B cell activation (E2)

Clonal expansion and development of effector function (F5)
Genes, T helper cells, cytokines and the neuroendocrine system (G5)

Selection and activation of B cells

When antigen is introduced into an individual, B cells with receptors for that antigen bind and internalize it into an endosomal compartment, and process and present it on MHC class II molecules to helper T cells (Topic E2). These B cells are triggered to proliferate, giving rise to clones of large numbers of daughter cells. Some of the cells of these expanding clones serve as memory cells, others differentiate and become plasma cells (Topic E2) that make and secrete large quantities of specific antibody. For example, on introduction of antigen 5 (Ag5) into a person (*Fig. 1*), more than 10^6 B cells have the opportu-

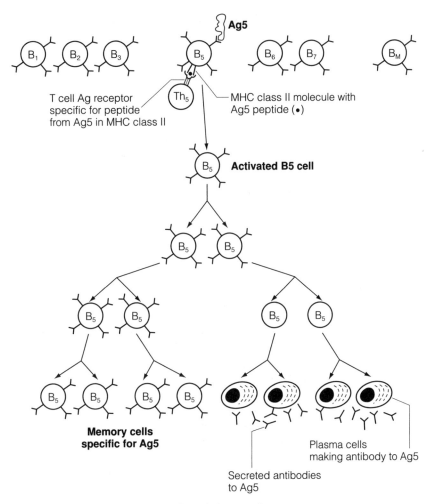

T cell Ag receptor specific for peptide from Ag5 in MHC class II

MHC class II molecule with Ag5 peptide (•)

Activated B5 cell

Memory cells specific for Ag5

Secreted antibodies to Ag5

Plasma cells making antibody to Ag5

Fig. 1. Clonal selection, memory cells and plasma cells.

nity to interact with it. Only a very few B cells (e.g. B5) have receptors specific for this antigen. B5 binds Ag5, internalizes, and processes and presents it on MHC class II molecules on the surface of this B cell. T helper cells with specific receptors for a peptide from Ag5 in MHC class II bind to this complex and stimulate this B cell to clonally expand and differentiate into memory B cells and plasma cells that produce soluble antibody to Ag5. In addition, direct T cell interaction with the B cell induces class switching, which depending on the type of helper cell (Th1 vs Th2) and the cytokines it secretes, will result in production of antibody of the IgG, IgA or IgE classes (Topic D3, G5).

Primary and memory responses

When introduced into an individual who has not previously encountered the antigen (e.g. microbe), a **primary** immune response will develop within 4–5 days (*Fig. 2*). This response results initially in the production of IgM and then IgG or other antibody isotypes directed toward the antigen, and has a duration and antibody isotype profile that depends on the quantity of antigen introduced

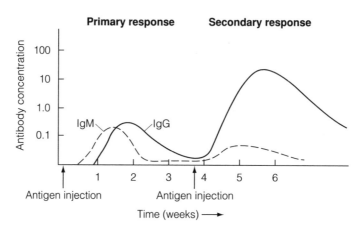

Fig. 2.   Kinetics of the immune response.

and its mode of entry. The antibody produced reacts with the remaining antigen, forming complexes and/or precipitates which are eliminated by phagocytes. Antibody is continually made by plasma cells during their short life span (3–4 days). If enough antigen is introduced initially, there could be restimulation of antigen-specific B cells, subsequent development of more plasma cells and thus increased production of antibody. Eventually, when all of the antigen has been removed and none remains to stimulate B cells, the antibody response will reach its peak and the concentration of antibody in the circulation will begin to decrease as a result of the normal rate of catabolism of the antibody.

At the time antigen is reintroduced, more antigen-specific B cells exist in the individual compared with the period before primary introduction of antigen. Moreover, these cells have differentiated to more antigen-responsive memory B cells. Thus, when antigen is reintroduced a secondary (**memory** or anamnestic) antibody response occurs which is characterized by:

- a much shorter lag period before significant levels of antibody are found in the serum,
- the presence of many more plasma cells,
- a higher rate of antibody production, and thus a much higher serum concentration of antibody,
- production mainly of antibodies of the IgG class,
- higher affinity antibodies.

Multiclonal responses

Although antibodies produced by a single cell and its daughter cells are identical (homogeneous or monoclonal), the response to a given antigen involves many different clones of cells and thus, overall, is very heterogeneous (multiclonal). Considering the size of an antigenic determinant, the number of determinants on a molecule, and the number of different molecules on a microorganism, the total response to a microorganism results in a large number of different antibodies (*Fig. 3*). Even antibodies against a single antigenic determinant are heterogeneous, indicating that the immune system is capable of producing many different antibodies, even to a single well-defined antigenic determinant. This heterogeneity is essential for many of the protective functions of antibodies (Topic D8).

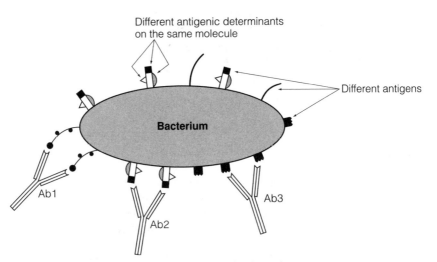

Fig. 3.   A heterogeneous antibody response against bacteria.

**Cross-reactive
responses**

Occasionally, a similar or identical antigenic determinant is found in association with widely different molecules or cells. This is termed cross-reactivity. Thus, the presence in most individuals of antibodies directed toward blood group carbohydrates other than their own is a result of the presence on certain microorganisms of carbohydrate antigens which are very similar, if not identical, to the blood group antigens. Infection with such an organism causes the production of antibodies directed toward the antigenic determinants of the microorganism including these carbohydrate antigens (*Table 1*).

Table 1.   Examples of clinically relevant cross-reactivity

Immunogen	Cross-reactive antigen	Importance
Tetanus toxoid	Tetanus toxin	Protection vs bacterial toxin
Sabin attenuated strain of polio virus	Poliomyelitis polio virus	Protection vs pathogenic virus
Various microorganisms	Type A and type B RBC carbohydrates	Transfusions
β-hemolytic *Streptococcus*	Heart tissue antigens	Rheumatic fever

The development of immunity to one organism could, in some instances, protect against infection by another organism with cross-reactive antigens. Many vaccines are effective because of similar or identical determinants expressed by: (a) both virulent and avirulent strains of the organism; or (b) toxic molecules and their non-toxic derivative. Natural or innate antibody to a wide variety of molecules is probably a result of the same phenomenon. In addition, certain kinds of autoimmune disease are due to infection by organisms bearing antigens that are cross-reactive with normal self antigens. Group A β-hemolytic streptococcal infections can lead to rheumatic fever as a result of the development of antibodies to the streptococcal determinants. Because of the similarity of the streptococcal antigens to molecules in heart tissue, the antibodies may then react with and damage not only the microorganism but also heart muscle cells (Topics K3 and L3).

E4 ANTIBODY RESPONSES IN DIFFERENT TISSUES

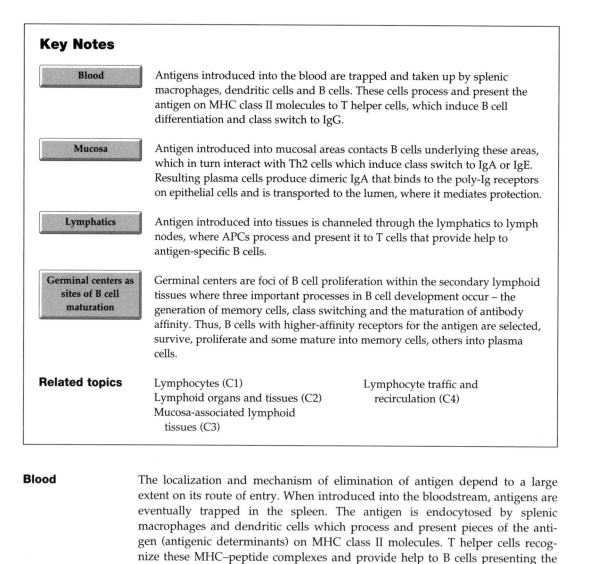

Key Notes

Blood

Antigens introduced into the blood are trapped and taken up by splenic macrophages, dendritic cells and B cells. These cells process and present the antigen on MHC class II molecules to T helper cells, which induce B cell differentiation and class switch to IgG.

Mucosa

Antigen introduced into mucosal areas contacts B cells underlying these areas, which in turn interact with Th2 cells which induce class switch to IgA or IgE. Resulting plasma cells produce dimeric IgA that binds to the poly-Ig receptors on epithelial cells and is transported to the lumen, where it mediates protection.

Lymphatics

Antigen introduced into tissues is channeled through the lymphatics to lymph nodes, where APCs process and present it to T cells that provide help to antigen-specific B cells.

Germinal centers as sites of B cell maturation

Germinal centers are foci of B cell proliferation within the secondary lymphoid tissues where three important processes in B cell development occur – the generation of memory cells, class switching and the maturation of antibody affinity. Thus, B cells with higher-affinity receptors for the antigen are selected, survive, proliferate and some mature into memory cells, others into plasma cells.

Related topics

Lymphocytes (C1)
Lymphoid organs and tissues (C2)
Mucosa-associated lymphoid
    tissues (C3)

Lymphocyte traffic and
    recirculation (C4)

Blood

The localization and mechanism of elimination of antigen depend to a large extent on its route of entry. When introduced into the bloodstream, antigens are eventually trapped in the spleen. The antigen is endocytosed by splenic macrophages and dendritic cells which process and present pieces of the antigen (antigenic determinants) on MHC class II molecules. T helper cells recognize these MHC–peptide complexes and provide help to B cells presenting the same antigen. These T helper cells also induce class switching to IgG.

Mucosa

On penetrating the mucosal epithelium, the antigen comes into contact with lymphocytes underlying the mucosal areas, including those in the tonsils and Peyer's patches. As in the spleen, B cells interact with antigen through cell-surface antibodies which function as their antigen-specific receptor. T cells interact with antigen that is processed and presented by B cells, and a humoral immune response is stimulated. In this case, the T helper cell population is a

Th2 cell that usually induces B cell class switch to IgA, but sometimes to IgE. Dimeric IgA (mainly of the IgA2 subclass: Topic D2) is released from plasma cells, binds to the poly-Ig receptor on epithelial cells and is transported through the cell to the lumen, where it has its primary protective role (*Fig. 1*).

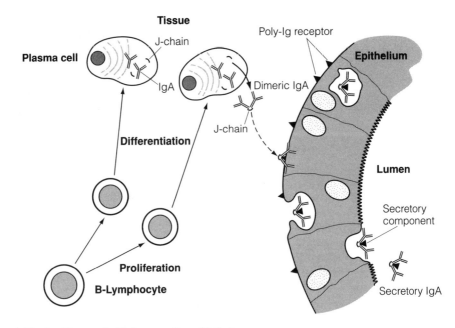

Fig. 1.   Transport of IgA across the epithelium.

Lymphatics

Antigen introduced into tissues is channeled through the lymphatics to the lymph nodes, where again, B cells, macrophages or dendritic cells trap, process the antigen and present it to T cells for initiation of specific immune responses. Antigen is also picked up by dendritic cells (Langerhans cells) in the dermis, processed and carried via the lymphatics to the draining lymph nodes where it is presented to T helper cells. B and T cells are concentrated in different parts of the lymph nodes, the B cells in follicles and the T cells in the paracortical areas. The center of each follicle is the germinal center and is made up of rapidly dividing B cells.

Germinal centers as sites of B cell maturation

Germinal centers are unique well-defined proliferating foci within the secondary lymphoid tissues where three important processes in B cell maturation occur – the generation of memory cells, antibody class switching and the maturation of antibody affinity (*Fig. 2*). Primary B cell follicles in secondary lymphoid tissues, e.g. lymph nodes and spleen, are made up of aggregates of B cells. When B cells in the primary follicle are stimulated by antigen and also receive T cell help, they proliferate, associate with dendritic cells in the follicle (FDC), and begin to form the germinal center. Germinal centers are formed from a small number of activated B cells. These B cells begin to lose their surface IgM and IgD, and switch to IgG (usually in the spleen or lymph nodes) or to IgA (usually in mucosal tissues). During this time, there is hypermutation of the variable region genes, and receptors with slightly different amino acid

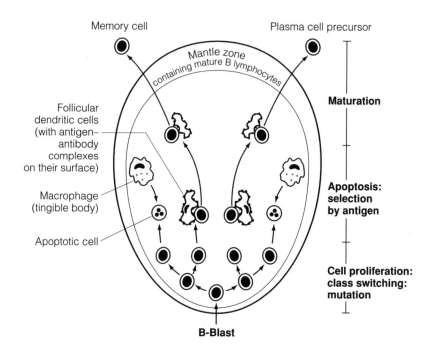

Memory cell   Plasma cell precursor

Mantle zone containing mature B lymphocytes

Follicular dendritic cells (with antigen–antibody complexes on their surface)

Macrophage (tingible body)

Apoptotic cell

Maturation

Apoptosis: selection by antigen

Cell proliferation: class switching: mutation

B-Blast

Fig. 2. B cell maturation in the germinal center (GC). A B cell in a primary follicle having been activated with T cell help (now a B cell blast), begins to proliferate and initiate GC formation. During proliferation the cells undergo somatic mutation of antibody V genes and class switching. B cells expressing new antigen receptors with the same or higher affinity for the same antigens will be selected for proliferation and differentiation. Those B cells with new receptors not able to bind the antigen will die by apoptosis and be taken up by tingible body macrophages. Those with antigen receptors with high affinity for the displayed antigen will survive to leave the GC either as memory cells or plasma cell precursors which either mature locally into plasma cells outside the GC or leave via the bloodstream to mature into plasma cells in bone marrow, lymph nodes, spleen and mucosa-associated lymphoid tissue depending on Ig class of the precursor and what secondary lymphoid site it was induced in.

sequences appear on the surface of these B cells. Some of these modified receptors are unable to bind the same antigen that triggered them and B cells with these receptors will therefore not be able to be restimulated by this antigen. However, some receptors will be able to bind more strongly to this same antigen, which is often found bound to the surface of the FDC in the form of antibody/antigen complexes. Thus, B cells with higher-affinity receptors for the antigen are selected (they compete best for antigen), survive, proliferate and some mature into memory cells that stay in the mantle of the germinal center or join the recirculating lymphocyte pool. Others mature into plasma cells each of which can only synthesize and secrete one class of specific antibody (Topic D3).

F1 THE ROLE OF T CELLS IN IMMUNE RESPONSES

Key Note

Overview	T cells have evolved to protect us against intracellular microbes (viruses and some bacteria) and to help B cell responses. The specific T cell antigen receptor (TCR) recognizes protein antigens that have been processed into peptides and bound to MHC molecules. Helper (CD4$^+$) T cells recognize peptide antigens in MHC class II molecules on dendritic cells, macrophages and B cells. Cytotoxic (CD8$^+$) T cells recognize peptides in MHC class I molecules. The T cell repertoire is generated and selected for survival in the thymus. Recognition of the peptide antigen by the TCR results in signaling leading to transcription of genes encoding cytokines and their receptors, e.g. IL-2, required for clonal expansion of specific T cells. Effector molecules such as IFNγ for activating macrophages are produced by Th1 cells. IL-4 is produced by Th2 cells and is important for B cell proliferation.
Related topics	Cell-mediated immunity in context (F6) Immunity to different organisms (H2)

Overview

Cell-mediated immunity is due to the direct action of T cells, which distinguishes it from immunity mediated by antibodies (humoral immunity). These terms evolved from the finding that immunity to certain antigens could be transferred to other animals by either cells, if they were of the same inbred strain, or antibodies. T cells have evolved to protect us against intracellular microbes (viruses and some bacteria) and to help B cell (antibody) responses against extracellular microbes. They do this by monitoring the cells of the body for foreign antigens.

Foreign antigens in host cells are broken up into linear peptides (processed) and displayed by major histocompatibility complex (MHC) molecules expressed on their cell surface. Unlike antibodies that recognize the three-dimensional shape of antigens, the T cell antigen receptor (TCR) only recognizes linear antigens (peptides) bound to MHC molecules, i.e. T cells cannot directly recognize or bind to microbes or their unprocessed molecules. Helper (CD4$^+$) T cells recognize peptide antigens in the context of MHC class II molecules that are expressed by dendritic cells, macrophages and B cells. Cytotoxic (CD8$^+$) T cells recognize peptides associated with MHC class I molecules. This differential requirement for CD4 and CD8 relates to the fact that CD4 and CD8 attach to the non-polymorphic (non-variant) part of the MHC class II and MHC class I molecules, respectively.

Association of antigens with the variable part of either of the two classes of MHC molecules is the result of the cellular pathways used to process the proteins into peptides. Each T cell recognizes only one specific foreign peptide and to do this a large TCR repertoire needs to be generated. This occurs during normal thymus development where the T cells are 'educated,' i.e. selected for survival or eliminated if self-reactive. There are two kinds of T helper cells, each with different functions in the immune response that are dictated by their cytokine profiles. Th1 cells help macrophages to get rid of intracellular microbes and help the development of cytotoxic T cells to kill virus-infected cells. Th2 cells are mainly involved in helping B cells to develop into memory cells and plasma cells that produce antibodies.

T cells need to be activated in order for them to carry out their function. Recognition of the peptide antigen by the TCR is not sufficient to activate the cells, as accessory molecules are also required together with co-receptors involved in signaling events. Signaling leads to transcription of genes coding for cytokines and their receptors, e.g. IL-2 is required for clonal expansion of the specific T cells. Effector molecules such as IFNγ, which activates macrophages, are produced by Th1 cells. IL-4 is produced by Th2 cells and is important for B cell proliferation. Enzymes and molecules involved in killing by CD8$^+$ cells are also induced during activation.

F2 T CELL RECOGNITION OF ANTIGEN

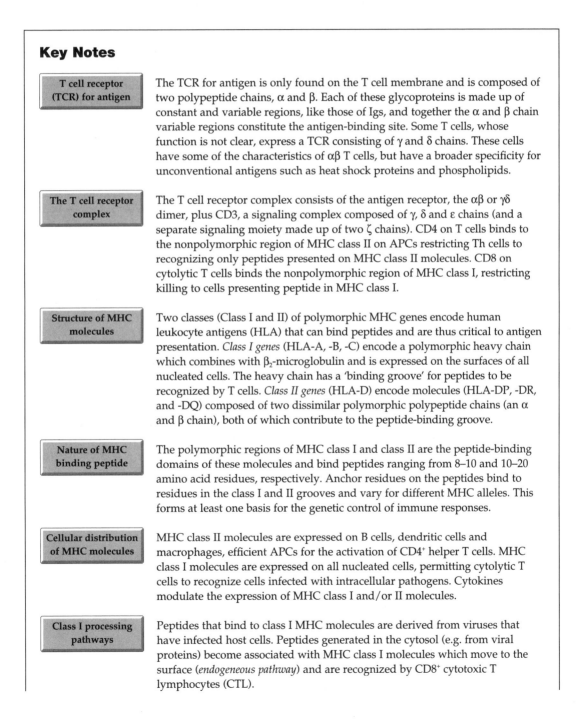

Key Notes

T cell receptor (TCR) for antigen	The TCR for antigen is only found on the T cell membrane and is composed of two polypeptide chains, α and β. Each of these glycoproteins is made up of constant and variable regions, like those of Igs, and together the α and β chain variable regions constitute the antigen-binding site. Some T cells, whose function is not clear, express a TCR consisting of γ and δ chains. These cells have some of the characteristics of αβ T cells, but have a broader specificity for unconventional antigens such as heat shock proteins and phospholipids.
The T cell receptor complex	The T cell receptor complex consists of the antigen receptor, the αβ or γδ dimer, plus CD3, a signaling complex composed of γ, δ and ε chains (and a separate signaling moiety made up of two ζ chains). CD4 on T cells binds to the nonpolymorphic region of MHC class II on APCs restricting Th cells to recognizing only peptides presented on MHC class II molecules. CD8 on cytolytic T cells binds the nonpolymorphic region of MHC class I, restricting killing to cells presenting peptide in MHC class I.
Structure of MHC molecules	Two classes (Class I and II) of polymorphic MHC genes encode human leukocyte antigens (HLA) that can bind peptides and are thus critical to antigen presentation. *Class I genes* (HLA-A, -B, -C) encode a polymorphic heavy chain which combines with β_2-microglobulin and is expressed on the surfaces of all nucleated cells. The heavy chain has a 'binding groove' for peptides to be recognized by T cells. *Class II genes* (HLA-D) encode molecules (HLA-DP, -DR, and -DQ) composed of two dissimilar polymorphic polypeptide chains (an α and β chain), both of which contribute to the peptide-binding groove.
Nature of MHC binding peptide	The polymorphic regions of MHC class I and class II are the peptide-binding domains of these molecules and bind peptides ranging from 8–10 and 10–20 amino acid residues, respectively. Anchor residues on the peptides bind to residues in the class I and II grooves and vary for different MHC alleles. This forms at least one basis for the genetic control of immune responses.
Cellular distribution of MHC molecules	MHC class II molecules are expressed on B cells, dendritic cells and macrophages, efficient APCs for the activation of CD4+ helper T cells. MHC class I molecules are expressed on all nucleated cells, permitting cytolytic T cells to recognize cells infected with intracellular pathogens. Cytokines modulate the expression of MHC class I and/or II molecules.
Class I processing pathways	Peptides that bind to class I MHC molecules are derived from viruses that have infected host cells. Peptides generated in the cytosol (e.g. from viral proteins) become associated with MHC class I molecules which move to the surface (*endogeneous pathway*) and are recognized by CD8+ cytotoxic T lymphocytes (CTL).

Class II processing pathways	Some pathogens replicate in cellular vesicles of macrophages, others are endocytosed from the environment into endocytic vesicles (*exogenous pathway*). In both cases peptides from proteins associated with these microbes are primarily presented on MHC class II molecules to CD4$^+$ helper T cells.
Related topics	Antigens (A4) Shaping the T cell repertoire (F3)
	Lymphocytes (C1) Transplantation antigens (M2)

T cell receptor (TCR) for antigen

There is as much diversity of TCR as of Ig receptors, but unlike the B cell antigen receptor (Ig), the TCR for antigen is only found on the T cell membrane and not in the serum or other body fluids. Two different groups of T cells can be defined based on their use of either α and β or γ and δ chains for their TCRs. Both develop in the thymus.

Alpha/beta (αβ) T cells
αβ T cells are the 'conventional' T cells that undergo positive and negative selection in the thymus (Topic F3) and make up the majority of human peripheral T cells. These αβ T cells complete their functional maturation in the secondary lymphoid tissues and provide protection against invading microbes. Some T cells reside, at least temporarily, in T-cell-dependent areas of tissues. These cells function to control intracellular microbes and to provide help for B cell (antibody) responses. Two different kinds of αβT cells are involved in these functions, T helper (Th) cells and T cytotoxic (Tc) cells.

The TCR of these cells is composed of two polypeptide chains, α and β, which have molecular weights of 50 and 39 kDa, respectively. Each of these glycoproteins is made up of constant and variable regions like those of Ig and together the α and β variable regions constitute a T cell antigen-binding site (*Fig. 1*). However, as previously indicated, TCR, unlike antibodies, do not recognize native antigen, but can only bind processed antigen presented in MHC molecules. The genes coding for TCR polypeptide chains are members of the Ig super family.

Gamma/delta (γδ) T cells
γδ T cells are similar in morphology to NK cells containing intracellular granules (Topic C1) and represent a subpopulation of thymocytes and a small group of peripheral T cells. They express a TCR consisting of γ and δ chains with V

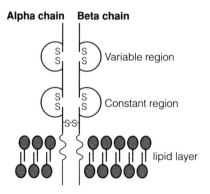

Fig. 1.   T cell antigen receptor αβ dimer.

and C regions that are similar to the αβ TCR. Unlike 'conventional' αβ T cells that have highly specific recognition structures, these cells appear to have a broader specificity for recognition of unconventional antigens such as heat shock proteins and phospholipids and do not recognize them in association with MHC molecules. However, since these cells are produced in the thymus, have a T cell receptor and express T-cell-associated molecules they are believed to represent a transition state between the innate and adaptive immunity. Although the function of these γδ-TCR-expressing T cells is not well understood, they are often found at epithelial surfaces and may control microbes at this location through cytotoxic activity and cytokine production.

The T cell receptor complex

The T cell receptor complex consists of the antigen receptor, the αβ or γδ dimer, associated with several other polypeptides important in T cell signaling and recognition. In particular, the TCR is associated with CD3, a signaling complex which is itself composed of several polypeptides including γ, δ and ε. ζ chains are also part of the signaling complex (*Fig. 2*). Two other molecules, CD4 and CD8, on T cells also play a role in T cell recognition of antigen. CD4 binds to the non-polymorphic region of MHC class II and restricts Th cells to recognizing only peptides presented on MHC class II molecules (*Fig. 3*). Similarly, CD8

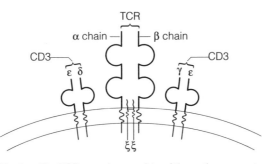

Fig. 2. The TCR complex consists of the antigen receptor, the αβ or γδ dimer, associated with several other polypeptides involved in T cell signalling. The signalling complex is composed of CD3-γ, δ and ε polypeptide chains and a separate homodimer of ξ chains.

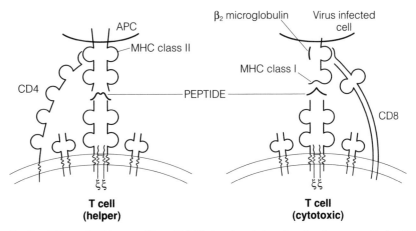

Fig. 3. CD8 and CD4 recognition of MHC class I and class II molecules, respectively. CD4 on T helper cells bind to the nonpolymorphic region of MHC class II; CD8 on cytolytic T cells binds the nonpolymorphic region of MHC class I.

on cytolytic T cells binds the nonpolymorphic region of MHC class I, restricting these killer T cells to recognize only cells presenting peptide in MHC class I molecules.

Structure of MHC molecules

Although molecules coded for by the MHC were originally identified based on their role in transplant rejection, they actually evolved to present foreign antigens to T cells. Two classes (class I and II) of MHC genes, closely linked on chromosome 6 in humans, code for human leukocyte antigens (HLA) which are the molecules critical to antigen presentation. There are many alternative forms of genes for each subregion of the MHC. This high degree of polymorphism in class I MHC and class II MHC molecules is *not* due to generation of diversity within the individual (as is the case for Ig molecules) but rather to the many alternative forms or alleles of MHC that exist in the species (Topic M2). These different alleles are not inherited entirely randomly as there is a variable distribution of determinants among different ethnic groups. Moreover, these alleles are inherited in groups. The combination of the encoded alleles at each of the loci within the MHC on the same chromosome is referred to as the haplotype (for haploid, as opposed to diploid). Since genes within the MHC are closely linked, haplotypes are usually inherited intact.

Class I genes (HLA-A, -B, -C)
Class I genes encode class I molecules that are expressed on the surfaces of all nucleated cells as two polypeptide chains. Only the H-chain is coded by the MHC, and contains regions of sequence variability that are the result of the many allelic forms of MHC class I molecules in the population. This accounts for the more than 35 million HLA phenotypes (Topic M2). The L-chain, β_2-microglobulin (different from κ and λ Ig L-chains), shows no polymorphism and is coded for on chromosome 15. The H-chain of these molecules has a region that forms a 'binding groove' for peptides, such that when the class I molecule is synthesized it is able to interact with and bind certain kinds of peptides. Only the H-chain is involved in this binding, with β_2-microglobulin stabilizing the molecule and permitting it to be displayed on the cell surface (*Fig. 4*).

Class II genes (HLA-D)
Class II genes encode structural glycoproteins found on B cells, macrophages and dendritic cells, as well as sperm, and vascular endothelial cells. This

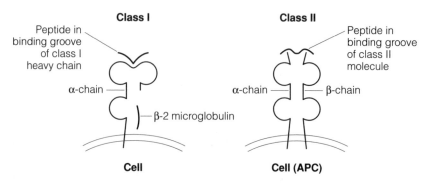

Fig. 4.   MHC class I and class II molecules binding peptide.

HLA-D region can be subdivided into sets of genes which encode different HLA-DP, -DR, and -DQ class II molecules. Class II molecules are composed of two dissimilar polypeptide chains (i.e. an α and β chain heterodimer). Both chains are encoded by the MHC and β_2-microglobulin is *not* involved. As with class I MHC molecules, class II MHC molecules are polymorphic due to their many different allelic forms (Topic M2) and are also able to bind peptides. In this case both the α and β chains of the class II molecule contribute to the binding groove (*Fig. 4*).

Nature of MHC binding peptide

The peptide-binding domains of MHC class I and class II molecules are different for each allelic form of the MHC molecules. That is, there are particular amino acid residues in the 'binding groove' that vary from one allelic form to another and thus from individual to individual. Polymorphic residues within the peptide-binding pocket of each of the molecules make contact with the antigenic peptide. The peptides that are bound by MHC class I and class II molecules are short, ranging from 8–10 amino acid residues (for MHC class I) to 10–20 amino acid residues (for MHC class II). The sites on the peptides that fasten the peptide to the MHC molecule are the **anchor residues** (Topic A4 *Fig. 2*). The peptide residues in the MHC-binding groove are the same for each allelic form of the MHC molecule. Therefore, each allelic form of MHC molecule is only able to bind peptides bearing specific anchor residues. Thus, depending on the MHC molecules that are inherited, a person might not be able to bind specific peptides from e.g. a virus. If the person's MHC molecules cannot bind the peptides generated from a specific virus, then they will be unable to mount a CD8 response to that virus. This forms at least one basis for the genetic control of immune responses. That is, the MHC molecules inherited by an individual ultimately determine to which peptides that individual can elicit T-cell-mediated immune responses, and at the population level, the polymorphism increases the chances of survival of at least some individuals.

Cellular distribution of MHC molecules

MHC class I and MHC class II molecules have a distinct distribution on cells (*Table 1*) that directly reflects the different effector functions that those cells play. Furthermore, under some conditions (e.g. cytokine activation) the expression of MHC class I and/or II molecules may be induced or enhanced (e.g. activated T cells become class II positive). Cells that express MHC class II molecules (B cells, dendritic cells, macrophages) are efficient antigen-presenting cells for the activation of CD4$^+$ helper T cells. In contrast, MHC class I molecules are expressed on virtually all cells in humans except for RBC. The expression of

Table 1. Expression of MHC class I and II molecules

Tissue	MHC class I	MHC class II
T cells	+++	–
B cells	+++	+++
Macrophages	+++	++
Dendritic cells	+++	+++
Neutrophils	+++	–
Hepatocytes	+	–
Kidney	++	–
Brain	+	–
Red blood cells	–	–

MHC class I molecules on all nucleated cells permits the immune system to survey these cells for infection by intracellular pathogens and allows their destruction via class I-restricted CTLs. It is interesting to note that the absence of class I MHC molecules on RBC may allow the unchecked growth of *Plasmodium*, the agent responsible for malaria.

Class I processing pathways

To a large extent, fragments of peptides that bind to class I MHC molecules are derived from viruses that have infected host cells (*Fig. 5*). Degraded viral proteins (peptides of 8–10 aa) are transported into the endoplasmic reticulum by specific transporter proteins (transporters associated with antigen processing; TAP). In this intracellular compartment linear peptides bind to class I MHC molecules (*endogeneous pathway*). The class I MHC–peptide complex is then exported to the cell surface. In general, peptides generated in the cytoplasm, i.e. the cytosol (as would be the case for cytosolic microbes), become associated with MHC class I molecules that move to the surface and can be recognized by cytotoxic T lymphocytes (CTL), which are distinguished by expression of CD8 (*Table 2*).

Class II processing pathways

While viruses and some bacteria replicate in the cytosol, several types of pathogens including mycobacteria and *Leishmania* replicate in cellular vesicles of macrophages. In addition, pathogens can be endocytosed from the environment into endocytic vesicles (*Table 2*). Thus, both pathogens in cellular vesicles and pathogens and antigens that come from outside the cell (*exogenous pathway*) are primarily presented on MHC class II molecules. Class II MHC molecules are present in the endocytic vesicles of macrophages, B cells and dendritic cells that present antigen to CD4+ helper T cells. Upon fusion with the endocytic vesicles, class II MHC molecules become loaded with linear peptides of 10–20 aa, and the class II–MHC peptide complex is transported to the cell surface where it can be recognized by CD4+ T cells (*Fig. 5*). CD4 T cells also assist in the destruction

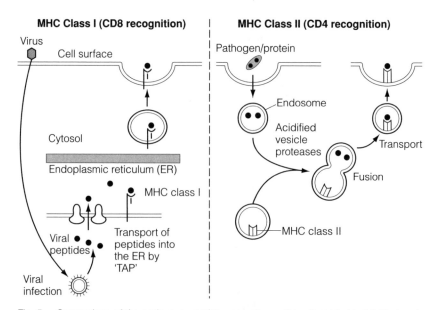

Fig. 5. Comparison of the pathways used to generate peptides that bind to MHC class I and class II molecules.

Table 2. MHC class I and II processing pathways

	Cytosolic pathogens	Intracellular pathogens	Extracellular pathogens
Degraded in:	Cytosol	Acidic vesicles	Acidic vesicles
Peptides presented by:	Class I MHC	Class II MHC	Class II MHC
Peptides presented to:	CD8 T cells (cytotoxic)	CD4 T cells (helper)	CD4 T cells (helper)
Effect on APC:	Cell death	Activation of macrophages to kill intracellular parasites	Activation of B cells to secrete Ig, to eliminate extracellular pathogens/toxins

of parasites in vesicular compartments, e.g. mycobacteria, by activating the cells that harbor these pathogens to kill them. For extracellular parasites, CD4 T cells can activate macrophages to endocytose and destroy the pathogens, as well as instruct B cells to produce antibody to opsonize the pathogens. There are two subsets of CD4⁺ cells potentially involved in these responses (Topic F5).

F3 SHAPING THE T CELL REPERTOIRE

Key Notes

Generation of T cell diversity

Multiple genes code for each of the two polypeptide chains (α and β or γ and δ) of the TCR. Each chain, like those of antibodies, is made up of a V (variable) and a C (constant) region. Three different gene segments – V, D and J – encode the V region of β and δ chains, whereas two different gene segments – V and J – encode the V region of α and γ chains. As with antibody genes, the T cell V gene segments rearrange in each developing T cell in the thymus, resulting in a breadth of T cell diversity similar to that for B cells. Allelic exclusion assures that each T cell will have a single specificity.

Selection of the T cell repertoire

In the thymus, those T cells that express a TCR that binds weakly to self MHC are positively selected. Of this group, those that express a TCR that binds strongly to self MHC are eliminated (negative selection). In addition, T cells that recognize self MHC plus self peptides are also removed (negative selection) leaving those T cells that recognize modified self MHC molecules – self MHC molecules plus foreign peptide – to survive, mature and become functional T cells in the peripheral lymphoid tissues.

Related topics   Lymphoid organs and tissues (C2)   Generation of diversity (D3)

Generation of T cell diversity

Each of the very large numbers of T cells produced in the thymus has only one specificity, defined by its antigen receptor. Millions of T cells, each with receptors specific for different antigens, are generated by gene rearrangement from multiple (inherited) germline genes. Multiple genes code for each of the two polypeptide chains (α and β or γ and δ) of the TCR. Each chain, like those of antibodies, is made up of a V (variable) and a C (constant) region. Three different gene segments – V, D and J – encode the V region of β and δ chains, whereas two different gene segments – V and J – encode the V region of α and γ chains (*Fig. 1*). The many

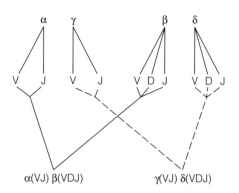

Fig. 1.   Gene segments involved in information of the V region of the different polypeptides of the TCR.

genes within each segment, i.e. V, D or J (for β and δ chains) and V and J (for α and γ chains), are separated by non-coding DNA in the germline.

During development of αβ T cells the V, D, and J gene segments are rearranged to form a complete V region gene for the β chain (*Fig. 2*) and V and J gene segments are rearranged to form a complete V region gene for the α chain. Variability in junction formation and random insertion of nucleotides contributes further to the diversity of variable region gene products (Topic D3). As in the case of immunoglobulin rearrangements, the expression of a complete α chain and a complete β chain by the T cell excludes further rearrangement (allelic exclusion). The cell thus becomes committed to the expression of a single V–C α-chain combination and a single V–C β-chain combination. Together these two chains form an antigen-binding site that determines the specificity of the T cell. Similarly, in some developing T cells, γ and δ gene rearrangements occur, resulting in the T cell expressing γδ TCRs. Since the rearrangements occur randomly in millions of T cells, considerable diversity of specificity is generated *prior* to antigen stimulation. Cells that fail to rearrange functional TCR genes die in the thymus.

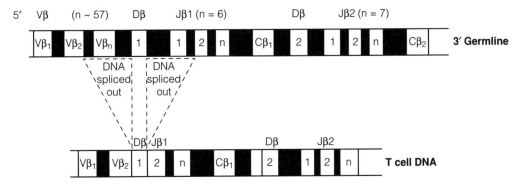

Fig. 2. V region gene for the human TCRβ chain. Similar to antibody genes in B cells, T cells rearrange their TCR genes during development. An example of a complete V region gene for β chain gene is shown as an example. The VDJ exon is transcribed and spliced to join the Cβ gene segment. The resulting mRNA is translated into a β chain of the TCR. There are approximately 57 genes in the Vβ segment and 2 Dβ genes. There are two sets of Jβ segments with 6 and 7 genes respectively and two Cβ segments. The Cβ genes do not appear to differ functionally from each other unlike the various immunoglobulin C region genes.

Selection of the T cell repertoire   Upon entry into the thymus, T cell precursors from the bone marrow begin TCR rearrangements and the receptor is expressed on thymocytes that bear both CD4 and CD8 markers (double-positive thymocytes). T cells that express a TCR that can bind *weakly* to self MHC are spared from death and are *positively selected* to survive (*Fig. 3*). Therefore, the T cell repertoire is first selected for cells that can bind self MHC. Of this group, those that express a TCR that binds *strongly* to self MHC are autoreactive and may cause problems if they enter the periphery. These cells are induced to die (are *negatively* selected). This positive and negative selection results in survival and maturation of T cells that recognize peptides in the context of self MHC (modified self MHC), but cannot react productively with self antigens (Topic G2). The failure to rearrange a functional TCR, negative selection or a lack of positive selection is responsible for the death of the majority (95%) of T cells in the thymus through apoptosis.

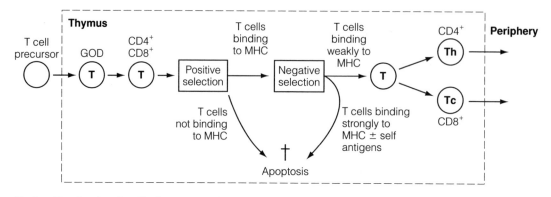

Fig. 3.   Thymic education. T cell precursors derived from lymphoid stem cells (LSC) enter the thymus where they develop T cell antigen receptors through multiple gene rearrangements, generation of diversity (GOD). They also acquire CD4 and CD8 molecules and undergo positive and negative selection. They leave the thymus as CD4+ helper or CD8+ cytotoxic T cells and migrate to the secondary lymphoid organs/tissues.

F4 T CELL ACTIVATION

Key Notes

Accessory molecules	Initial recognition of processed antigen by T cells is via the T cell antigen receptor. Accessory molecules further link the APC and the T cell leading to a stronger cell interaction. For example CD4 binds to the constant region domain of class II MHC molecules while CD8 binds to class I MHC molecules. Other ligand–receptor pairs such as LFA-1 and ICAM1 are also important.
Co-stimulatory molecules: two signals required for T cell activation	Full activation of antigen-specific T cells requires **two signals** – one signal coming via the TCR and the other signal through engagement of co-stimulatory molecules. T cells receiving one signal via their TCR are turned off (become anergic), while those also receiving the second signal, i.e. via T cell CD28 binding to B7 on the APC, induce T cell lymphokine production and T cell proliferation.
Th activation through superantigens	Some protein products of bacteria and viruses can initiate T cell activation by directly linking the TCR on T cells to the MHC class II–peptide complex on APCs without the need for antigen processing. These super-antigens include *staphylococcal enterotoxins (SE)* that cause common food poisoning and the toxic shock syndrome toxin (TSST).
Early signaling events through co-receptors	Contact between TCR, accessory and co-receptor molecules with antigen-presenting molecules and ligands on the APC is called the 'immunological synapse'. This specialized signaling domain conveys a signal to the nucleus resulting in specific gene transcription. This *signal transduction* is brought about by phosphorylation and dephosphorylation of particular amino acids thus activating them in a sequential fashion leading eventually to activation of specific transcription factors in the nucleus and production of functional proteins. CD45 (a phosphatase) on the APC initiates this process by activation of a CD4-associated kinase (lck), which together with Fyn then phosphorylates ITAMs on the zeta chain of the signaling complex. Binding of ZAP70 to the phosphorylated ITAMs initiates two biochemical pathways
Related topics	Lymphocytes (C1) Central and peripheral tolerance B cell activation (E2) (G2)

Accessory molecules

Pathogens or antigens infecting peripheral sites are typically trapped in the lymph nodes directly downstream of the site of infection. Bloodborne pathogens are trapped in the spleen. These secondary lymphoid organs contain APCs (dendritic cells and macrophages) that efficiently trap antigen for processing and presentation. Naive T cells recirculate through these sites looking for appropriately processed antigen. Initial recognition of processed antigen by T cells is via the T cell antigen receptor.

Accessory molecules provide additional linkages between the APC and the T cell to strengthen their cellular association (*Fig. 1*). CD4 binds to the constant

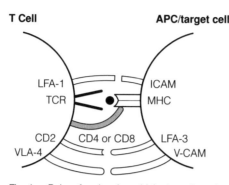

Fig. 1.   Pairs of molecules which strengthen the association of T cells with antigen presenting and target cells.

region domain of class II MHC molecules thereby strengthening the association of the TCR with peptide-class II MHC molecules. Likewise, CD8 binds to class I MHC molecules to strengthen the association of the TCR with class I MHC molecules. In addition to engagement of these ligand–receptor pairs (*Fig. 1*), additional adhesion molecules, integrins, become engaged. These include inter-cellular adhesion molecules (ICAMs) and lymphocyte function-associated anti-gens (LFAs). Some of these accessory molecules are also important in regulating early activation events through signaling, e.g. CD4 and CD8, and are sometimes termed co-receptors.

Co-stimulatory molecules: two signals required for T cell activation

Ligation of the TCR on its own does not stimulate T cell clonal expansion or lymphokine production. The full activation of antigen-specific T cells requires **two signals**. Signal one is provided by the engagement of the T cell antigen receptor and signal two is provided by engagement of a co-stimulatory mole-cule. The best-characterized co-stimulatory molecule is B7, which is on many APCs and binds to CD28 on the T cell. Signals emanating from the TCR and CD28 synergize to induce T cell lymphokine production and T cell proliferation. If the T cell receives signal 1 (TCR binding) and not signal 2 (co-stimulation) the T cell is turned off (*Fig. 2*; Topic G2).

Precursors of CD8[+] cytotoxic T cells also need to be activated to develop into mature CD8 effector T cells containing granzymes and perforin (Topic F5). This requires attachment of their TCR to MHC class I–peptide complexes on APCs (signal 1). In addition, a second co-stimulatory signal involving binding of B7 to

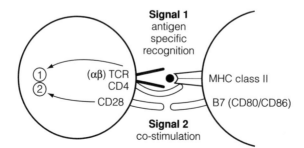

Fig. 2.   The role of co-stimulation in T cell activation.

CD28 on the CTL is required. Cytokines produced by Th cells and APCs and ligation of APC CD40 are important for enhancing expression of the co-stimulatory molecules. Of note, although other Th-cell-conditioned APCs may be able to provide the necessary signals for Tc (CTL) activation, dendritic cells are the only cells which have a significant cross-over of processed antigen between exogenous and endogenous pathways (Topics F2 and F6). Moreover, they are, in general, the most efficient of the antigen-presenting cells.

Once activated, mature CD8⁺ cytotoxic T cells do not, in most instances, need to be further activated to release granzyme and perforin. Thus, when activated CTLs come into contact with virus-infected cells, they appear to need, at least initially, only the first signal provided by TCR recognition of viral peptide plus MHC class I, although the interaction of LFA-1 on the cytotoxic cell with ICAM-I on the target cell is also important.

Th activation through superantigens

Some protein products of bacteria and viruses produce proteins known as **superantigens** that bind simultaneously to lateral surfaces of the MHC class II molecules (not in the peptide-binding groove) and the V region of the β subunit of the TCR. Superantigens are not processed into peptides as conventional antigens, but are able to bind to a specific family of TCR. In a sense they 'glue' T cells to APC (*Fig. 3*) and cause stimulation of the T cell. However, these T cells are not specific for the pathogen that produced the superantigen, since all members of a particular family of TCR are activated. The consequence of binding to a large percentage of the T cells is the massive production of cytokines leading, in some cases, to lymphokine-induced vascular leakage and shock. Among the bacterial superantigens are the *staphylococcal enterotoxins* (SE) that cause common food poisoning and the toxic shock syndrome toxin (TSST).

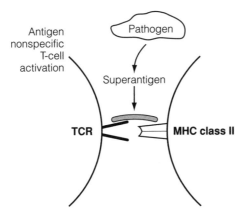

Fig. 3.   Superantigen activation of T cells by bridging TCR and MHC class II.

Early signaling events through co-receptors

The early signaling events are complex and therefore only a simplified outline will be presented. The area of contact between the TCR accessory and co-receptor molecules on the T cell surface with molecules and ligands on the APC is called the 'immunological synapse'. This is the specialized membrane region that conveys a signal from the T cell surface via the cytosol into the nucleus to give rise to specific gene transcription. This *signal transduction* is mediated by TCR molecules, co-receptors and enzymes that lie in cholesterol-rich areas of the membrane called 'lipid rafts' (*Fig. 4*).

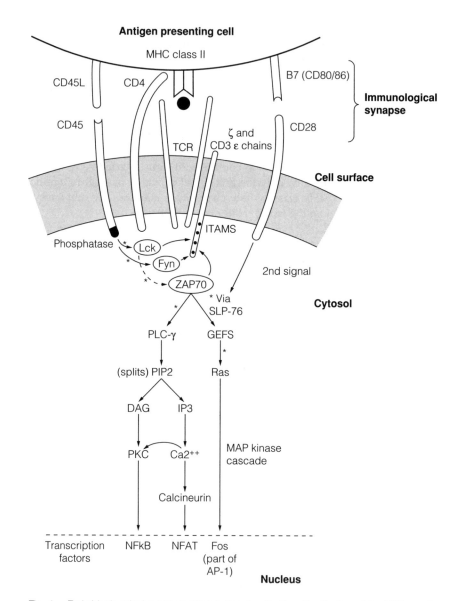

Fig. 4. *Early biochemical events leading to T cell activation. The ligation of the TCR results in the initiation of signaling pathways through the action of CD45, the kinases lck and Fyn and other kinases including ZAP70. These enzymes 'activate' their target molecules by removing or adding phosphates. Ligation of CD45 induces activation of lck and Fyn which these phosphorylate ITAMs on the ζ chain and CD3. Once phosphorylated ZAP70 binds to the ITAMs and is activated by lck to initiate two main biochemical pathways. One is via the phosphatidyl inositol pathway where phospholipase C-γ (PLC-γ) cleaves phosphatidylinositol bisphosphate (PIP2) to produce diacyl glycerol (DAG) and inositol trisphosphate (IP3). DAG activates protein kinase C (PKC) which activates NFκB that translocates to the nucleus. IP3 increases intracellular Ca²⁺ activating the phosphatase calcineurin that, in turn, activates NFAT (nuclear factor of activated T cells) and causes it to translocate to the nucleus. The second pathway involves the MAPkinase cascade initiated by RAS through GEFS activated via binding of SL76. This cascade leads to activation of Fos, a component of the AP-1 transcription factor. The second signal delivered via T cell CD28 interaction with CD80/CD86 on the antigen-presenting cell is required to activate the cell. It is thought that CD28 ligation (and indeed ligation of CTLA4) with CD80/CD86 modulates these biochemical pathways.*

Neither of the two chains of the TCR have intracytoplasmic tails of sufficient length or amino acid composition to act as signaling molecules. Therefore, T cell signaling is initiated through the longer tails of the ζ chains, and ε chains of the associated CD3 molecule that have sets of tyrosine molecules called ITAMS (immunoreceptor tyrosine activation motifs). On ligation of the TCR, CD45 (an endogenous phosphatase) activates (by removal of phosphates) two enzymes lck and Fyn that phosphorylate the ITAMs of the ζ chains. ZAP70 then 'docks' with the phosphorylated ITAMs and itself becomes activated leading to further phosphorylation events. Activation of phospholipase C-γ via the phosphatidyl inositol pathway leads to activation of the transcription factors NFAT (nuclear factor of activated T cells) and NFκB and their translocation into the nucleus. Another consequence of the phosphorylation mediated by ZAP70 is the activation of the MAP kinase cascade via SLP-76, Guanine nucleoside exchange factors (GEFS) and Ras which finally leads to activation of Fos – a component of the AP-1 transcription factor. This whole process is very rapid and the multiple phosphorylation and dephosphorylation events in the membrane take place within seconds of ligation of the TCR. The initial signal occurring within the lipid rafts is amplified via the molecules of the different biochemical pathways ('second messengers') leading finally to transcription of effector molecules, e.g. cytokines (IL-2, IL-4 and IFNγ) and cell cycle proteins (cyclins), required for clonal expansion.

F5 CLONAL EXPANSION AND DEVELOPMENT OF EFFECTOR FUNCTION

Key Notes

Clonal expansion

In addition to cell cycle proteins, cytokines and their receptors are produced following antigen activation of T cells. These are involved in the expansion and further differentiation of the T cells into memory and effector cells. IL-2 is an autocrine factor which leads to T cell proliferation. Other surface molecules induced following activation include CD40L (CD154) which interacts with CD40 on dendritic cells inducing them to produce cytokines (e.g. IL-12) required for T cell proliferation and differentiation into Th1 cells. This leads to the specific T cell priming and clonal expansion necessary for their effector function and the development of memory.

Helper T cells

T helper cells are divided into two main types dependent on their cytokine profiles. Th1 cells or inflammatory T cells produce high levels of IFNγ and TNFα which primarily act on macrophages to cause their activation. Th2 cells which are characterized by their production of IL-4, IL-5 and IL-6 are involved mainly in B cell differentiation and maturation.

Cytotoxic T cells

Cytotoxicity by Tc can be mediated through (a) lytic granule release of perforin and granzymes onto the surface of the target cell, and (b) interaction of FasL on the CTL with Fas on infected cells. Both mechanisms result in programed cell death (apoptosis) of the infected cell.

Related topics

Immune defense (A3)
Genes, T helper cells, cytokines and
   the neuroendocrine system (G5)

Immunity to different organisms
   (H2)

Clonal expansion

In addition to cell cycle proteins, cytokines and their receptors are produced following activation of T cells. These are involved in the expansion and further differentiation of the T cells into memory and effector cells. On stimulation, T cells produce IL-2, an autocrine growth factor important to T cell proliferation, and express IL-2 receptors. Other surface molecules induced by activation of T cells include CD40L (CD154), which interacts with CD40 on dendritic cells. Binding of CD40 induces dendritic cells to produce cytokines (e.g. IL-1, IL-12) required for T cell proliferation and differentiation into Th1 cells (*Fig. 1*). This leads to specific T cell priming, clonal expansion and development of memory cells. Cytokines produced by the Th1 cells (e.g. IFNγ) and by dendritic cells are important in development and clonal expansion of CD8+ CTL from their precursors (Topic F6). Thus, following activation by antigen, specific clones of T cells

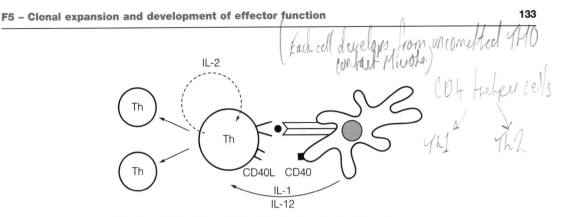

Fig. 1. Initial priming of helper T cells through dendritic cells.

are expanded to carry out their effector function and develop into memory cells.

Helper T cells

There are two kinds of CD4+ helper T cells (Th1 and Th2) with different functions. Each develops from uncommitted Th0 cells following initial contact with a microbe. Th1 cells are predominately involved in mediating inflammatory immune responses (through the activation of macrophages), while Th2 cells are primarily involved in the induction of humoral immunity (via the activation of B cells). In this regard, Th0 to Th1 cell development is encouraged when a Th0 cell recognizes a microbial peptide presented by an infected macrophage that is producing IL-12 (*Fig. 2*). In contrast, Th0 cells are encouraged to become Th2 cells under the influence of IL-4 released by B cells and other cells (e.g. mast cells). Thus, following activation by specific peptide antigen, Th1 cells derived from Th0 cells produce cytokines such as IFNγ and TNFα that primarily act on macrophages. Cytokines produced by Th2 cells (IL-4, IL-5, IL-6, and IL-13) are involved mainly in B cell differentiation and maturation. IL-10 is also produced

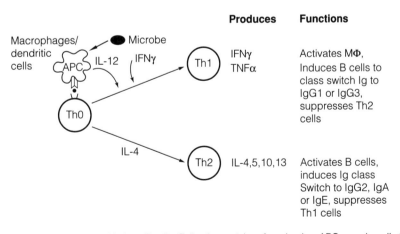

Fig. 2. Two types of helper T cells. Following uptake of a microbe, APCs produce IL-12, and present microbial-derived peptides to specific Th0 cells. In the presence of IL-12 and IFNγ, Th0 cells differentiate into Th1 cells whereas in the presence of IL-4 and other Th2 cytokines the Th0 cells differentiate into Th2 cells.

by Th2 cells and regulates the activity of Th1 cells (Topic G5). It is important to remember that in most cases, an immune response elicits both Th1 and Th2 activities, although there are some instances where one or the other is more effective in mediating protection (Topic H2).

Th2 cells

Participation of T cells is required for B cell responses to most antigens (Topic E2). T cells most effective in inducing the production of antibody from B cells, especially of the IgA and IgE isotype, are the helper CD4 Th2 cells. Th2 cells induce B cells to produce Ig, switch the isotype of Ig being produced, and induce affinity maturation of the Ig. This involves not only cytokines but direct engagement of surface molecules on the T and B cells (cognate interactions) which trigger their activation.

More specifically, Th2 cells recognize antigenic peptides in MHC class II molecules on the surface of antigen-specific B cells and through interaction with other surface molecules are activated (Topics F2 and F4). The interaction of CD40L on T cells with CD40 on B cells induces B cell proliferation and class switching to IgE- and IgA-producing cells (Topic D3, *Fig. 4*). Cytokines produced by Th2 cells, including IL-4, IL-5, and IL-6) act as growth and differentiation factors for B cells.

Th1 cells

Role of Th1 cells in macrophage recruitment and activation. The response to a variety of intracellular parasites is dependent upon functionally intact Th1 cells. For example, the immune responses to *Leishmania* and mycobacteria are severely diminished if the host cannot produce IFNγ and TNFα. This is because, in the absence of these mediators, infected macrophages cannot become activated to kill the pathogen. Although other cytokines can augment macrophage activities, both IFNγ and TNFα are critical for effective macrophage activation.

Th1 cells when activated also produce chemokines that assist in the recruitment of monocytes, and colony-stimulating factor (GM-CSF) that induces their differentiation into macrophages at the site of infection. In addition, IL-3 increases the production and release of monocytes from the bone marrow. Also, TNFα from Th1 cells alters the surface properties of endothelial cells to promote the adhesion of monocytes at the site of infection (Topic B4). The coordinated production of these mediators allows the infiltration of T cells and monocytes to the site of inflammation where their interaction leads to macrophage differentiation, activation and the elimination of the pathogen (*Fig. 3*).

Role of Th1 cells in isotype switching and affinity maturation. Th1 cells may also induce B cells to produce Ig, switch the isotype of Ig produced, and undergo affinity maturation of the Ig (Topic D3, *Fig. 4*). As with Th2 cells, the interaction of CD40L on Th1 cells with CD40 on B cells induces B cell proliferation and class switching. Cytokines are also important, but in this case IFNγ and TNFα are involved, resulting in signals and help for the development of B cells that produce primarily IgG antibodies.

Role of Th1 cells in induction of cytotoxicity by CD8⁺ CTLs. Antigen-presenting cells (APCs) initially process and present microbial peptides via the exogenous pathway in association with MHC class II molecules (Topic F2). Th1

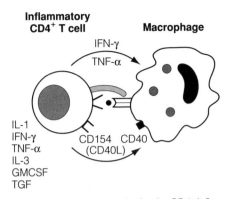

Fig. 3. *Macrophage activation by CD4⁺ inflammatory T cells. Cytokines released by Th1 cells, as well as signaling through direct contact of cell surface receptors, increase: (a) fusion of lysozomes and phagosomes; (b) production of nitric oxide and oxygen radicals for killing pathogens; and (c) expression of MHC class II molecules and TNF receptors by macrophages. Note that CD154/CD40 interactions are also important in activation of the macrophage .*

cells recognize and are activated by interaction with these cells, and in turn influence APC function. They do this by direct cell–cell interaction and signaling and through release of cytokines that act on APCs, including IFNγ. As a result of these interactions with specific Th1 cells, APCs become '**conditioned**' to more efficiently present peptides to CTLs via their MHC class I molecules and to Th cells through MHC class II (Topic F6, *Fig. 1*).

Cytotoxic T cells　*Recognition of antigen and activation*

Peptides derived from viral proteins are processed via the endogenous route and are presented on the cell surface by MHC class I molecules, marking this cell as infected and as a target for CTL killing. CTLs express cell surface CD8 which binds to the nonpolymorphic region of MHC class I (expressed on all nucleated cells), restricting these killer T cells to recognizing only cells presenting peptide in MHC class I molecules (Topic F2). This interaction also serves to stabilize the interaction of the T cell receptor with specific peptides bound to the polymorphic part of the MHC class I molecule (*Fig. 4*). Other surface co-stimulatory and adhesion molecules such as LFA-1 are important for close interaction of the CTL with the infected cell and for activating its cytotoxic

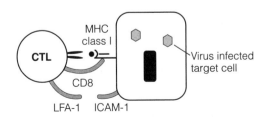

Fig. 4. *CTL recognize peptides associated with MHC class I molecules. CD8 binds to non-polymorphic MHC class I stabilizing this interaction and enhancing killing. The interaction of LFA-1 and ICAM-1 is also important in killing of the target.*

machinery (Topic F4). This activation step also induces the expression of FasL on the CTL, which can interact with Fas expressed on the surface of the virus-infected cell.

Mechanisms of cytotoxicity

Mature CTLs, generated with the help of Th1 cells, contain the cytotoxic machinery required to kill virus-infected cells. In particular, these CTLs are able to induce programed cell death (apoptosis) of the virus-infected cells through two distinct pathways: (a) release of lytic granules containing perforin and granzymes which enter the target cell; (b) interaction of FasL on the CTL with Fas on the target cell.

1. *Perforin-induced apoptosis.* CTL contain large cytolytic granules and are difficult to distinguish morphologically from NK cells (also called large granular lymphocytes; Topic B1). These intracytoplasmic granules contain proteases, granzyme A and granzyme B, and perforin, a molecule similar to C9 of the complement pathway (Topic D8). On interaction of the CTL with a virus-infected cell, the granules move toward the portion of the membrane close to the point of contact with the target cell. On fusion with the membrane, the granules release perforins which polymerize in the membrane of the infected cell creating pores that allow entry of the proteases (*Fig. 5*). These enzymes cleave cellular proteins, the products of which initiate induction of programed cell death (apoptosis). CTL then re-synthesize their granular contents in preparation for specific killing of another infected cell.

2. *Fas-mediated apoptosis.* Nucleated cells of the body infected with some viruses upregulate expression of Fas (CD95). CTL activated to release their granules by their first encounter with antigen presented by MHC class I molecules, are induced to upregulate FasL which then also allows them to kill specific virus-infected cells by an additional mechanism through interaction with surface CD95 (*Fig. 6*).

The importance of apoptosis as a killing mechanism used by the immune system is that targeted cells can be removed rapidly by phagocytes without

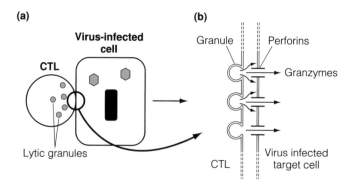

Fig. 5.   Apoptosis induced by release of lytic granules. (a) Lytic granules containing perforin and granzymes accumulate at the point of contact of CTL with virus-infected cell. (b) The granule contents are released and the perforins polymerize in the infected cell membrane allowing entry of granzymes into the target cell which induce apoptosis.

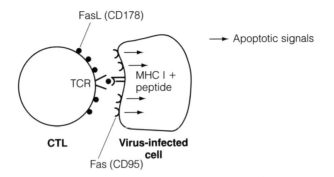

Fig. 6. *Apoptosis induced by Fas/FasL interactions. CTL have preformed FasL in their granules which is rapidly expressed on their surface when they attach via their TCR to the target cell. Ligation of Fas on the virus-infected cell by FasL on the CTL is an additional mechanism for induction of apoptosis.*

initiating inflammatory responses. Another mechanism of cell death – necrosis – results from tissue trauma or certain kinds of infection and leads to acute inflammation through the production of inflammatory cellular products.

F6 CELL-MEDIATED IMMUNITY IN CONTEXT

Key Note

Cell-mediated immunity in context	Antigen-presenting cells (APCs) initially process and present microbial peptides via the exogenous pathway in association with MHC class II. Specific Th cells are activated by interaction with these cells to produce cytokines, including IFNγ, that activate macrophages to kill pathogens. In addition, Th cells influence APC function, i.e. they 'condition' the APC. This occurs through direct cell–cell interaction and signaling and through the release of cytokines by the Th cell. These 'conditioned' APCs are then able to process the internalized antigen through the endogenous pathway and therefore are better able to present antigen in association with MHC class I to CD8$^+$ CTLs and to present antigen more efficiently via class II to CD4$^+$ Th cells. Specific CTLs activated by APCs in this way are able to kill infected cells expressing viral antigens in association with MHC class I.
Related topics	The role of T cells in immune responses (F1) Immunity to different organisms (H2)

Cell-mediated immunity in context

To understand and appreciate the various functional activities of the different T cell subpopulations, it is important to first put these cells and their properties into a relevant context, e.g. to consider the role of these cells in immunity to an infectious organism. Microbes first entering the body are taken up into dendritic cells or macrophages (antigen-presenting cells) through interaction with innate immune system receptors such as TLR and/or mannose receptors (Topic B3). If the microbe has been previously encountered, this uptake may be enhanced by opsonization of the microbe with antibody and/or complement and subsequent interaction with Fc and complement receptors, respectively. These antigen-presenting cells process microbial proteins via the exogenous pathway displaying peptides from these proteins on their surface in association with MHC class II molecules (*Fig. 1*). Th cells that recognize antigen on these APCs are activated (Topic F4) to produce cytokines, including IFNγ or IL-4.

In addition, the cell–cell interaction and signaling that occurs between the Th cell and the antigen-presenting cell, along with the cytokines produced by the Th cell, 'conditions' the antigen-presenting cell such that it can interact with, present antigen to, and thus prime precursor CD8$^+$ CTLs. Dendritic cells, in particular, when primed are able to pick up exogenous antigen and present it on MHC class I molecules to precursor CTLs, as well as on MHC class II molecules to Th cells (Topic F4). That is, there is some crossing of exogenous antigen into the endogenous pathway with the consequence that some peptides become associated with MHC class I molecules. Thus, in the presence of antigen and cytokines, specific Th *and* CTLs are generated. The 'primed' Th and CTLs are 'effector cells' which can then deal with infected cells. Specific Th1 cells activated by binding to macrophages that are presenting antigen in association with MHC class II molecules, produce IFNγ, resulting in activation of killing mechanisms in the macrophage. Other Th cells will interact with antigen presented by B cells and induce them to differentiate into plasma cells that produce antibodies to deal with those microbes accessible to antibody and complement (Topics D8 and F5). Conversely, specific CTLs attaching to virus-infected cells via antigen presented in MHC class I molecules will be activated to kill the infected cell either by release of perforins and granzymes or by FasL/Fas interactions.

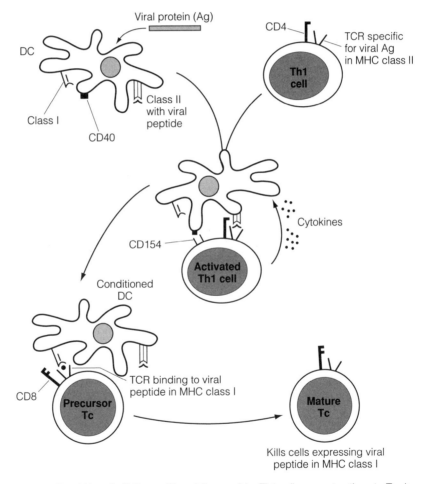

Fig. 1.   Dendritic cells (DC) conditioned (licensed) by Th1 cells present antigen to Tc via MHC class I. Interaction of specific Th1 cells with peptide (e.g. from a virus or tumor cell protein) presented in MHC class II on the DC involves adhesion molecules as well as binding of B7 to CD28. This series of interactions induces expression on the Th1 cells of CD154 which then binds CD40 on the DC. This triggering through CD40, in the presence of cytokines also released by Th1 cells, conditions the DC to present antigen in MHC class I to peptide specific Tc precursor cells, inducing their maturation into Tc cells.

G1 OVERVIEW

Key Notes

Overview	The immune system has to be tightly regulated, 'turned on' in response to a threat from a 'foreign' organism, fine tuned and 'turned off' again when the threat has been removed. In addition, the immune system components need to be regulated so that they do not respond against self (immunological tolerance).
Self, non-self discrimination by the innate immune system	In the innate immune system, phagocytes only recognize self cells if they are damaged or dying; natural killer cells are normally inhibited from killing self cells through inhibitory receptors; complement cannot be activated on the surfaces of normal body cells due to inhibitory molecules.
Regulation by the adaptive immune system	Antigen initiates and drives the immune response, the magnitude of which is under genetic control (e.g. MHC locus genes). Removal of the antigen results in the response subsiding. Helper T cells (through their cytokines and cell interactions) are involved in regulating the immune response and in modulating the functions of other cells. IgG antibodies can inhibit (negative feedback) further antibody production. Tolerance to self of lymphocytes and antibodies is initiated at the level of development (central tolerance) and in the periphery mainly through the lack of co-stimulatory signals and through activation-induced cell death. The neuroendocrine system also plays an important role in modulating immune responses.
Related topics	Cells of the innate immune system (B1) Recognition of microbes by the innate immune system (B3) Molecules of the innate immune system (B2)

Overview

It is essential that the immune system be tightly regulated. It has to be 'turned on' following a threat from a 'foreign' organism, fine tuned to give an optimum and appropriate response and 'turned off' again when the threat has been removed. In addition, since self antigens are ubiquitous and would continuously drive the immune response, the cells and molecules playing a role in the immune system need to be regulated so that they respond only against foreign organisms and not against self. This unresponsiveness to self is termed 'immunological tolerance'. The main 'switch' to turn on the immune response is the presence of antigen (Topic A4). This drives the immune response, the magnitude of which is under genetic control (e.g. MHC locus genes).

Self, non-self discrimination by the innate immune system

In the case of the cells and molecules of the innate immune system that have evolved to be aggressive towards microbes there are two ways in which self reactivity is prevented: lack of recognition (ignorance) of self cells unless they change their surface structure; and the presence of inhibitory structures/receptors on the nonimmune cells.

Phagocytes
Phagocytic cells of the innate system, including macrophages and neutrophils, do not normally 'recognize' or phagocytose living self cells. However, aging (erythrocytes), dying or dead cells express new surface molecules that are recognized by phagocytes, which results in the removal of these altered self cells. Phagocytes recognize microbes through pattern recognition receptors, including sugars, e.g. mannose (Topic B3). Target molecules on the surface of mammalian cells that might be recognized by these receptors are either absent or concealed by other structures, e.g. sialic acids. When an erythrocyte ages, it loses sialic acid exposing N-acetyl glucosamine which the phagocyte now recognizes as non self and phagocytoses (*Fig. 1*). When nucleated cells die, a large number of surface molecules are exposed which are recognized by phagocytes. One of these molecules, phosphatidyl serine (PS) – a membrane phospholipid, is normally restricted to the inner surface of the cell membrane. When the cell begins to die through apoptosis PS 'flips' onto the surface and is recognized by the phagocytes.

Self cells

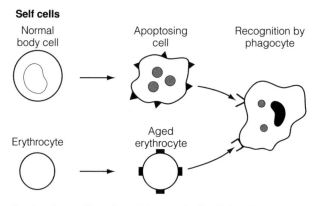

Fig. 1.   Recognition of aged/damaged self cells by phagocytes.

Natural killer cells
These cells play an important role in killing virus-infected cells. They are prevented from killing the non-infected nucleated cells of the body through a balance in signaling involving killer activation receptors (KAR) and killer inhibitory receptors (KIR) that recognize molecules on self cells. The inhibitory receptors recognize MHC molecules on normal cells and prevent their killing by NK cells (Topics B1, F2 and N3). However, when certain viruses infect cells they downregulate expression of molecules (MHC class I) recognized by KIR giving rise to an overriding activation through KAR leading to death of the infected cells (*Fig. 2*).

The complement system
C3 is activated through the alternative pathway by stabilization of appropriate enzymes on the surface of some microorganisms (Topic B2). This cannot occur

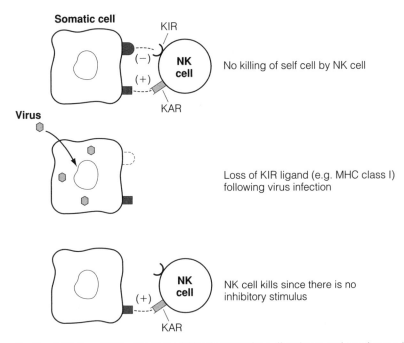

Fig. 2.   Inhibition of NK cell activity. NK cells recognize self-antigens and travel around the body in search of aberrant self-cells. When they come into contact with a healthy cell they receive two signals – a positive signal to kill via their KAR (killer activation receptors) and a negative signal via their KIR (killer inhibitory receptors). These two signals cancel each other out and the NK cell goes on its way. Some viruses inhibit expression of the self-molecules recognized by the KIR (e.g. MHC class I, HLA-A, B, C in man) which means that the negative signal is absent and the NK cell carries out its lethal duty.

on the body's cells since they all have inhibitory molecules (Topic D8) on their surface membranes (*Fig. 3*).

Regulation by the adaptive immune system

Tolerance to self of lymphocytes and antibodies of the adaptive system is initiated at the level of development of T and B cells (Topics A5, C1, F3 and G2) in the primary lymphoid organs (central tolerance). Those lymphocytes escaping elimination at this stage are prevented from responding to self through lack of co-stimulatory signals (e.g. those provided by CD80 or CD86 on APC that are necessary for T cell activation) resulting in anergy or activation-induced cell death by T cells (peripheral tolerance).

The nature of the antigen is also important, since its size, state of aggregation, composition (e.g. protein vs carbohydrate), etc., significantly influence the type of response and its strength (Topic A4). Removal of the antigen and therefore the stimulus results in the response subsiding. Helper T cells are involved in regulating this response and in modulating the functions of other cells, including dendritic cells, NK cells, macrophages, and cytotoxic T cells. Although this modulation is often mediated through cytokines, it may also involve direct cell–cell interactions. The influence of Th cells can significantly affect the type of response depending at least partly on the kinds of cytokines produced and the particular cell participating in the response. Antibody itself can, in some

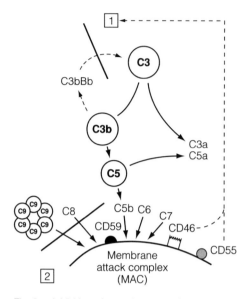

Fig. 3. *Inhibition of complement activation on self-cell surfaces by regulatory proteins.* ⎡1⎤ *Inhibition of C3 convertase by membrane cofactor proteins (CD46) and decay accelerating factor (CD55).* ⎡2⎤ *Blocking by CD59 of attachment of C8 and C9 of MAC to membrane, inhibits active lysis.*

instances, either enhance (IgM) and complement or inhibit (IgG: negative feedback; Topics E2 and G4) further antibody production.

It is also important to note that the immune system does not function in isolation, but rather is influenced by other body systems. In particular, the neuroendocrine system plays an important role in modulating immune responses.

G2 CENTRAL AND PERIPHERAL TOLERANCE

Key Notes

Central tolerance

Central tolerance is the process whereby immature T and B cells acquire tolerance to self antigens during maturation within the primary lymphoid organs/tissues (thymus and bone marrow, respectively). It involves the elimination of cells with receptors for self antigens.

Peripheral tolerance

Since not all self-reactive lymphocytes are eliminated by central tolerance mechanisms (due primarily to the absence of most self antigens in the primary lymphoid organs), self reactive lymphocytes are anergized or deleted in the peripheral tissues. Peripheral T cells are made unresponsive (anergic) through the absence of the second signal (essential for T cell activation) given by co-stimulatory molecules (i.e. B7) on antigen-presenting cells (APCs). Peripheral B cells may become anergic and unable to develop into plasma cells as a result of the absence of co-stimulatory signals from T cells. Moreover, under appropriate conditions, activated T cells expressing Fas Ligand (FasL) may kill Fas-expressing B cells (and, perhaps, other T cells) through **activation-induced cell death** (AICD).

Related topics

Generation of diversity (D3)
B cell activation (E2)
Shaping the T cell repertoire (F3)

T cell activation (F4)
Autoimmune diseases –
  mechanisms of development (L3)

Central tolerance

The fundamental basis for central tolerance is that interaction of antigen with immature clones of lymphocytes already expressing antigen receptors, would result in an unresponsive state. This theory, for which Burnet and Medawar received the Nobel Prize in 1960, is now recognized to involve a mechanism that causes self-reactive lymphocytes to be eliminated (**clonal deletion**) on contact with self antigens. Immature precursor cells derived from bone marrow stem cells migrate to the thymus to mature into immunocompetent T cells or mature in the bone marrow to become B cells. T cells with specificity for self appear during normal development in the thymus as the result of the expression of combinations of V segment genes (Topics D3, E3 and F3). These self-reactive T cells must be eliminated to prevent autoimmunity.

T cells with receptors with weak binding to MHC class I and II antigens are permitted to survive, **positively selected** (see Topic F3 *Fig. 3*). T cells which bind with high affinity to MHC class I and II, alone or carrying self peptides (Topics F2, F3), are induced to die through the process of apoptosis. This **negative selection** leads to elimination of some but not all self-reactive T cells. Cortical epithelial cells are the main players in the positive selection process whereas macrophages and interdigitating dendritic cells play a leading role in negative selection. This 'education' process within the thymus leads to suicide of greater than 90% of the T cells. Thus, only a small percentage of the T cells generated survive to emigrate to the peripheral tissues. These T cells are the ones capable of recognizing foreign non self peptide antigens in the context of self MHC molecules.

A similar process of negative selection occurs during B cell development in the bone marrow. As in the thymus, receptor diversity for antigen is created from rearrangement of V segment genes resulting in some B cells having membrane antibodies with self reactivity. **B cell tolerance** occurs as a result of clonal deletion, through apoptosis, of immature B cells reactive to self antigens (*Fig. 1*). Immature B cells expressing surface IgM that react with self antigens are rendered unresponsive or anergic. Thus, only those B cells that do not react with self antigens in the bone marrow are allowed to mature and migrate to the periphery where further maturation occurs.

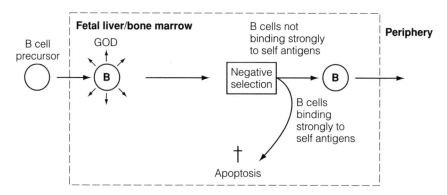

Fig. 1.   Central tolerance: B cells. B cell precursors develop diverse antigen receptors (GOD). They undergo negative selection and the surviving cells migrate to peripheral (secondary) lymphoid organs/tissues.

Peripheral tolerance

Most self-reactive lymphocytes cannot all be eliminated in the primary lymphoid organs for two reasons. Firstly, many self antigens are neither present in the primary lymphoid organs nor supplied to them via the bloodstream. Moreover, with the exception of self antigens that do not normally come into contact with the immune system ('sequestered antigens' such as lens proteins in the eye), most self antigens expressed as the result of differentiation of cells and tissues in the major organs of the body do not 'pass through' the primary lymphoid organs. Certainly, lymphocytes in the periphery do come into contact with these antigens. Secondly, different receptor specificities may be generated as the consequence of somatic mutation of the antibody genes in B cells. This occurs within the germinal centers of secondary lymphoid organs/tissues (Topics C2, D3 and E4). Unlike B cell antigen receptors, it is believed that TCRs do not normally mutate.

T cell anergy

Peripheral self-reactive T cells can be deleted or anergized. The main mechanism preventing autoreactivity in the periphery involves development of anergy. Naive T cells require two main signals to respond to an antigen. One comes via the TCR, the other comes from co-stimulatory molecules. The glycoproteins B7.1 (CD80) and B7.2 (CD86) are essential co-stimulatory molecules, found almost exclusively on professional antigen-presenting cells (APCs). Interaction of these B7 molecules on APCs with CD28 on T cells is required for T cell activation (*Fig. 2*). Thus, in the absence of professional presentation of self antigens and engagement of co-stimulatory molecules (signal 2), the binding of self antigens presented in MHC molecules to the TCR on naive T cells, results in anergy. Moreover, if naive T cells do become activated they express an additional receptor called CTLA-4 which has a greater binding affinity for the B7 molecules than CD28. Binding of CTLA-4 to B7 results in a negative signal to the T cells resulting in inhibition of T cell activity (Topic F4).

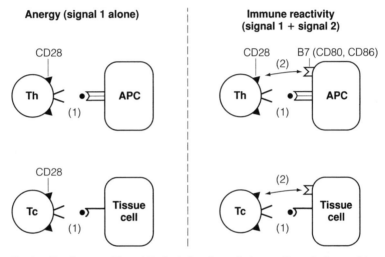

Fig. 2. T cell anergy. Th and Tc (including those that are self reactive) cannot be activated by one signal. Binding of B7 (CD80, CD86) on the APC/tissue cell to CD28 provides a second signal to the T cells leading to their activation.

B cell anergy
Self-reactive B cells require T cell help in order to respond to T-dependent antigens. Since most self-reactive T cells have been deleted during thymic maturation, self-reactive B cells on contact with self antigens do not receive the required co-stimulatory signals (signal 2) from T helper cells and consequently become anergic (*Fig. 3*). Engagement of the B cell co-stimulatory molecules CD40 and B7 by CD154 and CD28 on T cells, as well as certain cytokines (IL-2, IL-4, IL-5, IL-6), are required for activation (Topic E2).

Activation-induced cell death
Fas/FasL (CD95/CD95L) interaction is directly responsible for AICD. This is important in maintaining immunological as well as physiological homeostasis by eliminating unnecessary cells through apoptosis. Activated T lymphocytes can express both the receptor protein Fas and its ligand (FasL), whereas B cells mainly express Fas. Peripheral tolerance may be facilitated by interaction between activated T cells and B cells (and, perhaps under certain conditions, other T cells) resulting in apoptosis (*Fig. 4*). In addition, T cells activated to kill

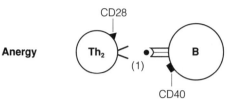

Anergy

No help from T cells (no signal 2)

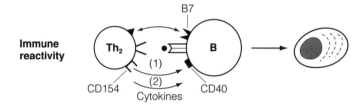

Immune reactivity

Help from T cells (signal 1 + signal 2)

Fig. 3. B cell anergy. B cells require triggering through their CD40 molecules to progress through activation and maturation. Interaction of CD28 on T cells with B7 on B cells is necessary to induce expression of CD154 (CD40 ligand). This binds to CD40 on the B cell, acting as the second signal for activation.

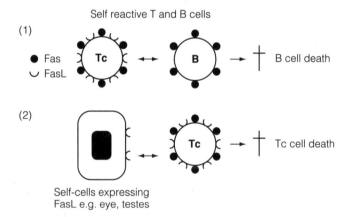

Fig. 4. Activation-induced cell death (AICD) in peripheral tolerance. Tc cells may kill self-B cells expressing Fas(1) and because Tc can also express Fas on activation, may themselves be killed by tissue cells expressing FasL:CD178(2).

self cells may themselves be killed by interaction with FasL expressed by certain somatic cells, e.g. those in the eye and testis (Topic L3) thus preventing killing of these self cells. This may also be a strategy used by tumor cells to prevent their demise by cytotoxic T cells.

G3 ACQUIRED TOLERANCE

Key Notes

Introduction	That tolerance can be induced to certain antigens under appropriate conditions has considerable importance to immune defense as well as to modulating immunity to self antigens. Acquired tolerance is primarily associated with tolerance to non-self antigen and may involve anergy, deletion and active suppression by Th2 cells. These mechanisms are influenced by the nature of antigen, its route of administration and concentration and the maturity of the immune system.
Nature of antigen	The chemical makeup and complexity of the antigen, as well as how similar it is to the species into which it is being introduced determines its ability to induce tolerance or immunity. The closer the similarity with self the easier it is to induce tolerance.
Maturity of the immune system	Tolerance is easier to achieve before birth or in early neonatal life, perhaps related to immaturity of T, B and/or antigen-presenting cells. It is easier to tolerise T cells than B cells. It is difficult to induce tolerance to a specific antigen to which there is already an ongoing immune response.
Route of administration	The route of administration may determine whether tolerance is induced or not. Certain antigens introduced intraperitonealy or intravenously are often more tolerogenic than when the same antigens are given subcutaneously or intramuscularly. Exposure to antigens via the oral route can result in both immunity or peripheral tolerance. Immunity to an antigen may, in some instances, be prevented by feeding these antigens orally.
Dose of antigen	Low or high doses of antigen may induce systemic tolerance, whereas intermediate doses may elicit an immune response. Larger doses are needed for tolerance in adults compared to neonates.

Related topics

Antigens (A4)
Molecules of the innate immune
  system (B2)
Mucosa-associated lymphoid tissues
  (C3)
Central and peripheral tolerance
  (G2)

Secondary (acquired)
  immunodeficiency (J3)
Diagnosis and treatment of
  autoimmune disease (L5)

Introduction

Under appropriate conditions tolerance can be induced to certain non-self antigens. This has considerable importance to immune defense as acquired tolerance to critical epitopes on microbes may compromise protective immune responses to the organism. Acquired tolerance also has the potential for modulating immunity to self antigens (e.g. MHC molecules, permitting grafting of

MHC-incompatible organs) or allergens. The mechanisms that lead to the induction of acquired tolerance to foreign antigens are not clearly understood. Three basic mechanisms have been suggested based on experimental data. These include active suppression by Th2 cells, anergy and deletion.

- Active suppression requires the production by Th2 cells of inhibitory cytokines such as TGFβ and IL-10 and can be adoptively transferred by lymphocytes from one animal to another (using inbred strains of mice).
- Anergy results when an antigen-sensitive cell becomes unresponsive and goes into a resting state.
- Deletion involves the removal of an antigen-reactive cell by apoptosis.

There are many factors that may influence the induction of tolerance systemically, including:

- Nature of the antigen
- Maturity of the immune system (age of host)
- Route of immunization with the antigen
- Dose of antigen

Moreover, T and B cell tolerance may differ. The genetic background of the host may also influence the development of tolerance as the immune response is under the control of immune response genes (IR genes, Topics F2 and G5).

Nature of antigen

The more dissimilar and complex the foreign antigen is in composition and structure to the host, the more difficult it is to induce tolerance. The closer the composition and structure of the antigen is to self antigens, the easier it is to induce tolerance. Aggregated antigens or antigens with multiple different epitopes are usually good 'immunogens' (i.e. able to induce immunity) but poor tolerogens, whereas soluble antigens are poor immunogens but good tolerogens.

Maturity of the immune system

Tolerance is easier to achieve before birth or in early neonatal life. This may be related to the immaturity of both T and B cells and/or APCs. It is also easier to induce tolerance in immune-compromised individuals, e.g. immunodeficient individuals or animals that are recovering from irradiation (Topic J3). Moreover, it is easier to induce tolerance in T cells than in B cells and, once attained, this tolerance lasts longer. Relative to B cell tolerance, T cell tolerance is achieved with lower doses of antigen and occurs more quickly after exposure. It is difficult to induce tolerance to a specific antigen to which there is an ongoing immune response. This is presumably because the immune cells are relatively long-lived and memory T and B cells are more difficult to tolerise, e.g. in autoimmune diseases (Topic L5).

Route of administration

The route of administration of antigen may influence the nature of the immune response. Certain antigens given subcutaneously or intramuscularly may be more immunogenic than when given intravenously or intraperitoneally.

Antigens introduced into an individual by the oral route (feeding) can induce oral tolerance. At least three mechanisms are involved, including active suppression, clonal anergy and deletion. Active suppression probably involves the release of inhibitory cytokines such as TGFβ and IL-10 and can be adoptively transferred. In animal models of oral tolerance, active suppression can be adoptively transferred by both CD4 and CD8 cells. Clonal anergy is usually induced by exposure to low or high doses of antigen. Thus, in the absence of co-stimulatory accessory signals, T or B cells may undergo anergy. Deletion results when high doses of antigen are fed, which has been shown to induce lymphocytes to undergo apoptosis in the Peyers patches. The requirements for tolerance induction may be different for different antigens and may also depend on the context of the stimulus. Antigens seen in the context of microbial infection may induce immune reactivity instead of tolerance.

Dose of antigen   Tolerance, rather than immunity is induced by extremes in antigen dose. The tolerance induced by the administration of high doses of antigen is called 'high zone tolerance'. In mature animals, a much larger dose is required than may be necessary in neonates. Tolerance can also be induced by extremely low doses of antigen, so called 'low zone tolerance'.

G4 REGULATION BY ANTIGEN AND ANTIBODY

Key Notes

Initiation of the response	Antigen initiates the immune response via presentation of its peptides by antigen-presenting cells (dendritic cells and macrophages) to antigen-specific Th cells. Th cells then help B cells produce antibody, or CTLs develop. The physical state (e.g. aggregation) and composition (e.g. protein) of the antigen are also important.
Removal of antigen	Removal of antigen by antibody, and ultimately through phagocytic cells, is the most effective means of regulating an immune response, since in its absence, the restimulation of antigen-specific T and B cells stops. Thus, maternal IgG in the newborn may bind antigen and remove it, thereby interfering with development of active immunity to this antigen. Furthermore, therapy with passive antibodies may interfere with the development of active immunity. For example, antibodies to Rhesus D (RhD) given to RhD negative mothers inhibit their production of anti-RhD antibodies in future pregnancies. Persistent antigen, as found with some viruses and bacteria, maintains production of specific immune responses.
Positive effects of antibodies	Antibodies of the IgM class may regulate the immune response through complement activation. Thus, interaction of antigen–IgM–complement complexes with complement receptors (CD21) on antigen-specific B cells may enhance the response.
Negative feedback by IgG	IgG-antigen complexes may specifically inhibit further responses by antigen-specific B cells as a result of a negative signal transduced by FcγRII (CD32) on binding of the Fc region of the IgG component of the complex.
The idiotype network	The ability of the immune system to produce anti-idiotypic responses (immune responses to the variable region of immunoglobulin molecules) has been proposed as a mechanism by which immune responses can be regulated.

Related topics	Antigens (A4)	The cellular basis of the antibody response (E3)
	Molecules of the innate immune system (B2)	Immunization (I2)
	Adaptive immunity at birth (C5)	IgG- and IgM-mediated (type II) hypersensitivity (K3)
	Antibody classes (D2)	
	Allotypes and idiotypes (D4)	
	The B cell receptor complex, co-receptors and signaling (E1)	

Initiation of the response

Antigen is an absolute requirement for the initiation of an immune response. Recognition of microbes as foreign or non-self is initially mediated through microbe pattern recognition by receptors of the innate immune system or antigen-specific receptors on lymphocytes (Topics B3, E1, F2). The nature of the antigen is also important in that particulate antigens produce stronger immune responses than soluble forms of the same antigen. This may in part be due to the ability of soluble antigens to produce a tolerogenic response rather than an immune response. Aggregated antigens are also more likely to be taken up and processed by antigen-presenting cells.

Removal of antigen

The successful generation of an antigen-driven cell-mediated and/or antibody response, leads in most cases to removal of the invading microbes. Microbial debris and dead virus-infected cells are cleared by the phagocytic system, thus removing the antigenic source and therefore the stimulus. In particular, as a result of elimination of antigen by antibody, restimulation of antigen-specific T and B cells stops, preventing more specific antibodies from being made at a time when antigen is being effectively cleared from the system. The ability of preformed antibodies to inhibit specific unwanted host responses to antigens has been shown clinically by passive immunization. Injection of antibodies to RhD into RhD– mothers before or immediately after birth of an RhD+ infant removes RhD+ erythrocytes that may have passed into the maternal circulation. This prevents the development of hemolytic disease of the newborn from occurring as a result of future pregnancies (Topic K3). This results from the simple removal of antigen (RhD+ erythrocytes), such that the mother never develops a memory response to RhD antigen.

Similarly, unresponsiveness of the newborn to certain antigens may be related to the passive immunity acquired from the mother (Topic C5). Due to transfer of maternal IgG across the placenta during fetal life, the infant at birth has all of the IgG-antibody-mediated humoral immunity of the mother. Furthermore, maternal IgA obtained by the infant from colostrum and milk during nursing coats the infant's gastrointestinal tract and supplies passive mucosal immunity (Topics C5, D8 and E4). Thus, until these passively supplied antibodies are degraded or used up, they may bind antigen and remove it, thereby interfering with development of active immunity.

Of note, some microbes persist and continuously stimulate specific T and B cells. For example, Epstein–Barr virus, which causes glandular fever, persists for life at low levels in the pharyngeal tissues and B cells, continually restimulating immunity to the virus.

Positive effects of antibodies

Antibodies of the IgM class appear to be important in enhancing humoral immunity. In particular, antigen–IgM–complement complexes that bind to the B cell antigen receptor stimulate the cell more efficiently than antigen alone (*Fig. 1*). This is probably the result of simultaneous interaction of the C3b component of complement with the CD21 molecule of the antigen receptor complex, which then transduces a positive signal to the B cell.

Negative feedback by IgG

The interaction of IgG–antigen complexes with antigen-specific B cells through the simultaneous binding of both the B cell antigen receptor and the FcγRII molecule of the B cell receptor complex can deliver a negative signal to the B cell (*Fig. 1*). Thus, IgG, which is produced later in the antibody response, could interact with antigen (if present) forming a complex that, on binding to antigen-specific B cells, may provide feedback inhibition mediated via FcγRII, decreasing the amount of antigen-specific antibody being produced.

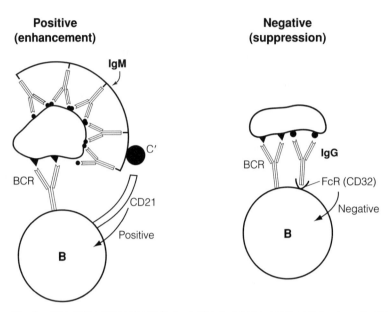

Fig. 1.   Regulation of B cell activity by antibody. IgM bound to antigen recognized by the BCR fixes complement which then interacts with CD21 giving a positive signal to the B cell. However, IgG bound to antigen attached to the BCR binds to FcγR (CD32) and delivers a negative signal to the B cell.

The idiotype network

The hypervariable region, the idiotype, of the immunoglobulin molecule (Topic D4) is immunogenic, and thus antibody and T cell responses can be produced to this region. It has been suggested that these immune responses to idiotypes have an immunoregulatory role. That is, antibodies or T cells directed to the idiotype of an antigen-induced antibody may, by interacting directly with the B or T cell, regulate its further proliferation and differentiation. Anti-idiotypic antibodies or T cells may thus form networks of connectivity and act as inducers and regulators of their own responses. In the absence of antigen, B cells or T cells with idiotypic and anti-idiotypic antigen receptors may directly anergize other B and T cells through direct contact of the antigen receptors.

Furthermore, two different sets of antibodies can be produced against the idiotype of an antibody molecule. One set of antibodies may express anti-idiotype binding sites that resemble the antigenic determinant on the original antigen. Thus, for example, an antibody directed against an antigenic determinant on a microbe may stimulate an immune reaction that results in anti-idiotypic antibodies with variable regions that resemble the antigenic determinant on the microbe. Anti-idiotypes so produced can potentially act as surrogate antigens. For example, antibodies to hepatitis B antibodies have been used as vaccines for hepatitis B. Anti-idiotype antibodies behaving as surrogate antigens may permit the immune system to boost its own response during infection. In this way, during an immune response to a microbe, anti-idiotypic antibodies that mimic microbial antigens may amplify the immune response against the microbes.

It is also possible that anti-idiotypic antibodies which mimic self molecules may cause enhanced autoimmune responses. For example, antibodies made against a hormone may induce anti-idiotypic antibodies that mimic the hormone and thus bind to and stimulate the hormone receptor (Topic L3).

G5 GENES, T HELPER CELLS, CYTOKINES AND THE NEUROENDOCRINE SYSTEM

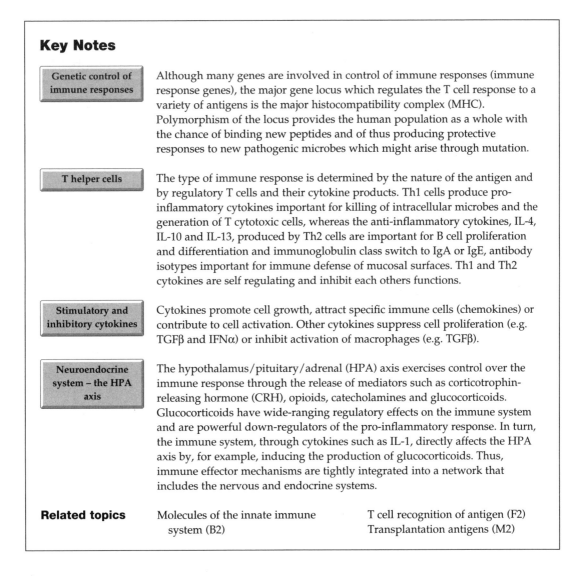

Key Notes

Genetic control of immune responses

Although many genes are involved in control of immune responses (immune response genes), the major gene locus which regulates the T cell response to a variety of antigens is the major histocompatibility complex (MHC). Polymorphism of the locus provides the human population as a whole with the chance of binding new peptides and of thus producing protective responses to new pathogenic microbes which might arise through mutation.

T helper cells

The type of immune response is determined by the nature of the antigen and by regulatory T cells and their cytokine products. Th1 cells produce pro-inflammatory cytokines important for killing of intracellular microbes and the generation of T cytotoxic cells, whereas the anti-inflammatory cytokines, IL-4, IL-10 and IL-13, produced by Th2 cells are important for B cell proliferation and differentiation and immunoglobulin class switch to IgA or IgE, antibody isotypes important for immune defense of mucosal surfaces. Th1 and Th2 cytokines are self regulating and inhibit each others functions.

Stimulatory and inhibitory cytokines

Cytokines promote cell growth, attract specific immune cells (chemokines) or contribute to cell activation. Other cytokines suppress cell proliferation (e.g. TGFβ and IFNα) or inhibit activation of macrophages (e.g. TGFβ).

Neuroendocrine system – the HPA axis

The hypothalamus/pituitary/adrenal (HPA) axis exercises control over the immune response through the release of mediators such as corticotrophin-releasing hormone (CRH), opioids, catecholamines and glucocorticoids. Glucocorticoids have wide-ranging regulatory effects on the immune system and are powerful down-regulators of the pro-inflammatory response. In turn, the immune system, through cytokines such as IL-1, directly affects the HPA axis by, for example, inducing the production of glucocorticoids. Thus, immune effector mechanisms are tightly integrated into a network that includes the nervous and endocrine systems.

Related topics

Molecules of the innate immune system (B2)

T cell recognition of antigen (F2)
Transplantation antigens (M2)

Genetic control of immune responses

It has been well established that many genes are involved in regulation of immune responses (immune response genes). Many of these undoubtedly code for the large number of receptors, signaling proteins, etc., that are critical to the specific immune response. However, the major gene locus which regulates the T cell response to most antigens is the major histocompatibility complex (MHC). This complex, which is composed of six major loci (Topics F2, M2) is polymorphic with allelic forms which encode different amino acids within the peptide-binding region of the MHC class I and class II molecules. This polymorphism is believed to provide the human population as a whole with the chance of binding any new peptides which might arise through mutations of microbes. Those individuals who have MHC molecules able to bind peptides from a new peptide would be selected to survive in a Darwinian way.

T helper cells

Th cells are an absolute requirement for immune responses to protein antigens in general, and for helping B cells to make the different classes of antibodies. The type of response is, in some instances, determined by the nature of the antigen and its mode of entry as well as the effect of regulatory CD4+ T helper subsets, Th1 and Th2, and their cytokine products (Topic F5). The pro-inflammatory cytokines, IL-2, TNFα and IFNγ, produced by Th1 cells are important for killing of intracellular microbes and the generation of T cytotoxic cells, whereas the anti-inflammatory Th2 cytokines, IL-4, IL-10 and IL-13, are important for B cell proliferation and differentiation and immunoglobulin class switch to IgA and IgE as well as the IgG2 response to the polysaccharide antigens associated with encapsulated bacteria such as *Pneumococcus*. Th2 cytokines are also important in helping to eradicate parasitic infections as they lead to the production of IgE and the recruitment of eosinophils which have powerful anti-parasitic functions (Topic H2). Th1 and Th2 cytokines are self regulating and also inhibit each other's functions (*Fig. 1* and Topic B2). For example, IL-4 and IL-10 downregulate Th1 responses whereas IFNγ has an antagonistic effect on Th2 cells. Downregulatory mechanisms are necessary to prevent collateral damage as well as being energy conserving. Patients with atopy, i.e. with a genetic predisposition to having high levels of IgE, are believed to poorly regulate their Th2 cells (Topic K2). In addition, in AIDS there is some suggestion that the response is biased in favor of a Th2 rather than Th1 response (Topic J3).

Stimulatory and inhibitory cytokines

Most cytokines promote growth of particular cell lineages, attract specific immune cells (chemokines) or contribute to cell activation. Other cytokines can be suppressive. TGFβ inhibits activation of macrophages and the proliferation of B and T cells. IFNα also has cell growth inhibitory properties. The action of these suppressive cytokines is a primary way that T cells and macrophages

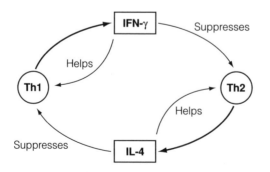

Fig. 1.   Reciprocal regulation of Th1 and Th2 cells. Th1 cells release IFNγ which suppresses proliferation of Th2 cells and their IL-4 production. Th2 cells release IL-4 (and IL-10) which suppresses IFN-γ production by Th1 cells and their proliferation.

regulate immune responses. In addition, the stimulatory and inhibitory action of cytokines produced by Th1 and Th2 cells on each other also plays a major role in determining the type and extent of an immune response (Topic B2).

Neuroendocrine system – the HPA axis

The activity of the immune system is influenced by other systems and perhaps most importantly by the neuroendocrine axis. Thus, lymphocytes are not only susceptible to regulation by cytokines of the immune system but also by hormones and neurotransmitters. The hypothalamus/pituitary/adrenal (HPA) axis exercises powerful control over the immune response through the release of mediators such as corticotrophin-releasing hormone (CRH), opioids, catecholamines and glucocorticoids (*Fig. 2*). While the effector mechanisms for some of these mediators are not fully understood, it is known that they act on both the sensory (mast cells) and cognitive (lymphocytes) cells of the immune system.

Glucocorticoids have wide-ranging regulatory effects on the immune system, including: reducing the number of circulating lymphocytes, monocytes and eosinophils; suppressing cell-mediated immunity by inhibiting the release of the pro-inflammatory cytokines IL-1, IL-2, IL-6, IFNγ and TNFα; decreasing antigen presentation; and inhibiting mast cell function. Growth hormone and prolactin, which are produced by the pituitary, are apparently also able to modulate the activity of the immune system. It has been shown that rats which undergo hypophysectomy (destruction of the pituitary) have prolonged allograft survival that is reduced on the reintroduction of prolactin or growth hormone.

Neurotransmitters including adrenaline (epinephrine), noradrenaline (norepinephrine), substance P, vasoactive intestinal peptide (VIP) and 5′-hydroxytrypt-

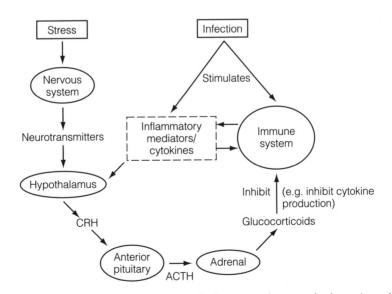

Fig. 2.   The interconnectivity between the immune and neuroendocrine systems. Infection or stress can affect, either directly or indirectly, both the immune and the nervous systems. Inflammatory mediators/cytokines released in response to infection not only are involved in the development and regulation of immune responses, but also stimulate the release of immune modulators such as glucocorticoids, which downregulate immune responses. Stress and inflammatory mediators cause the release of corticotrophin releasing hormone (CRH) by the hypothalamus, which stimulates the pituitary to release ACTH. ACTH causes the adrenal gland to release glucocorticoids, which in turn downregulate the immune system.

amine (5HT) can also have both wide-ranging and specific effects on immune function.

Interestingly, the HPA axis is also directly influenced by the immune system as evidenced by the fact that the cytokines IL-1, TNFα and IL-6, which are released during the inflammatory response, directly affect the hypothalamus, anterior pituitary and adrenal cortex. Thus, immune effector mechanisms are tightly integrated into a network that includes the nervous and endocrine systems.

H1 THE MICROBIAL COSMOS

Key Notes

Infection and its consequences	In the past, epidemics caused by plague and influenza have caused the deaths of large numbers of people as well as causing changes in social structures and behavior. Today, diseases such as those caused by the human immunodeficiency virus (HIV), *Legionella*, *Helicobacter pylori* as well as the emergence of multi-drug-resistant tuberculosis (TB) and SARS virus, present new challenges to the immune system and man's inventiveness.
Microbe habitat and immune defense	Microbes that live outside the cells of the body (e.g. many bacteria and fungi) are usually dealt with by phagocytes, complement and specific antibodies. However, those having an intracellular habitat (e.g. viruses, some bacteria and protozoa) are controlled by neutralizing antibodies, cytotoxic T cells or NK cells.
Pathogen protective mechanisms	Microbes have evolved ways to evade the multiple defenses of the body's immune system and thus cause infection. First, they may avoid recognition by having an intracellular habitat, by molecular mimicry (antigens of the infectious agent are antigenically indistinguishable from host antigens) and by antigenic variation. Second, they may down-modulate the effector arm of the immune response.
Damage caused by pathogens	Pathogens can cause tissue damage directly by production of toxins but also through an overzealous immune response. Mechanisms of immune-mediated damage to the host include anaphylaxis, immune complex disease, necrosis and apoptosis.
Related topics	Cells of the innate immune system (B1) Antibody functions (D8) Molecules of the innate immune system (B2) Clonal expansion and the development of effector function (F5)

Infection and its consequences

As well as being useful, microbes (and larger parasites) are still one of man's greatest threats to survival. In the past, diseases such as tuberculosis (TB) and epidemics caused by plague and influenza have caused the deaths of large numbers of people and changed social structures and behavior. It is estimated that the 1918 flu epidemic killed between 40 and 100 million people and it is suggested that more people died from TB as a result of the Second World War than from the war alone. Today, diseases such as those caused by the human immunodeficiency virus (HIV), *Legionella*, *Helicobacter pylori* as well as the emergence of multi-drug resistant TB and the severe acute respiratory syndrome (SARS) virus, present new challenges to the immune system and man's inventiveness.

Microbe habitat and immune defense

Microbes can invade the host through mucosal surfaces, skin, bites and wounds. Such invasion is usually countered by innate defense mechanisms, which act rapidly. In the event that the infectious agent still survives these first lines of defense, the adaptive immune system responds more specifically, but more slowly, in an effort to eliminate the pathogen. In this way the adaptive and nonadaptive immune systems can be considered as brain versus brawn, respectively. The final pathway of defense usually results in immunological memory so that repeated infection with the causative microbe or parasite is minimized or, as is the case with infectious agents such as smallpox and measles, prevented.

The immune responses to bacteria, viruses, fungi, protozoa and worms differ in the variety of defensive mechanisms used. In general, microbes (e.g. many bacteria and fungi) living outside the cells of the body are more likely to be opsonized by specific antibodies and engulfed by phagocytes or destroyed by the alternative or classical complement pathway, whereas those having an intracellular habitat (e.g. viruses, some bacteria and protozoa) may require the presence of antibodies (neutralization), as well as cytotoxic T cells or NK cells to provide effective protection. The immune response to fungi is poorly understood, and while antibodies may play a role in their elimination, the major mechanism of protection against these microorganisms appears to be through a cell-mediated response (T cells and macrophages). Both humoral and cellular responses are required for protection against protozoa, which are difficult to immunize against. Immune protection against helminths (worms) is difficult to achieve because of size and complexity. The major response mechanisms include the production of antibodies, especially immunoglobulin (IgE), and a cellular response including eosinophils, mast cells, macrophages and CD4 T cells. Both mast cells and basophils degranulate in the presence of IgE antigen complexes; IgA complexes also cause eosinophils to degranulate. Mast cells release histamine, which causes gut spasms and, whereas eosinophils release cationic protein and neurotoxins, helminth antigens direct the immune system to develop a Th2 response that results in the preferential production of IgE.

Pathogen protective mechanisms

Many microbes have evolved ways to evade the multiple and overlapping human immune defense mechanisms and of causing infection. Microbial strategies of escape from immune surveillance are essentially of two kinds. First, some are able to avoid recognition. They do this by having an intracellular habitat, by molecular mimicry (where critical antigens of the infectious agent are antigenically indistinguishable from host antigens) or by antigenic variation. Second, some microbes may modulate the effector arm of the immune response by interference with complement activation, by inhibiting phagocytosis, by decreasing antibody responses and/or by influencing the Th1 vs Th2 nature of the immune response.

Damage caused by pathogens

Pathogenic organisms can cause tissue damage and disease directly through the production of toxins. For example, bacteria and protozoa produce exotoxins and endotoxins. In addition, most viruses have a lytic stage resulting in tissue damage. On the other hand, the immune response to certain infectious microbes may be more destructive than the offending pathogen itself, especially in persistent states (Section K). Some examples are listed in *Table 1*. Mechanisms of immune-mediated damage to the host include anaphylaxis, immune complex disease, necrosis and apoptosis.

Table 1. *Pathogens and hypersensitivity*

Type I	Echinococcus – hydatid cyst, when it bursts it produces an anaphylactic response
Type II	Cross-reactions of antibodies to shared antigens, e.g. streptococci and heart tissues in rheumatic fever
Type III	Immune complex deposition in kidney, lung, blood vessel or joint causing glomerulonephritis (e.g. streptoccocal infection), bronchiectasis, vasculitis or arthritis, respectively
Type IV	Granuloma formation, e.g. TB and leprosy

H2 IMMUNITY TO DIFFERENT ORGANISMS

Key Notes

Immunity to bacteria	Extracellular bacteria may be killed directly through the alternative complement pathway or, after activation by antibody binding to the microbe, through the classical complement pathway. Antibodies and complement also act as opsonins facilitating engulfment and killing by phagocytes. For intracellular bacteria, e.g. TB bacilli, that evade the immune system by surviving in host cells such as monocytes and macrophages, a cell-mediated immune (CMI) response is required. This results in the release of cytokines such as IL-12 and IFNγ that enhance monocyte/macrophage killing of intracellular bacteria.
Immunity to virus	The innate immune system inhibitors of viral infection are IFNα and β. However when viruses replicate in host cells, a CTL response is required for their eradication. After infection, viral-specific peptides become expressed on the cell surface in MHC molecules and become targets for CTLs. Antibodies can neutralize free virus (prevent its attachment to, and infection of, target cells) and enhance phagocytosis of the virus.
Immunity to fungi	The immune response to fungal infections (mycoses) is poorly understood. While antibodies may have some role in their eradication, immunity principally involves T cells and macrophages.
Immunity to protozoa	Protozoa infections such as malaria, trypanosomiasis, leishmaniasis and toxoplasmosis are a major threat to health in the tropics and in the developing world. Protozoa are difficult to immunize against and protection is thought to require both cellular and humoral immunity.
Immunity to worms	Immune protection against helminths (worms) is difficult to achieve because of their size and complexity. The response mechanisms include the production of antibodies, especially IgE, and a cellular response including eosinophils, mast cells, macrophages and CD4 T cells. Degranulation of mast cells and eosinophils through IgE-antigen and IgA-antigen complexes results in acute inflammation and the release of cationic proteins and neurotoxins.
Related topics	Cells of the innate immune system (B1) Molecules of the innate immune system (B2) Innate immunity and inflammation (B4) Antibody functions (D8) Clonal expansion and the development of effector function (F5) The microbial cosmos (H1) Deficiencies in the immune system (J1)

Immunity to bacteria

A summary of the main effector defense mechanisms against extracellular bacteria is shown in *Fig. 1*. Bacteria that avoid destruction by the classical or alternative complement pathways may be opsonized by acute phase reactants or specific antibodies and engulfed by phagocytes expressing receptors for the Fc region of these antibodies. Both PMNs and macrophages express receptors for IgG as well as IgA. Inflammatory cytokines such as IFNγ can dramatically upregulate expression of these receptors and the efficiency of killing by these effector cells. In addition, the innate pattern recognition receptors expressed by macrophages and dendritic cells are important in cytokine production and initiating responses against bacteria (and other microbes) by the adaptive immune system (Topic B3).

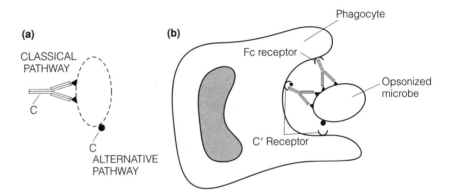

Fig. 1.   Defense mechanisms against extracellular bacteria. Bacteria can be killed by (a) complement-dependent lysis with or without antibodies and (b) phagocytosis following opsonization with complement and/or antibody alone.

Some bacteria invade host cells and survive in them, including TB bacilli, *Listeria monocytogenes*, *Salmonella typhi* and *Brucella* species. These **intracellular** bacteria evade the immune system's surveillance by surviving in host cells such as monocytes and macrophages. The immune system counteracts them by mounting a cell-mediated immune (CMI) response to the infection. Cells involved in the CMI response include Th1 and Th2 CD4 cells, CD8 cells, monocytes/macrophages and NK cells. Th1 cells release IFNγ, which makes the monocytes/macrophages more potent at killing intracellular bacteria and also enhances their antigen-presenting capabilities (*Fig. 2*). This CMI response is important not only in the protection against diseases such as TB, but also some viral and fungal infections.

Immunity to viruses

Natural immunity to viral infections is associated with interferons (especially IFNα and β) so called because of their interference with viral replication (Topic B2). IFNγ is probably most effective in protecting against extracellular bacteria through its ability to enhance immune-mediated mechanisms. Since viruses require attachment to host cells before they can replicate and cause infection, antibodies to the virus that prevent attachment represent an important mechanism that protects against viral infection. These protective antibodies may be IgG or IgA as in the case of polio prevention.

Since viruses replicate in cells where they are no longer exposed to circulating antibodies, their eradication depends upon killing the infected host cells.

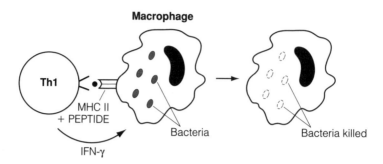

Fig. 2. Defense mechanisms against intracellular bacteria. Macrophages containing intracellular bacteria present microbial peptides on their MHC class II molecules to specific Th1 cells which produce IFNγ. This 'activates' the macrophage resulting in enhanced intracellular killing.

This of course would require a CTL response. As virally infected cells usually express viral peptides in MHC class I on their surface, they become targets for destruction by cytotoxic CD8 T cells. Cells infected by virus also become susceptible to killing by NK cells (Topic B1). In this way, viral replication is prevented and the viral infection eliminated (*Fig. 3*).

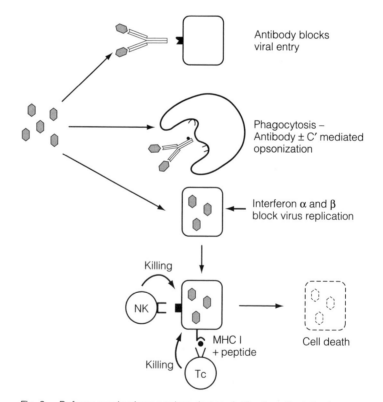

Fig. 3. Defense mechanisms against viruses. Antibodies attach to viruses preventing their entry into cells and opsonize them for phagocytosis. Interferons α and β block viral replication in infected cells. NK cells can kill virus infected cells if they have little or no expression of MHC class I. Tc cells kill virus-infected cells expressing viral peptides in MHC class I.

Immunity to fungi

Fungal diseases (mycoses) are common but are most problematic when associated with immunocompromised individuals (Topic J1). Although the immune response to fungal infections is poorly understood, it is clear that neutrophils and other phagocytic cells are important in removing infections caused by some fungi and that antibodies may have some role in their eradication. It also seems clear that protective immunity is principally cellular, especially in those infections deep within the body. This is particularly evidenced by studies of acquired immune deficiency syndrome (AIDS) patients where low T cell counts are commonly associated with fungal infections.

Immunity to protozoa

Protozoa infections such as malaria, trypanosomiasis, toxoplasmosis, leishmaniasis and amoebiasis are a major threat to health in the tropics and in particular in the developing world. Protozoa are difficult to immunize against and protection is thought to require both cellular and humoral immunity, although the humoral response, and in particular the IgG response, may be the most important.

In malaria, antibodies appear to protect against infection by preventing the merozoites (blood stage) from gaining entrance to red cells. However, there are several different strains of malaria and immunity to one strain or species may not be protective against others. Other innate or nonadaptive immune mechanisms may also be involved in protection against certain malaria infections. For example, individuals lacking the Duffy blood group antigen Fy (a-b-) are immune to *Plasmodium vivax* infection. Also, the hemoglobin structure associated with sickle cell anemia appears to be inhibitory to the intracellular growth of *P. falciparum*.

Trypanosomes continuously challenge the immune system by producing progeny with different antigens. Thus, as the immune system develops a response to antigens on these microbes, they change the structure of some of their surface proteins (switch antigenic coats) such that the antibodies produced in the initial response are no longer reactive or effective in mediating protection against this modified trypanosome. This leads to wave after wave of infection and response.

Toxoplasma acquire protection from the immune system by coating themselves with laminin, an extracellular matrix protein, which prevents phagocytosis and oxidative damage. The cellular response to *toxoplasma* appears to be most effective in combating infection, since patients with low T cell counts, as in HIV infection, are more at risk from infection with *toxoplasma*. Other protozoan diseases such as leishmaniasis have a predilection for infecting macrophages and require a cellular response for eradication. Moreover, a Th1 response seems to be essential for protection, since IFNγ appears to be the most important cytokine for parasite killing.

Immunity to worms

An immune response to worms (helminths) is difficult to achieve and not very effective, probably as a result of the size and complexity of these microbes. Thus, diseases such as those caused by *Schistosoma mansoni* (schistosomiasis) and *Wuchereria bancrofti* (lymphatic filariasis, elephantiasis) represent major problems, especially in the developing world. Although PMNs, macrophages and NK cells may be involved, the main protective mechanism against helminths appears to be mediated by eosinophils and mast cells. While worms are too large to be phagocytosed, they can be coated with IgE, IgA and IgG antibodies. In the event that this happens, the major phagocytic cells as well as eosinophils and mast cells will bind to the parasite's surface through their Fc receptors for these molecules and release their toxic cellular contents. Both mast cells and eosinophils degranulate in the presence of IgE–antigen complexes. When mast cells degranulate they release histamine, serotonin and leukotrienes. These vasoactive amines are neurotransmitters and cause neurovasculature as well as neuromuscular changes resulting in gut spasm diarrhea and the expulsion of material from the intestine. Eosinophils also have IgA receptors and have been shown to release their granule contents when these receptors are cross-linked. On degranulation, eosinophils release powerful antagonistic chemicals and proteins including cationic proteins, neurotoxins and hydrogen peroxide, which also probably contribute to a hostile environment for worm habitation. Helminth infections usually direct the immune system towards a Th2 response and the production of IgE, IgA and Th2 cytokines as well as the chemokine eotaxin. The Th2 cytokines IL-3, IL-4 and IL-5 as well as the chemokine eotaxin are chemotactic for eosinophils and mast cells. *Fig. 4* summarizes the major immune mechanisms for removal of helminths.

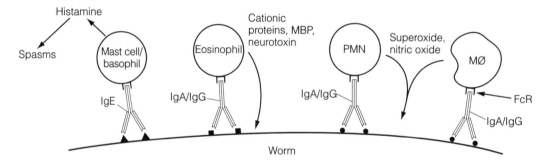

Fig. 4. Defense mechanisms against worms. Worms are usually too large to phagocytose, but coated with specific antibodies they can activate a number of 'effector' cells via their Fc receptor (FcR). IgE-mediated degranulation of mast cells/basophils results in production of histamine, which causes spasms in the intestine where these worms are often found. Eosinophils attach to the worm via IgG/IgA antibodies and release cationic proteins, major basic protein and neurotoxin. PMNs and macrophages attach via IgG or IgA antibodies and release superoxide, nitric oxide and enzymes which kill the worm.

H3 PATHOGEN DEFENSE STRATEGIES

Key Notes

The battle to stay ahead	Over time, microbes have developed strategies to circumvent and/or inactivate host immune defense mechanisms. Some pathogens avoid immune recognition by intracellular habitat, mimicking of self-antigens, encapsulation or by changing their surface antigens (antigenic variation). Other pathogens compromise effector mechanisms by inhibiting complement activation, phagocytosis and/or cytokine production, and through superantigens or immunosuppression.
Avoidance of recognition	The intracellular habitat of viruses, some bacteria and protozoa prevents recognition by innate and adaptive immune systems. Other microbes can change their antigens by mutation (drift), by nucleic acid recombination (antigenic shift) and by switching genes encoding cell surface antigens. Still other microbes express antigens very similar to self antigens (molecular mimicry), while others wear the antigens of the host they are infecting. Furthermore, distraction of lymphoid cells may be achieved through poly- or oligoclonal activation by microbial products.
Inactivation of immune effector mechanisms	Some microbes can inhibit phagocytosis, a critical mechanism for killing extracellular microbes. Viruses such as hepatitis B inhibit the production of IFNα by infected cells. Low-affinity antibodies are produced to some organisms, e.g. treponemes, while others inactivate the antibodies by production of proteases. Complement activation is also blocked by some viruses and bacteria. CD4$^+$ T cells are inactivated by HIV and some viruses decrease expression of MHC class I molecules by infected cells, blocking the activity of cytotoxic T cells. Other microbes produce endotoxins that channel the immune response toward one that is ineffective, e.g. inducing a humoral response when a cellular response is required for protection.
Related topics	The microbial cosmos (H1) Immunity to different organisms (H2)
	Autoimmune diseases – mechanisms of development (L3)

The battle to stay ahead

Immune defense against pathogens is dependent on first being able to recognize the intruder as a threat, and second being able to eliminate it. While the physical and mechanical barriers as well as the adaptive and nonadaptive immune systems are powerful in the prevention of infection, microbes have developed ways of both avoiding recognition and of inactivating components used for their elimination (*Table 1*). Some pathogens avoid immune recognition by intracellular habitat, mimicking of self-antigens, encapsulation or by changing their surface antigens (antigenic variation). Other pathogens compromise effector mechanisms of immunity by inhibiting complement activation, phagocytosis and/or cytokine production. They can release soluble neutralizing antigens,

Table 1. Pathogen defense strategies

Avoidance of recognition	
Intracellular habitat	Viruses, mycobacteria, *Brucella*, *Legionella*
Antigenic variation	
Drift	Viruses undergo mutation to alter antigens, e.g. influenza, HIV
Shift	Recombination with animal viral nucleic acids, e.g. influenza pandemics
Gene switching	Expression of a sequence of different surface antigens, e.g. *Borellia*, *Trypanosoma*
Disguise	
Molecular mimicry	Microbes have antigens in common with self, e.g. *Streptococcus*, bacteroides
Coating with self proteins	Covering of surface with serum proteins, e.g. *Schistosoma*, *Toxoplasma*
Immune distraction	Some microbes, e.g. *Staphylococcus*, produce superantigens which stimulate many different B and T cells, diluting the effects of specific antigens
Inactivation of host immune effector mechanisms	
Phagocytosis	Encapsulation of some bacteria inhibits phagocytosis e.g. *Pneumococci*, *H. influenzae* and *E. coli*.
Cytokines	Inhibition of interferon production e.g. Hepatitis B
Antibodies	Low-affinity antibody production e.g. treponemes
	Neutralization of antibody by large amounts of soluble antigens, e.g. *Streptococcus pneumoniae*, *Candida* sp.
	Release of proteases that cleave IgA e.g. *Pseudomonas* sp., *Neisseria gonorrhoeae*, *H. influenzae*
	Production of proteins that bind to the IgG Fc region and prevent opsonization, e.g. *Staphylococcus* protein A
Complement activation (classical pathway)	Inhibition by incorporation of host complement regulatory proteins into microbial cell wall, e.g. HIV
T cells	CD4 T cells infected and killed, e.g. HIV
Antigen processing and presentation	Inhibition of antigen processing, e.g. measles virus
Regulatory mechanisms	Endotoxins released by some microbes induce a Th2 response that is ineffective against intracellular microbes e.g. *Salmonella typhi*

produce enzymes capable of destroying antibodies or complement, produce superantigens or induce overall immunosuppression.

Avoidance of recognition

Intracellular habitat

Viruses, some bacteria (e.g. mycobacteria, listeria, *Salmonella typhi* and *Brucella* species) and certain protozoa (i.e., malaria-causing *Plasmodium falciparum*, *P. malariae*, *P. ovale* and *P. vivax*) are obligate intracellular organisms, thus evading direct recognition by, and the effects of, the innate and adaptive immune systems.

Antigenic variation

Alteration of cell surface antigens through mutation (**antigenic drift**) is achieved by some viruses, e.g. influenza. This makes it very difficult for the immune system to keep up, as a continuous primary response would need to be generated. The recombination of nucleic acids from human and animal viruses can lead to major **antigenic shifts**, and is known to be responsible for pandemics, e.g. influenza. Other organisms can produce continuous changes in their antigenic coat distracting the immune system, e.g. trypanosomes, *Borrelia recurrentis*. In the case of trypanosoma, at least 100 different surface coats can be expressed in sequence.

Disguise

Some microbes use antigens common or cross-reactive with self to try to look like self antigens (**molecular mimicry**) so as to appear nonimmunogenic. For example, the hyaluronic acid capsule of some streptoccocal species is the same as that of host connective tissue. While this seems an excellent strategy, it can lead to the development of autoimmune disease (Topic L3). *Schistosoma* wears the antigens of the host that it infects, again trying to look like self. In other cases, specific T cells and B cells can be 'distracted' through poly- or oligoclonal activation by microbial products. For example, an enterotoxin of *Staphylococcus* (a 'superantigen'), activates large numbers of T cells independent of their specificity. Similarly, Epstein–Barr virus activates most B cells but they only produce low-affinity IgM antibodies and few are directed to the virus.

Inactivation of immune effector mechanisms

In this approach the microbe attempts to create at least a partial state of immunodeficiency or immunosuppression in the host in order to allow it to survive.

Phagocytosis

Phagocytes play a critical role in the killing of extracellular microbes and do this primarily through phagocytosis. Microbes use different strategies to inhibit several of the stages of phagocytosis (Topic B1). Virulent strains of *Pneumococcus*, *H. influenzae* and *E. coli* are encapsulated making them difficult to phagocytose. Once engulfed, microbes are normally killed in phagolysosomes through oxygen-dependent and oxygen-independent mechanisms. Some microbes have developed enzymes that inhibit the oxygen burst, an essential event leading to killing. Certain strains of staphylococci have a protein coat (protein A) that can also inactivate IgG and IgA antibodies by binding to their Fc fragment thereby preventing them from acting as opsonins.

Inhibition of cytokines

Some viruses inhibit the production of IFNα by infected cells. This is seen in hepatitis B infection of hepatocytes.

Antibodies

Some organisms, e.g. treponemes, induce low-affinity antibodies, while others, e.g. *Streptococcus pneumoniae* and *Candida*, release large amounts of soluble antigens that bind to antibodies and block their binding to the microbe. In another strategy, microbes produce proteases that destroy antibodies. Bacteria associated with mucosal infections such as *Neisseria gonorrhoeae* and *Pseudomonas* species produce protease enzymes that can destroy IgA, the antibody associated with mucosal protection. Pseudomonas also produces an elastase that inactivates C3b and C5a inhibiting opsonization and chemotaxis.

The complement system

Some organisms block complement activation and the lytic effects of complement. For example, HIV incorporates host complement regulatory proteins in its outer membranes to counteract the activation of complement.

T cells

HIV targets CD4 T cells, infecting and destroying them, effectively disarming the immune system and leaving the host immunodeficient. Some viruses decrease the expression of MHC class I on infected cells thus making it difficult for cognate interactions and killing of the infected cell by CD8$^+$ cytotoxic T cells.

Antigen processing

Measles virus, as well as infecting human T cells, inhibits antigen processing required to generate an immune response against it.

Regulatory mechanisms

Microbes such as S. typhi produce endotoxins that predispose the immune system to develop a Th2 response and thus primarily humoral immunity to the pathogen. However, eradication of these organisms requires a cellular response.

I1 PRINCIPLES OF VACCINATION

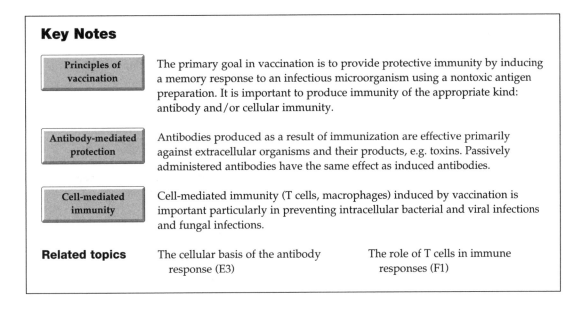

Key Notes

Principles of vaccination	The primary goal in vaccination is to provide protective immunity by inducing a memory response to an infectious microorganism using a nontoxic antigen preparation. It is important to produce immunity of the appropriate kind: antibody and/or cellular immunity.
Antibody-mediated protection	Antibodies produced as a result of immunization are effective primarily against extracellular organisms and their products, e.g. toxins. Passively administered antibodies have the same effect as induced antibodies.
Cell-mediated immunity	Cell-mediated immunity (T cells, macrophages) induced by vaccination is important particularly in preventing intracellular bacterial and viral infections and fungal infections.
Related topics	The cellular basis of the antibody response (E3) The role of T cells in immune responses (F1)

Principles of vaccination

Edward Jenner, a country physician in England, noticed that dairymaids who frequently contracted cowpox often were immune to the ravages of smallpox, leading him to develop an approach whereby cowpox was used to vaccinate people against smallpox. The term vaccination is derived from the Latin word 'vaccinus' meaning 'from cows'. Vaccination eventually resulted in the complete eradication of smallpox (in 1980) and has been generalized as a reliable method of protection against many pathogens.

The aims of vaccination are to induce memory in T and/or B lymphocytes through the injection of a nonvirulent antigen preparation. Thus, in the event of an actual infection, the infectious agent and/or its toxin is met by a secondary rather than a primary response. The ideal vaccine would protect the individual and ultimately eliminate the disease, but most vaccines simply protect the individual. A more or less standard set of vaccines are now in use worldwide, some of which are (or should be) given to everyone and others to those particularly at risk (*Table 1*). The timing of vaccination depends on the likelihood of infection; vaccines against common infections being given as early as possible, allowing for the fact that some vaccines do not work properly in very young infants.

Antibody-mediated protection

Antibodies either produced as a result of immunization or passively introduced into the host are very effective means of preventing infection. They will be ready and able to bind the infectious agent at the time of infection instead of waiting for the host's immune system to respond. Antibodies can either block

Table 1.   *Vaccine recommendations*

Recommended for	Vaccine	When given/to whom
All	Measles Mumps Rubella	From 1 year (6 months in tropics) boost at 10–14 yrs
	Diphtheria Tetanus Pertussis	From 2–3 months old dip/tet boost at 5 yrs
	Polio (Sabin) (or *Salk)	2–6 months (oral) parenterally
All, unless Mantoux +	BCG	10–14 yrs (at birth in tropics)
Those at risk	Hepatitis B	1–6 months/12 intervals (childhood in tropics)
	Hepatitis A Influenza Rabies Meningococcus Pneumococcus Haemophilus Varicella-zoster	Institutions, nurses etc., annual boost needed Travel, post-exposure: vaccine + antibody Epidemics Elderly Children Children with leukaemia
At risk (travel)	Typhoid Cholera Yellow fever	Travelers Travelers Travelers: boost 10 intervals

* The Salk is the polio vaccine of choice in Holland and Scandinavia.

viral or bacterial antigens from entering host cells by preventing adherence or prevent damaging effects on other cells by neutralizing toxins such as those produced by *Diphtheria* or *Clostridium* species (Topic H2). IgA plays an important role at the mucosal surfaces where it helps to prevent viral or bacterial access to the mucosa lining cells. This is the mechanism by which polio vaccination works.

IgG antibodies are usually effective in the blood. Antibodies can also be transferred across the placenta to provide **passive immunity**. Mothers transfer their preformed IgG antibodies across the placenta to their newborn in order to protect them during the first months of life (Topic C5). This passive transfer can be of a disadvantage in that the presence of the maternal antibody inhibits effective immunization. Thus, immunization has to be delayed until after most of the maternal antibodies have been catabolized.

In pre-antibiotic days, it was common to treat or prevent infection by injecting antibody preformed in another animal, usually a horse or a recently recovered patient. This principle is still in use for certain acute conditions where it is too late to induce active immunity by vaccinating the patient (see Topic J4).

Cell-mediated immunity

While antibodies may play a major role in combating infections, cell-mediated immunity is essential for eradicating certain bacteria, fungi and protozoa (Topic F1): vaccination should therefore be aimed at inducing both cellular and humoral responses to the infectious agent. In certain instances not only are CD4 and CD8 lymphocyte responses desired but it may be more advantageous to specifically target Th1 or Th2 responses e.g., infections with helminths might favour a Th2 type immunity via induction of IgE antibodies, whereas protection against mycobacterial infections may be better obtained by a Th1 response, by producing macrophage activation factors (e.g. IFNγ). CD8 cytotoxic T lymphocytes find and kill infected cells which express proteins that are components of pathogens. The cell that is targeted is determined by the presence of the foreign protein in association with MHC class I molecules. The CD8 T cells lyse the infected cell; hopefully before progeny infectious organisms are fully developed. The CD4 cells are basically the directors of the immune response. These cells interact with foreign antigen expressed with MHC class II molecules and then provide soluble or membrane bound signals for B cells, macrophages or CD8 T cells to help them obtain their full effector cell functions: Ig production by B cells, killing by macrophages and CD8 T cells. Some diseases only require an antibody response for protection or clearance, while others require a cell-mediated immune response. Still other diseases are only resolved if both forms of protection are present.

12 IMMUNIZATION

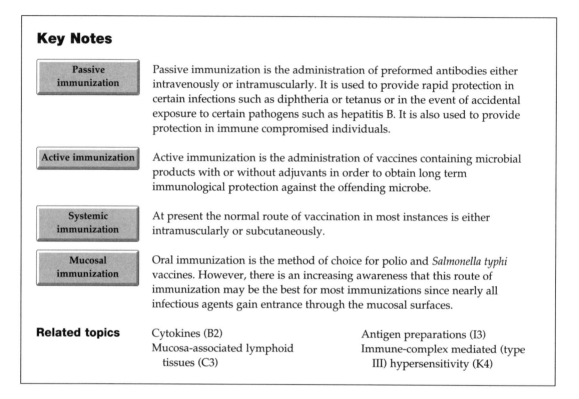

Key Notes

Passive immunization

Passive immunization is the administration of preformed antibodies either intravenously or intramuscularly. It is used to provide rapid protection in certain infections such as diphtheria or tetanus or in the event of accidental exposure to certain pathogens such as hepatitis B. It is also used to provide protection in immune compromised individuals.

Active immunization

Active immunization is the administration of vaccines containing microbial products with or without adjuvants in order to obtain long term immunological protection against the offending microbe.

Systemic immunization

At present the normal route of vaccination in most instances is either intramuscularly or subcutaneously.

Mucosal immunization

Oral immunization is the method of choice for polio and *Salmonella typhi* vaccines. However, there is an increasing awareness that this route of immunization may be the best for most immunizations since nearly all infectious agents gain entrance through the mucosal surfaces.

Related topics

Cytokines (B2)	Antigen preparations (I3)
Mucosa-associated lymphoid tissues (C3)	Immune-complex mediated (type III) hypersensitivity (K4)

Passive immunization

Passive immunization is the administration of preformed antibodies, usually IgG, either intravenously or intramuscularly. These antibodies may be derived from individuals who have high titres to particular microbes and are used to provide rapid protection in certain infections such as *Diphtheria*, *Clostridium* species, rabies etc., or in the event of accidental exposure to certain pathogens such as hepatitis B. Passive immunization is also used to provide protection in immune compromised individuals who are unable to make the appropriate antibody response or in some instances incapable of making any antibody at all, i.e., severe combined immunodeficiency. Antibodies given to immune deficient patients are usually IgG-derived from pooled normal plasma. These antibodies have to be given on a continuous basis, ideally every three weeks, since they are being continuously catabolized and only effective for a short period. Antibodies preformed in animals, notably horses, are also administered for some diseases. However, it is important that with repeated injections of horse antibody, there is the danger of immune complex formation and serum sickness (Topic K4). Antisera are usually injected intramuscularly, but can be given intravenously in extremely acute conditions. Indications for the use of passive immunization by the injection of preformed antibody are shown in *Table 1*.

Table 1. *Passive immunization*

Infection	Source of antiserum	Indications
Tetanus	Immune human; horse	Post exposure (plus vaccine)
Diphtheria	Horse	Post-exposure
Gas gangrene	Horse	Post-exposure
Botulism	Horse	Post-exposure
Varicella-zoster	Immune human	Post-exposure in immunodeficiency
Rabies	Immune human	Post-exposure (plus vaccine)
Hepatitis B	Immune human	Post-exposure Prophylaxis
Hepatitis A	Pooled human Ig	Prophylaxis
Measles	Immune human	Post-exposure in infants
Snakebite	Horse	Post-bite
Some autoimmune diseases	Pooled human Ig	Acute thrombocytopenia and neutropenia

Active immunization

Administration of vaccines containing microbial products with or without adjuvants in order to obtain long term immunological protection against the offending microbe is termed active immunization. Immunization can be given via two different routes.

Systemic immunization

Systemic immunization is the method of choice at present for most vaccinations. This is usually carried out by injecting the vaccine subcutaneously or intramuscularly into the deltoid muscle. Ideally all vaccines would be given soon after birth, but some are deliberately delayed, for various reasons. The common systemic vaccines for measles, mumps and rubella are usually given at 1 year of age because, if given earlier, maternal antibody would decrease their effectiveness. The carbohydrate vaccines for *Pneumococcus*, *Meningococcus* and *Haemophilus* infections are usually given at about 2 years of age as before this age they respond poorly to polysaccharides unless they are associated with protein components that can act to recruit T cell help for the development of anti-polysaccharide antibody, e.g. hen egg albumin (Topic I3).

Mucosal immunization

Recent vaccination approaches have focused on the mucosal route as the site of choice for immunization either orally or through the nasal associated immune tissue (NALT: Topic C3). This is because most infectious agents gain entry to the systemic system through these routes and the largest source of lymphoid tissue is at the mucosal surfaces. Moreover, if successful it would obviate the need for, in some instances, painful injections and allow for the self-administration of certain vaccines such as those used for immunization against influenza. Adjuvant vaccines and live vectors have been used to target the mucosal immune system with some success. Attenuated strains of salmonella can act as a powerful immune stimulus as well as acting as carriers of foreign antigens. This approach has been used to immunize mucosal surfaces against herpes simplex virus and human papilloma virus. Furthermore, bacterial toxins, e.g. those derived from cholera, *E. coli* and *Bordetella pertussis*, have immunomodulatory properties and are thus being exploited in the development of mucosally active adjuvants. Pertussis toxin has been shown to augment the costimulatory molecules B-7 on B cells and CD28 on T cells (Topic F4) as well as increasing IFNγ production. Hopefully, oral and nasal vaccines may soon be available to obviate the need for the invasive techniques that are currently in use.

13 ANTIGEN PREPARATIONS

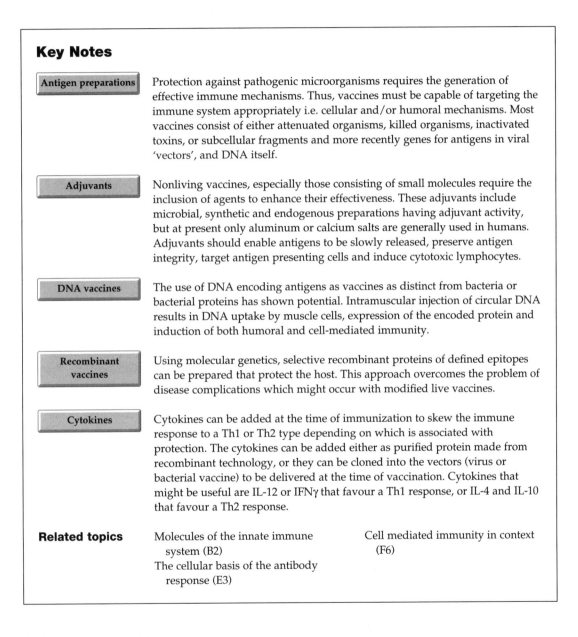

Key Notes

Antigen preparations
Protection against pathogenic microorganisms requires the generation of effective immune mechanisms. Thus, vaccines must be capable of targeting the immune system appropriately i.e. cellular and/or humoral mechanisms. Most vaccines consist of either attenuated organisms, killed organisms, inactivated toxins, or subcellular fragments and more recently genes for antigens in viral 'vectors', and DNA itself.

Adjuvants
Nonliving vaccines, especially those consisting of small molecules require the inclusion of agents to enhance their effectiveness. These adjuvants include microbial, synthetic and endogenous preparations having adjuvant activity, but at present only aluminum or calcium salts are generally used in humans. Adjuvants should enable antigens to be slowly released, preserve antigen integrity, target antigen presenting cells and induce cytotoxic lymphocytes.

DNA vaccines
The use of DNA encoding antigens as vaccines as distinct from bacteria or bacterial proteins has shown potential. Intramuscular injection of circular DNA results in DNA uptake by muscle cells, expression of the encoded protein and induction of both humoral and cell-mediated immunity.

Recombinant vaccines
Using molecular genetics, selective recombinant proteins of defined epitopes can be prepared that protect the host. This approach overcomes the problem of disease complications which might occur with modified live vaccines.

Cytokines
Cytokines can be added at the time of immunization to skew the immune response to a Th1 or Th2 type depending on which is associated with protection. The cytokines can be added either as purified protein made from recombinant technology, or they can be cloned into the vectors (virus or bacterial vaccine) to be delivered at the time of vaccination. Cytokines that might be useful are IL-12 or IFNγ that favour a Th1 response, or IL-4 and IL-10 that favour a Th2 response.

Related topics
Molecules of the innate immune system (B2)
The cellular basis of the antibody response (E3)

Cell mediated immunity in context (F6)

Antigen preparations

The protective immune response to pathogenic microorganisms requires the generation of specific T and B cell responses and appropriate effector mechanisms. In order to do this, vaccines must be capable of targeting the immune system appropriately. In principle anything from whole organisms to small peptides can be used, but in practice most vaccines consist of either attenuated organisms, killed organisms, inactivated toxins, or subcellular fragments (*Table 1*).

Table 1. Antigen preparations used in vaccines

Type of antigen	Examples	
	Viruses	Bacteria
Normal heterologous organism	Vaccinia (cowpox)	
Living attenuated organism	Measles	BCG
	Mumps	Typhoid (new)
	Rubella	
	Polio: Sabin	
	Yellow fever	
	Varicella-zoster	
Whole killed organism	Rabies	Pertussis
	Polio: Salk	Typhoid
	Influenza	Cholera
Subcellular fragment		
Inactivated toxin (toxoid)		Diphtheria
		Tetanus
		Cholera (new)
Capsular polysaccharide		*Meningococcus*
		Pneumococcus
		Haemophilus
		Typhoid (new)
Surface antigen	Hepatitis B	

There is also a fundamental distinction between live and dead vaccines. Living and nonliving vaccines differ in many important respects, notably safety and effectiveness. Live ones consist of organisms (nearly always viruses) that have been attenuated by growth in unfavourable conditions, forcing them to mutate their genes; mutants that have lost virulence but retain antigenicity are repeatedly selected. Nowadays, mutation is usually 'site-directed' by recombinant DNA technology. Such organisms, which are essentially new strains, can sometimes regain virulence by back-mutation, and can also cause severe disease in immunocompromised individuals. On the other hand they often induce stronger and better localized immunity, do not often require adjuvants or 'booster' injections and provide the possibility of 'herd' immunity in that mutated nonvirulent virus could be transferred to nonimmunized individuals in a local community. Moreover, the immunity induced is usually more appropriate for protection against the pathogenic strain of the organism, e.g. Th1 vs Th2 responses.

Killed organisms or molecules derived for these organisms are used when for some reason stable attenuated organisms cannot be produced. These antigens may however induce weak and/or inappropriate (e.g. antibody vs CTL) responses. Immune memory may be variable or poor, but they are usually safe if properly inactivated. In only one case (polio) is there a choice between effective live and killed vaccines. Recently, it has been shown that the genes for one or more antigens can be inserted into a living vaccine (usually virus) 'vector', and experiments are being performed with totally synthetic peptides, the idiotype network, and even DNA itself.

Adjuvants

Nonliving vaccines, especially those consisting of small molecules, are not very strong antigens, but can be made stronger by injecting them along with some other substance such as aluminum hydroxide, aluminum phosphate, calcium phosphate or hen egg albumin; such substances are called adjuvants. The properties of adjuvants should include the following: (i) the ability to enable antigens to be slowly released so as to prolong antigen exposure time to the immune system; (ii) preserve antigen integrity; (iii) target antigen presenting cells; (iv) induce cytotoxic lymphocytes; (v) produce high affinity immune responses; and (vi) have the capacity for selective immune intervention. A variety of microbial, synthetic, and endogenous preparations have adjuvant activity, but at present only aluminum and calcium salts are approved for general use in man.

Combinations of macromolecules (oils and bacterial macromolecules) are commonly used as adjuvants in experimental animals to promote an immune response. The oil in the adjuvants increases retention of the antigen, causes aggregation of the antigen (promoting immunogenicity), and inflammation at the site of inoculation. Inflammation increases the response of macrophages and causes local cytokine production, which can modulate the costimulatory molecules, needed for T cell activation. Microparticles have also been used as adjuvants in the experimental model; these include latex beads and poly (lactide-co-glycolide) microparticles. Adjuvants are now being designed and tested to determine how to selectively drive Th1 or Th2 responses. Some experimental adjuvants currently under investigation are shown in *Table 2*.

Table 2. *Experimental adjuvants currently undergoing assessment*

Experimental, but likely to be approved
Liposomes (small synthetic lipid vesicles)
Muramyl dipeptide, an active component of mycobacterial cell walls
Immune-stimulating complexes (ISCOMS) (e.g. from cholesterol or phospholipids)
Bacterial toxins (*E. coli*, pertussis, cholera)

Experimental only
Cytokines: IL-1, IL-2, IFNγ
Slow-release devices; Freunds adjuvant
Immune complexes

DNA vaccines

A few years ago an exciting discovery was made when it was shown that 'naked' cDNA that encoded the hemagglutinin of the flu virus could be inoculated into muscle tissue to stimulate both antibody production and a CTL response that was specific for the flu protein. The potential for this is still unknown, but if this can become a routine method of immunization, then the cost of generating and transporting vaccines should be very low. Other uses of recombinant DNA technology are the cloning of defined epitopes into viral or bacterial hosts. Typically well characterized infectious agents such as vaccinia, polio, or *Salmonella* are used. DNA sequences are cloned into the genome of these agents and are expressed in target structures that are known to be immunogenic for the host. This way the antigen is presented for optimal recognition by the host. Inclusion of cytokines with the vaccine vectors may prove to be an efficient method for ensuring the correct cytokine environment to steer the immune response accordingly. DNA vaccines have potentially a number of advantages over traditional methods of vaccination. These include specificity, the induction of potent Th1 and cytotoxic T lymphocyte responses similar to those observed with attenuated vaccines but without the potential to revert to overt infection.

Recombinant vaccines

Advances in molecular virology and bacteriology have provided the immunologist with many new targets for vaccine development. The last 20 years of study of viral and bacterial pathogenesis have identified the components of the immune system that are protective for many infectious agents. The use of defined epitopes that are protective for vaccines is now possible. The idea is that certain parts of an infectious disease causing organism, such as herpes virus glycoprotein D (glyD), stimulate CTL that are protective. If the host is inoculated with the defined peptide of glyD, they develop CTL responses to the epitope and do not have to worry about resulting disease from vaccination with a modified live vaccine. This approach is also possible for protection to infectious agents that is provided by antibody. In this scenario, both a B cell epitope (the site that the antibody binds to on the infectious agent) and a T cell epitope (the peptide that binds to the MHC Class II to stimulate the CD4 helper cells) must be present, so as to select the appropriate B cells, and to stimulate the specific T cell help.

Cytokines

The effects of cytokines can influence the function of professional antigen presenting cells (APC) enabling these cells with much greater efficiency. Thus, IFNγ and IL-4 causes increased levels of class II molecules to be expressed thereby enhancing their antigen presentation abilities. The use of such effector cytokines is being considered as a useful adjunct in vaccination, as polarization of the immune system to a Th1 or Th2 response may be preferable in some instances, e.g. a Th1 response is the preferred response in tuberculosis whereas a Th2 response is important in protecting against polio. Since Th1 and Th2 responses are mutually inhibitory manipulation of these responses may open up avenues of selective intervention.

14 VACCINES TO PATHOGENS AND TUMORS

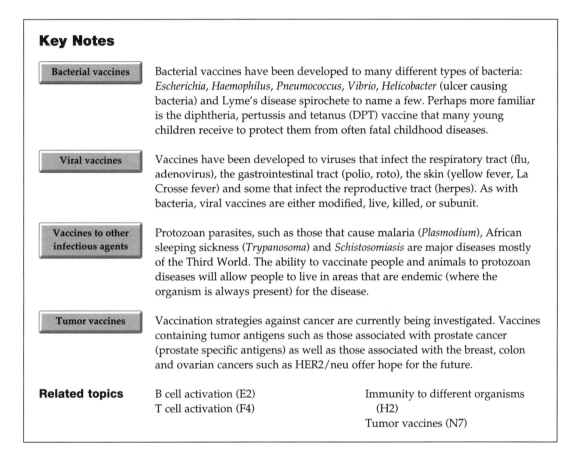

Key Notes

Bacterial vaccines	Bacterial vaccines have been developed to many different types of bacteria: *Escherichia, Haemophilus, Pneumococcus, Vibrio, Helicobacter* (ulcer causing bacteria) and Lyme's disease spirochete to name a few. Perhaps more familiar is the diphtheria, pertussis and tetanus (DPT) vaccine that many young children receive to protect them from often fatal childhood diseases.
Viral vaccines	Vaccines have been developed to viruses that infect the respiratory tract (flu, adenovirus), the gastrointestinal tract (polio, roto), the skin (yellow fever, La Crosse fever) and some that infect the reproductive tract (herpes). As with bacteria, viral vaccines are either modified, live, killed, or subunit.
Vaccines to other infectious agents	Protozoan parasites, such as those that cause malaria (*Plasmodium*), African sleeping sickness (*Trypanosoma*) and *Schistosomiasis* are major diseases mostly of the Third World. The ability to vaccinate people and animals to protozoan diseases will allow people to live in areas that are endemic (where the organism is always present) for the disease.
Tumor vaccines	Vaccination strategies against cancer are currently being investigated. Vaccines containing tumor antigens such as those associated with prostate cancer (prostate specific antigens) as well as those associated with the breast, colon and ovarian cancers such as HER2/neu offer hope for the future.
Related topics	B cell activation (E2) Immunity to different organisms T cell activation (F4) (H2) Tumor vaccines (N7)

Bacterial vaccines

Bacterial vaccines have been developed to many different types of bacteria: *Escherichia, Haemophilus, Pneumococcus, Vibrio, Helicobacter* (ulcer causing bacteria) and Lyme's disease spirochete to name a few. Perhaps more familiar is the diphtheria, pertussis and tetanus (DPT) vaccine that many young children receive to protect them from often fatal childhood diseases. Some bacterial vaccines are specific for proteins on the bacteria that are required for their attachment and subsequent invasion of the host. Vaccines can be used to induce immunity to endo- or exotoxins. Vaccines, as typified by BCG (*Mycobacterium tuberculosis*) are used to protect against tuberculosis. Modified, live, killed, and subunit vaccines have been developed for various bacteria. The difference in the forms will be discussed below. T-independent vaccines to carbohydrates such as the capsule of *Pneumococcus* or *Haemophilus* are in use. These vaccines are effective but have limitations because T cell help is not provided for affinity maturation and isotype switching.

Viral vaccines   Vaccines to viruses that infect the respiratory tract (flu, adenovirus), that infect the gastrointestinal tract (polio, roto), that infect the skin (yellow fever, La Crosse fever) and some that infect the reproductive tract (herpes) have been developed. As with bacteria, viral vaccines are either modified-live, killed, or subunit. The recent emergence of HIV virus as a world-wide health hazard has focused the world's attention on viral vaccine development. In fact, some viral vaccines have been developed for viruses that are in the same genetic classification group as HIV. These have proven to be effective, but why not for HIV? This question highlights an important issue in vaccine development. What is a good vaccine? They must be safe, effective, cheap to make and distribute, stable for long-term storage or transport, be insensitive to major changes in temperature and they should provoke an immune response that lasts for a long period of time.

Vaccines to other infectious agents   Protozoan parasites, such as those that cause malaria (*Plasmodium*), African sleeping sickness (*Trypanosoma*) and *Schistosomiasis* are very important diseases mostly of the Third World. The ability to vaccinate people and animals to protozoan diseases will allow people to live in areas that are endemic (the organism is always present) for the disease. Parasites express many antigens which are usually immunogenic, but most do not consistently stimulate protective responses. Of note, parasites have evolved defense mechanisms that allow a continual evolution of the immunogenic epitopes. This is best typified by *Plasmodium* that continually and rapidly develops variants with different surface proteins so that the current immune response is no longer effective. Parasites have also developed mechanisms to shift the focus of the immune response by altering the cytokine profile during the induction phase to one that is not protective (e.g. from Th1 to Th2 as in the case of *Mycobacterium lepri*) (Topic H3).

Tumor vaccines   These vaccines are in their infancy. In principle, the immune system should be able to recognize tumors which may have foreign antigens associated with them through immune surveillance. This works in part, but most tumor associated antigens are either absent or weakly immunogenic through being expressed at low levels. In experimental animals, tumors that are induced by chemicals are more likely to have new or neo-antigens that are immunogenic and are characteristic of the individual tumors. Most new approaches to both direct therapy and vaccines is through targeting the overexpressed products of protooncogenes which have been found in a variety of tumors. For example, the HER2/neu antigen is overexpressed by many prostate and breast tumors. The major challenge for immunologists is to optimize the routes of delivery of these antigens to maximize induction of protective immunity (Topic N7). Clearly of importance is the role of CTLs in immunity to tumors and recently immunogenic peptides have been isolated from class I molecules expressed on myeloma tumor cells which are effective at inducing tumor specific immunity.

J1 DEFICIENCIES IN THE IMMUNE SYSTEM

Key Notes

Components of the immune system

Each of the four components of the immune system (T cells, B cells, phagocytes, and complement) has its domain of function important to protection against certain pathogens. These components are intimately integrated into a program of immune defense that could be severely compromised if even one were absent or deficient.

Defects in specific immune components

The occurrence of repeated or unusual infections in a patient is a primary indication of immunodeficiency. Although a deficiency may compromise several components of the immune system, in most instances the deficiency is more restricted and results in susceptibility to infection by some but not all microbes. For example, defects in T cells tend to result in infections with intracellular microbes, whereas those involving other components result in extracellular infections.

Classification of immunodeficiencies

Immunodeficiencies are either primary (mostly congenital/inherited), or secondary (acquired as the consequences of other diseases and their treatments). These can be defined on the basis of the specific immune component that is abnormal.

Related topics

Hemopoiesis – development of blood cells (A5)
Cells of the innate immune system (B1)
Molecules of the innate immune system (B2)

Antibody functions (D8)
Clonal expansion and the development of effector function (F5)

Components of the immune system

The multiple interactive cellular and molecular components making up the immune response usually provide sufficient protection against bacterial, viral or fungal infections. However, any situation that results in impaired immune function may contribute to a spectrum of disorders referred to as immunodeficiency diseases. In particular, immunodeficiency is defined as an increased susceptibility to infection.

It is evident from a consideration of the disorders and infections in individuals with selective immunodeficiency that each component of the immune response (T cells, B cells, phagocytes and complement) has its domain of function. These four systems, although somewhat independent, are intimately integrated into a program of immune defense that could be severely compromised if even one were absent or deficient. In particular, the requirements for cell cooperation, the importance of chemotactic stimuli and activating factors emphasize the interdependence of these systems and the potential consequences of an abnormality in any of these systems. However, although the absence of, or an abnormality in one domain may compromise the individual, they need not be life threatening if other components of the immune system can compensate for this deficiency.

Defects in specific immune components

The occurrence of repeated or unusual infections in a patient is a primary indication of abnormalities in immune function and of immunodeficiency. A variety of circumstances may be involved in this impairment of immune function including genetic, tumors, irradiation, cancer chemotherapy, malnutrition, aging, etc. Although it is possible that the deficiency could be global and thus effect several components of the immune system (e.g. as in the case of severe combined immunodeficiency), in most instances the deficiency is restricted to a single component. Such deficiencies result in susceptibility to infection by some but not all microbes. For example, diseases involving defects in T cells predispose to infections with intracellular organisms including mycobacteria, some fungi and viruses, whereas those involving the other components of the immune response tend to result in infections by bacteria that have an extracellular habitat. In other words, infections with particular microbes are a reflection of which components of the immune system are defective. Moreover, it is often possible to define the abnormal immune component in an immune deficiency disease and in the process, discover a considerable amount about the importance of that component in normal immune defense and in its interrelationships with the other components of the immune system. Furthermore, it is important to recognize such abnormalities and to pinpoint them as accurately as possible since correction, if possible, must be tailored to the specific abnormality.

Classification of immuno-deficiencies

The immunodeficiency diseases can be classified as either primary – usually **congenital** (the result of a failure of proper development of the humoral and/or cellular immune systems), or secondary – **acquired** (the consequences of other diseases and their treatments). A large number of specific congenital or acquired abnormalities in the immune system have been identified which contribute to patient susceptibility to recurrent infections. These abnormalities range from those that affect the immune system at a very early level, and thus compromise the immune response to many antigens, to those that affect the final stages of differentiation of particular immune cells and hence lead to very selective abnormalities. The primary diseases are very rare whilst the secondary diseases are relatively common. A more pathophysiological description characterizes the specific immune component that is abnormal by defining quantitative or qualitative abnormalities of the cells (lymphocytes, phagocytes) and/or molecules (antibodies, cytokines, complement components) of the immune system.

J2 PRIMARY/CONGENITAL (INHERITED) IMMUNODEFICIENCY

Key Notes

Complement

Patients deficient in certain complement components (especially C3) are prone to recurrent infections with encapsulated organisms (*Pneumococcus* and *Streptococcus*) and *Neisseria*. Opsonization of these pathogens by C3b is important for their removal by phagocytosis. Deficiencies in membrane attack complex (MAC) components and in complement regulatory molecules also result in increased susceptibility to certain infections or to inflammation, respectively.

Phagocytosis

Intrinsic defects include those associated with differentiation, chemoattraction, and intracellular killing of the microbe. Extrinsic or secondary defects (not an inherent phagocytic defect) may result from antibody or complement deficiency or suppression of phagocytic activity.

Humoral immunity

Primary antibody deficiency may result from abnormal development of B cells or from lack of T helper activity. Patients suffer from recurrent extracellular bacterial infections. Those with severe combined immunodeficiency (SCID) and Bruton's disease have few or no B lymphocytes and no antibodies. In hyper-IgM syndrome, CD40 signaling is defective and there is no class switch from IgM. Common variable immunodeficiency (CVID) may result from lack of B cell terminal differentiation or absence of T cell help.

Cellular immunity

Most T cell deficiencies result in severely compromised humoral as well as cellular immunity. These patients have recurrent life-threatening viral, fungal, mycobacterial, and protozoan infections. In Di George syndrome, thymus embryogenesis is defective and few T cells develop. SCID may result from defects in the cytokine receptor γ chain or adenosine deaminase enzyme or purine nucleoside phosphorylase deficiency.

Related topics

Hemopoiesis – development of blood cells (A5)
Molecules of the innate immune system (B2)
Innate immunity and inflammation (B4)

Antibody functions (D8)
B cell activation (E2)
Clonal expansion and development of effector function (F5)

Complement

Primary immune deficiencies of the complement system have been described for many of the 21 different complement components and their inhibitors, some in terms of specific gene mutations. Patients with a deficiency of certain of these complement components (especially C3) are prone to recurrent infections with both encapsulated organisms such as *Pneumococcus* and *Streptococcus,* as well as with *Neisseria* (*Table 1*). The attachment of complement to the surface of some of

Table 1.   Complement deficiencies

Component deficient	Disease caused/common infections seen
Regulatory components	
C1q inhibitor	Hereditary angiedema (continuous complement activation and consumption)
Decay accelerating factor DAF (CD55)	Paroxysmal nocturnal hemoglobulinuria (lysis of red blood cells)
Complement components	
C1, C2 or C4	Immune complex disease (unable to remove Ag-Ab complexes); C2 deficiency associated with SLE
C3	The most serious; repeated infections with pyogenic bacteria
MAC complement component deficiencies C5–8	Meningococcal infections, e.g. *Neisseria*
component deficiency C9	None

these organisms is clearly important for their removal by phagocytic cells. Deficiencies in the later complement components and in the regulatory molecules of the complement system also result in increased susceptibility to certain infections (by meningococcus, e.g. *Neisseria*) or to inflammation, respectively.

Phagocytosis

Defects in phagocytic function can be classified as either intrinsic (related to the inherent properties of the phagocyte) or extrinsic (not the result of an inherent phagocytic defect). Intrinsic disorders related to different stages of phagocyte differentiation and function have been identified, including those associated with stem cell differentiation, chemoattraction to the site of microbial assault, and to intracellular killing of the microbe (*Table 2*). Extrinsic defects may result

Table 2.   Phagocytic defects

Defect in	Disease/mechanism
Stem cell differentiation/early development	Neutropenia: too few neutrophils Adhesion to endothelium for margination; leukocyte adhesion deficiency (LAD); due to a lack of expression (through specific gene mutation) of the critical surface adhesion molecule CD18, a leukocyte function associated (LFA) molecule.*
Phagocytosis	Chediak–Higashi syndrome: lack of fusion of phagosome with lysosomes
Defective intracellular killing	Chronic granulomatous disease: defect in genes encoding the four proteins making up the NADPH oxidase system, involved in oxygen-dependent killing within the phagolysosome
IFNγ or IL-12 receptors	Mycobacterial infections; failure to activate NADPH oxidase

*CD18, with CD11 form the C3bi receptor (CR3) that is necessary for binding C3b and thus for binding opsonized microbes, a critical step in the cell's attempt to engulf a bacterium. LFA molecules are present on all effector cell populations (including cytotoxic T cells) and are important in linking effector and target cells as an initial step in cytotoxicity or phagocytosis. Thus, the function of more than just phagocytes is affected by this defect. NADPH, reduced nicotinamide adenine dinucleotide phosphate.

from: (i) deficiency of antibody or complement, i.e. other primary defects; or (ii) suppression of phagocytic activity (e.g. by glucocorticoids or autoantibodies), i.e. secondary defects, to be discussed later.

Humoral immunity

Primary antibody deficiency mainly results from abnormal development of the B cell system. Any of the steps involved in B cell maturation may be blocked or abnormal (*Table 3*). The overall lack of antibodies means that the patients suffer from recurrent bacterial infections, predominately by *Pneumococcus*, *Streptococcus* and *Haemophilus*. Patients with severe combined immunodeficiency and Bruton's disease have few or no B lymphocytes and therefore few if any antibodies in their circulation. Thus, they are unable to coat the surface of (opsonize) bacteria for which phagocytosis is the primary defense.

Table 3. B cell deficiencies

Stage of differentiation/maturation	Disease
Lack of stem cells	Severe combined immunodeficiency (SCID), also affects T cell development
B cells fail to develop from B cell precursors	Bruton's disease: congenital agammaglobulinemia – mostly X-linked (XLA); due to a defective gene coding for a tyrosine kinase (btk) involved in activation of the pre-B cell to immature B cell (Topic E2); patients have normal T cells
B cells do not switch antibody classes from IgM	Hyper-IgM syndrome: increased IgM but little or no IgG in the circulation, due to defective gene coding for either CD40 on B cells or CD40L on activated T cells (Topic F4)
Common variable immunodeficiency (CVID)	IgG/IgA deficiency 1) B cells do not undergo terminal differentiation; IgA deficiency most common (1/700 people) 2) B cells normal; T cell signaling defective
Transient hypogammaglobulinemia	B cells normal; no CD4$^+$ T cell help early in life

Although some of these disorders are related to basic biochemical abnormalities of the B cell lineage, others are the result of defective regulation by T cells. Thus, humoral immune deficiency may result from the absence of T helper activity. This is seen as one form of common variable immunodeficiency (CVID). Another form of CVID involves B cells that do not respond to signals from other cells. It is also possible that monocyte presentation and/or IL-1 (or other cytokine) production abnormalities may contribute to, or be responsible for, some of these disorders. Moreover, since different classes of immunoglobulin are regulated by different T helper cell subpopulations (e.g. Th1 cells help IgG1 and IgG3 responses; Th2 cells help IgA and IgE responses) selective antibody class (IgA or IgG) deficiencies may result from abnormalities in the number or activities of these T cell subpopulations.

Cellular immunity

Deficiencies caused only by the loss of cellular immunity are very rare, as most T cell deficiencies result in severely compromised humoral immunity as well. T cell defects occurring during development are shown in *Table 4*. Deficiencies in cellular immunity may relate to T effector cells (e.g., cytotoxic T cells), whereas the T helper population may be normal. Children have also been described with an inability to produce or respond to IFNγ. In general, children with T cell deficiencies have recurrent viral, fungal, mycobacterial and protozoan infections.

Table 4. T cell deficiencies during development

T cell deficiency	Disease
Lack of a thymus	Di George syndrome; defect in thymus embryogenesis
Stem cell defect	SCID; 50% have a defect in γ chain used by many cytokine receptors including the IL-2 receptor
Death of developing thymocytes	SCID; 25% have adenosine deaminase enzyme deficiency or purine nucleoside phosphorylase deficiency; toxicity due to build up of purine metabolites which inhibit DNA synthesis

J3 SECONDARY (ACQUIRED) IMMUNODEFICIENCY

Key Notes

Factors causing acquired immunodeficiency	Secondary or acquired immunodeficiency, mainly affecting phagocytic and lymphocyte function, is the most common immunodeficiency. It may result from infection (HIV), malnutrition, aging, cytotoxic therapy, etc.
HIV and AIDS	Acquired immune deficiency syndrome (AIDS) is caused by human immunodeficiency virus, (HIV)-1 or HIV-2. The virus enters the body via infected body fluids and exhibits trophism for monocytes/MØ (primary reservoir for the virus) and helper T cells, gaining entry through the CD4 molecule on these cells. Chemokine receptors are also involved in HIV gp120 binding to these cells and critical to infection. Loss of CD4+ T cells eventually compromises the ability of the immune system to combat opportunistic infections.
Immune senescence: consequences of aging	With aging, memory T cells increase but become less able to expand. Moreover, fewer new (naive) T cells enter the pool due to thymic involution, diminishing the immune repertoire and the quality of T and B cell responses. B cell development in the bone marrow may also decrease. As a result of this reduction in immune capability, the elderly respond less well to vaccination.
Trauma	Patients suffering trauma (e.g., associated with burns or major surgery) are less able to deal with pathogens, perhaps as a result of the release of factors that dampen immune responses.
Related topics	Cells of the innate immune system (B1) Shaping of the T cell repertoire (F3)
	Molecules of the innate immune system (B2) T cell activation (F4)
	The cellular basis of the antibody response (E3) Clonal expansion and development of effector function (F5)
	Aging and the immune system (immunosenescence) (P1)

Factors causing acquired immunodeficiency

Secondary or acquired immunodeficiency is by far the most common immunodeficiency and contributes a significant proportion to hospital admissions. Factors causing secondary immunodeficiency mainly affect phagocytic and lymphocyte function and include the following (*Table 1*).

HIV and AIDS

Acquired immune deficiency syndrome (AIDS) is caused mainly by the retrovirus human immunodeficiency virus (HIV)-1 but also by HIV-2. The virus enters the body via infected body fluids and exhibits trophism for T cells, in particular the T helper population, and for monocytes and macrophages. It

Table 1. Factors causing secondary immunodeficiency

Factor	Components affected
Malnutrition	Protein–calory malnutrition and lack of certain dietary elements (e.g. iron, zinc); world-wide the major predisposing factor for secondary immunodeficiency
Tumors	Direct effect of tumors on the immune system by effects on immunoregulatory molecules or release of immunosuppressive molecules, e.g. TGFβ
Cytotoxic drugs/irradiation	Widely used for tumor therapy, but also kills cells important to immune responses, including stem cells, neutrophil progenitors and rapidly dividing lymphocytes in primary lymphoid organs
Aging	Increased infections; reduced responses to vaccination; decreased T and B cell responses and changes in the quality of the response
Trauma	Increased infections probably related to release of immunosuppressive molecules such as glucocorticoids
Other diseases (e.g. diabetes)	Diabetes is often associated with infections but the mechanism is unclear
Immunosuppression by microbes	Examples include malaria, measles virus but especially HIV; mechanisms involve decreased T cell function and antigen processing/presentation

binds and gains entry into T cells and monocytes (the primary reservoir for the virus) through the CD4 molecule on these cells. Other accessory receptors (chemokine receptors – Topic B2) are involved in viral gp120 binding to T lymphocytes and monocytes, and individuals lacking functioning chemokine receptors do not progress from HIV infection to AIDS. In particular, the chemokine receptors CXCR4 and CCR5 are coreceptors for HIV and are required for productive HIV infection of CD4$^+$ cells including monocytes, macrophages and T helper cells.

The development of AIDS is defined as the occurrence of opportunistic infections (e.g. pneumocystis) or Kaposi's sarcoma (caused by HHV8) in an individual who has been infected with HIV. This is a direct result of the loss of CD4$^+$ helper cells. Damage to the pivotal CD4$^+$ T cell has major effects on the functions of other cells of the immune system (Fig. 1). Infection of monocytes and antigen-presenting cells is also likely to be important in the speed of progression of the disease.

Immune senescence: consequences of aging

As one ages, changes occur in immune status (Section P). Reduced responses to vaccination and increased risk of infectious disease in the elderly are the result of reductions in immune function. Most striking of these changes is the involution of the thymus and the subsequent loss of T cell production. Thus, the host is dependent on the pool of T cells generated earlier in life. As one ages, memory T cells increase and naive cells decrease, suggesting that there is an accumulation of activated T cells and fewer naïve cells entering the pool. In addition, the ability of T cells from aged individuals to expand is limited, thus further diminishing cell-mediated immune responses.

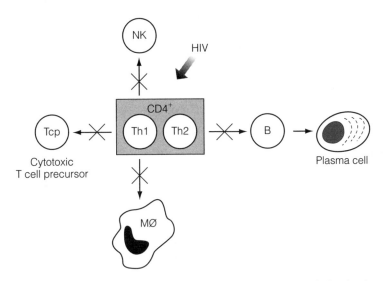

Fig. 1.   HIV infection of CD4⁺ Th cells compromises their ability to help other immune cell populations.

There is also an age-associated reduction in humoral immunity, at least one part of which results in reduced B cell development in the bone marrow and thus B cell diversity. This is manifest as a change in the quality of the antibody response, including a decrease in antibody affinity, a diminished response to vaccines and an increase in autoantibody production (Topic P5). Some of these alterations in humoral immunity may be due to the impaired capacity of T cells to induce the maturation of B cells to produce high-affinity, isotype-switched antibody.

Overall, the immune system appears to shift with age from one dependent primarily on adaptive immune responses to one somewhat more dependent on innate immunity.

Trauma

After significant trauma including that associated with burns or major surgery, the immune system seems less able to deal with pathogens. Although the basis for this apparent immunodeficiency is not understood, it is possible that these traumatic events induce release of other immunomodulatory factors (e.g. gluco-corticoids), which dampen immune responses (Topic G5).

J4 DIAGNOSIS AND TREATMENT OF IMMUNODEFICIENCY

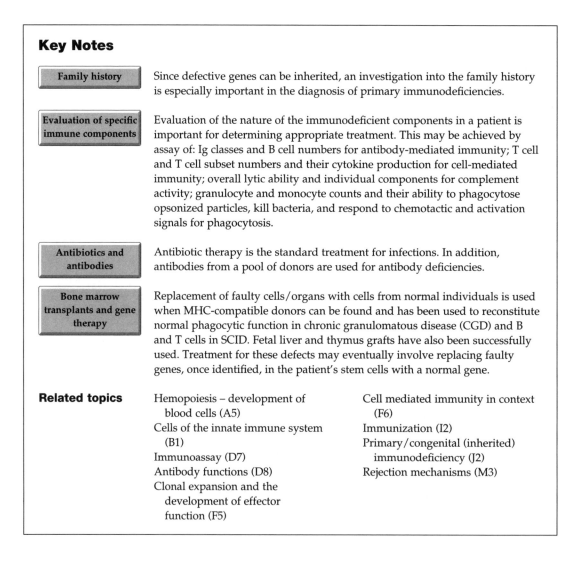

Key Notes

Family history

Since defective genes can be inherited, an investigation into the family history is especially important in the diagnosis of primary immunodeficiencies.

Evaluation of specific immune components

Evaluation of the nature of the immunodeficient components in a patient is important for determining appropriate treatment. This may be achieved by assay of: Ig classes and B cell numbers for antibody-mediated immunity; T cell and T cell subset numbers and their cytokine production for cell-mediated immunity; overall lytic ability and individual components for complement activity; granulocyte and monocyte counts and their ability to phagocytose opsonized particles, kill bacteria, and respond to chemotactic and activation signals for phagocytosis.

Antibiotics and antibodies

Antibiotic therapy is the standard treatment for infections. In addition, antibodies from a pool of donors are used for antibody deficiencies.

Bone marrow transplants and gene therapy

Replacement of faulty cells/organs with cells from normal individuals is used when MHC-compatible donors can be found and has been used to reconstitute normal phagocytic function in chronic granulomatous disease (CGD) and B and T cells in SCID. Fetal liver and thymus grafts have also been successfully used. Treatment for these defects may eventually involve replacing faulty genes, once identified, in the patient's stem cells with a normal gene.

Related topics

Hemopoiesis – development of blood cells (A5)
Cells of the innate immune system (B1)
Immunoassay (D7)
Antibody functions (D8)
Clonal expansion and the development of effector function (F5)

Cell mediated immunity in context (F6)
Immunization (I2)
Primary/congenital (inherited) immunodeficiency (J2)
Rejection mechanisms (M3)

Family history

Since defective genes can be inherited, e.g. defective CD40 and/or CD40 ligand in hyper-IgM syndrome (Topic J2, *Table 3*), it is important to establish any history of family members with similar recurrent episodes of infection. This information on family history is especially important in the diagnosis of primary immunodeficiencies and is valuable for genetic counseling.

Evaluation of specific immune therapy

Recognizing immune defects and pinpointing them is critical, since correction must be tailored to the abnormality. Although the nature of an infection or disorder will provide clues to which immune component is at a disadvantage, in many instances it is not clear which subcomponents are compromised. It is important, therefore, to apply a systematic evaluation of immune function to individuals suspected of immune abnormalities (*Table 1*).

Humoral (antibody) immunity may be initially evaluated by determining the presence and levels of the different antibody classes and subclasses in the serum of a patient using serum immunoelectrophoresis, radial immunodiffusion and/or radioimmunoassay (Topics D6 and D7). Detection of specific antibodies can be determined using skin tests (Topic K5), by agglutination (e.g. for IgM antibodies to blood group substances A and B) and/or enzyme-linked immunosorbent assay (ELISA) (e.g. for specific antibodies after immunization with killed vaccines). It is also important to determine B cell numbers and functional properties using mAbs to surface immunoglobulin and B cell differentia-

Table 1. *Evaluation of the different components of the immune system*

Evaluation of antibody-mediated immunity
Serum immunoelectrophoresis
Quantitate antibodies in serum and secretions by ELISA or radial immunodiffusion
Assay for specific antibodies:
  Assay by agglutination for IgM antibodies to blood group substances A and B
  Before and after immunization with killed vaccines
Quantitate circulating B cells by flow cytometry with mAbs to surface Ig
Evaluate induction of B cell differentiation *in vitro*
Evaluate the presence of B cells and plasma cells in lymph nodes (biopsy)

Evaluation of cell-mediated immunity
DTH skin tests to common antigens – candida, streptokinase, streptodornase
Determine:
  Total lymphocyte count (60–80% of blood lymphocytes are T cells)
  T cell number in blood (using mAb to CD3 and flow cytometry)
  T cell subpopulation percentages (using mAbs to CD4 and to CD8)
Evaluate lymphocyte proliferation to lectins (PHA, Con A) and alloantigens (MLR)
Analyse T-lymphocyte function:
  Lymphokine production: IFNγ, IL-2, etc
  Helper cell activity and cellular cytotoxicity

Evaluation of the complement system
Assay for total hemolytic complement – CH_{50}, a functional assay
Quantitate individual complement components by immunoassay
Assay neutrophil chemotaxis using C in patient's serum as a chemoattractant

Evaluation of phagocyte function
Determine total granulocyte and monocyte count
Assay for:
  Chemotaxis – using a Boyden chamber
  Phagocytosis – using opsonized particles
  Superoxide generation using nitroblue tetrazolium (NBT) reduction
  Bacterial killing
  Individual enzymes and for cytokines (IL-1 and IL-12)
  Response to activation by IFNγ, GM-CSF, etc
Evaluate ability to process and present antigen

PHA, phytohemagglutinin; Con A, concanavalin A; MLR, mixed lymphocyte reaction.

tion assays, respectively. Lymph node biopsy is used to determine the presence and numbers of B cells and plasma cells in the tissues.

Cell-mediated immunity is often evaluated by skin tests (delayed-type hypersensitivity, DTH, Topic K5) to common antigens (e.g. candida, streptokinase, streptodornase). Total lymphocyte, T cell (CD3+) and T cell subpopulation (CD4+ or CD8+) numbers are also useful in evaluating the potential for cell-mediated immune responses (Topic D7). However, normal numbers of T cells and T cell subpopulations in a patient do not mean that they function normally. Thus, lymphocyte proliferation to lectins (PHA and Con A) and alloantigens (MLR), lymphokine production (e.g. IFNγ, IL-2) and helper and killer cell activities may also need to be carried out.

Both classical and alternative pathways of the complement system can be evaluated for their overall functional activity in red cell lysis assays that determine total hemolytic complement (CH_{50}). Immunoassays can then be used to determine the concentration of individual complement components including those associated with the alternative pathway. Neutrophil chemotaxis assays using complement from a patient's serum as a chemoattractant can be used to evaluate complement chemotactic factors (Topics B2 and D8) such as C5a.

Cells of the phagocyte system are able to respond to chemotactic stimuli and migrate toward a pathogen, recognize the pathogen and mediate its phagocytosis and/or killing. These cells are involved in immune defense both as a result of their own recognition of microbe molecular patterns (Topic B3) and as a result of direction by the humoral, cellular and/or complement systems. Total granulocyte and monocyte blood counts permit determination of their presence in normal numbers. Chemotaxis assays (using Boyden chambers) evaluate their response to chemotactic molecules such as C5a. Assays for phagocytosis (using antibody and/or complement opsonized particles), for superoxide generation (using the reduction of nitroblue tetrazolium (NBT) test), and for bacterial killing are important in determining the functional capability of these cells. Assays for individual enzymes and for cytokines (IL-1 and IL-12) indicate their ability to produce molecules critical to microbe killing and in recruiting other cells and immune mechanisms. Their response to activation by IFNγ, GM-CSF, etc., indicates their ability to be induced to a higher level of cytotoxic ability. Finally, as many of these cells (monocytes, macrophages, dendritic cells) process and present antigen, it may be important to assay their ability to trigger T cells and thus to initiate specific immune responses.

One of the best ways to evaluate immune function involves looking at both the afferent (initiation) and efferent (effector) limb of the immune system of an individual. This can be done by injecting antigen into an individual and determining if a normal response develops. If it does, all of the T and B cell systems are probably intact. Another even more definitive evaluation procedure might be to use a live attenuated vaccine, e.g. polio virus, as this would permit evaluation of the immune response in a very real setting. However, this would never be done as even an attenuated live pathogen could cause a lethal infection in an immunodeficient individual (Topic I3).

Antibiotics and antibodies

Antibiotic therapy is the standard treatment for infections. Children whose immune system produces no antibodies begin to experience recurrent infections after maternal antibody from placental transfer *in utero* has been depleted. These individuals are treated with antibiotics and intravenously with periodic injections of pooled immunoglobulins from normal human serum.

Contamination of immunoglobulin preparations with viruses including HIV and hepatitis B and C must be excluded.

Bone marrow transplants and gene therapy

Replacement of faulty cells/organs with cells and organs from normal individuals is now commonly used when MHC-compatible donors can be found. In particular, bone marrow transplantation has been successfully used for reconstitution of normal phagocytic function in chronic granulomatous disease (CGD) and of B and T cells in SCID. Fetal liver and thymus grafts have also been successfully used. In most cases, such transplants carry the risk of rejection (Topic M3) and require appropriately regulated immunosuppression for their survival. Transplantation of stem cells from normal donors (stem cell therapy) is another very promising approach to the treatment of some of these diseases, and is being aggressively explored at the present time.

A number of genes have already been identified as faulty (Topic J2, *Tables 2–4*) in patients with primary immunodeficiency diseases. Thus, a definitive treatment for these defects may well be gene replacement therapy, in that faulty genes will be replaced in the patient's stem cells with a 'normal' gene. This approach has already been tried for adenosine deaminase (ADA) deficiency and is currently being tried for several of other disorders for which a faulty gene has been identified. The difficulty thus far appears to be in appropriately expressing the normal gene.

K1 DEFINITION AND CLASSIFICATION

Key Notes

Introduction

Damage to host tissue can occur as an overreaction by the immune system to a variety of both inert antigens and infectious organisms. This hypersensitivity occurs only after antigen sensitization of the host and is therefore the effect of the adaptive immune system. Overreaction to microbial antigens can occur in the natural immune system although these reactions are not currently classified as hypersensitivity reactions.

Classification

Hypersensitivity reactions have long been classified into four types, with an additional type recently added. Types I, II, III and V depend on antibodies, alone or with complement, and because they are evident within hours, are termed immediate hypersensitivities. Type IV is mediated by T cells and the cytokines they produce when activated. As this response requires at least a day to develop, it is termed delayed hypersensitivity.

Related topics

Molecules of the innate immune
   system (B2)
Antibody functions (D8)

The role of T cells in immune
   responses (F1)
Clonal expansion and development
   of effector function (F5)

Introduction

The immune system normally responds to a variety of microbial invaders with little or no damage to host tissues. However, in some situations, immune responses (especially to some antigens) can lead to more severe tissue damaging reactions (immunopathology). This 'overreactivity' by the immune system to antigens is often referred to as hypersensitivity and is by no means restricted to antigens of microbial origin since it also includes both inert and self antigens (autoimmunity). Hypersensitivity reactions are antigen specific and occur after the immune system has already responded to an antigen (i.e. the immune system has been primed). The adverse reactions are therefore mainly the result of antigen-specific memory responses. It is important to note that these responses are part of normal immune defense mechanisms and occur daily as immune cells and molecules come in contact with antigens and/or pathogens that had previously induced an immunity. What is unusual about hypersensitivities is that these normal responses become clinically evident because they are localized and/or involve interactions between large amounts of antigen with antibodies or immune cells. In addition, genetics plays a role in some types of hypersensitivity reactions. Moreover, some antigens can induce more than one type of tissue damaging reaction (hypersensitivity) and penicillin can induce types I, II, III and IV reactions.

Classification

Hypersensitivity reactions occur at different times after coming into contact with the offending antigens, within a few minutes (i.e. immediate), minutes to hours (intermediate) or after many hours (delayed). Generally, the delayed responses are mediated by the cellular components of the immune system (i.e. T cells) whilst the former are the result of the humoral arm of the immune response which includes antibodies and the complement system. The original classification by Gell and Coombs was into four main types, a fifth has since been added. *Table 1* summarizes the main immune system components which contribute to tissue damage. It should be stressed that more than one of these mechanisms can contribute to any one particular disease process.

Table 1.   Classification of hypersensitivities

Time of appearance	Type	Immune mechanism
2–30 min (immediate)	I	IgE antibodies (enhancement of acute inflammatory response)
5–8 h (cytotoxic)	II	Antibody and complement
2–8 h (immune complex)	III	Antibody/antigen complexes
24–72 h (delayed)	IV	T cell mediated (can be granulomatous)
(Stimulatory)	V	Antibody mediated

K2 IgE-MEDIATED (TYPE I) HYPERSENSITIVITY: ALLERGY

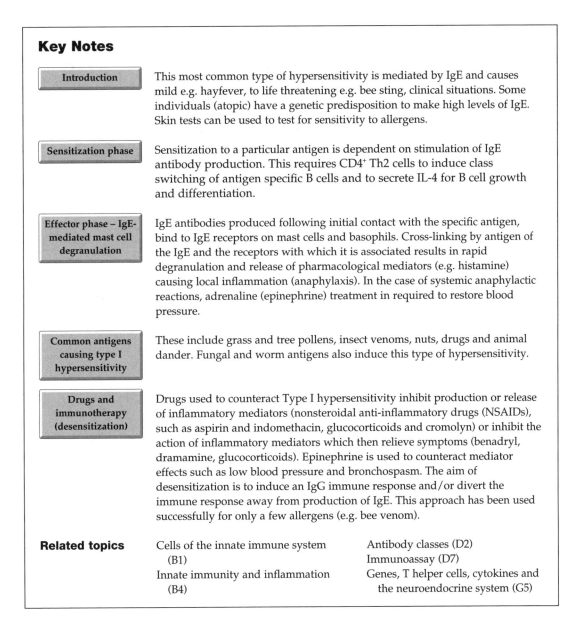

Key Notes

Introduction	This most common type of hypersensitivity is mediated by IgE and causes mild e.g. hayfever, to life threatening e.g. bee sting, clinical situations. Some individuals (atopic) have a genetic predisposition to make high levels of IgE. Skin tests can be used to test for sensitivity to allergens.
Sensitization phase	Sensitization to a particular antigen is dependent on stimulation of IgE antibody production. This requires CD4$^+$ Th2 cells to induce class switching of antigen specific B cells and to secrete IL-4 for B cell growth and differentiation.
Effector phase – IgE-mediated mast cell degranulation	IgE antibodies produced following initial contact with the specific antigen, bind to IgE receptors on mast cells and basophils. Cross-linking by antigen of the IgE and the receptors with which it is associated results in rapid degranulation and release of pharmacological mediators (e.g. histamine) causing local inflammation (anaphylaxis). In the case of systemic anaphylactic reactions, adrenaline (epinephrine) treatment in required to restore blood pressure.
Common antigens causing type I hypersensitivity	These include grass and tree pollens, insect venoms, nuts, drugs and animal dander. Fungal and worm antigens also induce this type of hypersensitivity.
Drugs and immunotherapy (desensitization)	Drugs used to counteract Type I hypersensitivity inhibit production or release of inflammatory mediators (nonsteroidal anti-inflammatory drugs (NSAIDs), such as aspirin and indomethacin, glucocorticoids and cromolyn) or inhibit the action of inflammatory mediators which then relieve symptoms (benadryl, dramamine, glucocorticoids). Epinephrine is used to counteract mediator effects such as low blood pressure and bronchospasm. The aim of desensitization is to induce an IgG immune response and/or divert the immune response away from production of IgE. This approach has been used successfully for only a few allergens (e.g. bee venom).
Related topics	Cells of the innate immune system (B1) Antibody classes (D2) Innate immunity and inflammation (B4) Immunoassay (D7) Genes, T helper cells, cytokines and the neuroendocrine system (G5)

Introduction

Allergy affects about 17% of the population through mild e.g. hayfever, to life threatening conditions e.g. bee sting allergy. It is mediated by IgE which is normally found in very small amounts in the circulation (Topic D2) and has probably evolved to protect us against worm infestations (Topics B4, H2). Allergic reactions can occur to normally harmless antigens (such as pollen or foodstuffs) and microbial antigens (fungi, worms). Some individuals in the population are genetically predisposed to respond to certain antigens by producing IgE to these antigens and are said to be atopic. Testing for allergy (Prausnitz-Kustner test) involves introduction of the allergen intradermally. A positive skin test occurs in the form of a wheal (fluid accumulation) and flare (redness) reaction at the site of injection.

Sensitization phase

Sensitization to a particular antigen is dependent on stimulation of IgE antibody production. Thus, B cell antigen receptors specific for the allergen bind, internalize, process and present the antigen in MHC class II molecules. CD4$^+$ Th2 cells recognize the antigen presented by these B cells and induce class switching of antigen-specific B cells. These T cells also secrete IL-4 which is important for B cell growth and differentiation (Topics B2, E3 and F5) (*Fig. 1*). Why certain individuals become sensitized to particular antigens by producing IgE is unclear, but the possibilities include: (i) the genetics of the individual; (ii) environmental factors (pollution) that condition mucosal tissues of the immune system to produce IL-4 which then predisposes a Th2 response; and (iii) that regulation of the response through Th1 cells is defective (Topics F5, G5).

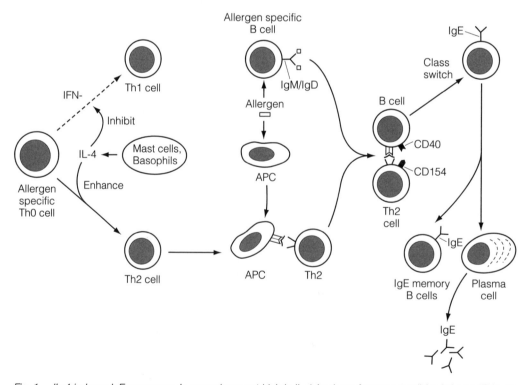

Fig. 1.   IL-4 induces IgE responses. In an environment high in IL-4 (perhaps from mast cells) relative to IFNγ, an allergen-specific Th0 cell differentiates into a Th2 cell rather than a Th1 cell. APCs present allergen peptides to this Th2 cell, inducing its activation and proliferation. An allergen specific B cell which has internalized allergen then presents allergen peptides in MHC class II to this Th2 cell. The Th2 cell stimulates antibody class switch (through triggering of b cell CD40 by CD154 on the T cell) and releases IL-4 which induces class switch to IgE antibodies. The IgE producing b cell proliferates and differentiates into IgE expressing B memory cells and IgE producing plasma cells.

Effector phase – IgE-mediated mast cell degranulation

Specific IgE antibodies produced as a result of previous contact with antigen (allergen) diffuse throughout the body, eventually coming in contact with mast cells and basophils. These cells have high affinity receptors for the Fc region of IgE and therefore bind to these antibodies. This does not have any effect on the mast cells directly until the specific antigen (allergen) is reintroduced into the body and comes into contact with the mast cell bearing the IgE antibodies in sufficient numbers to crosslink the antibodies on the cell surface (*Fig. 2*). The mast cells now immediately release granules (degranulate) which contain large amounts of pharmacological mediators (*Table 1*). These substances have a direct effect on nearby blood vessels causing vasodilation and an influx of eosinophils, which in turn release mediators that cause a prolonged 'late phase' reaction. Locally, e.g. in the nose, mediator release results in the symptoms of redness, itching and increased secretions by mucosal epithelial cells leading to a runny nose. Systemic release of histamine and other substances released by mast cells can lead to severe vasodilation and vascular collapse resulting in life-threatening systemic anaphylactic reactions which require treatment with epinephrine to restore blood pressure.

Leukotrienes, histamine, prostaglandins and platelet activating factor released from mast cells are key mediators of type I hypersensitivity. One way of classifying this growing body of inflammatory mediators is by their effects on target cells and tissues (*Table 1*).

Common antigens causing type I hypersensitivity

There are many antigens which can cause allergic (type I hypersensitive) reactions (*Table 2*). The most common allergic response is probably to pollens (allergic rhinitis: hayfever). Antigens from some invading organisms can also give rise to allergic reactions. These include fungal spores, viruses and worms. Systemic release of worm antigens from hydatid cysts binding to serum IgE can

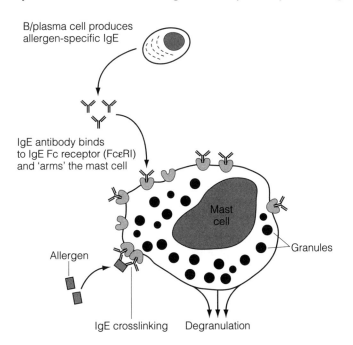

Fig. 2. IgE-mediated mast cell degranulation. Allergen binds to and crosslinks cytophilic (cell bound) IgE, signaling FcεR to trigger mast cell activation and degranulation with release of histamine, leukotrienes, etc.

Table 1.   Inflammatory mediators classified by their effects on target cells

Mediators with pharmacologic effects on smooth muscle and mucous glands
1. *Histamine*. Binds to two types of receptors on target cells, H1 and H2 receptors. Acting on H1 receptors, histamine contracts smooth muscle (e.g. in airways), increases vascular permeability and mucous secretion by goblet cells. Via H2 receptors, histamine increases gastric secretion, and feeds back to decrease mediator release by basophils and mast cells
2. *Slow reacting substance of anaphylaxis (SRS-A)*. These cysteinyl-leukotrienes (LTC$_4$, LTD$_4$, LTE$_4$), are potent constrictors of peripheral airways (i.e., bronchoconstrictors) and also cause leakage of post capillary venules, leading to edema. Leukotrienes are derived from the membrane fatty acids of mast cells, neutrophils and macrophages
3. *Prostaglandins*. A variety of effects are manifested by this large family of related compounds. Prostaglandin D$_2$ is produced by mast cells and causes bronchial constriction. Prostaglandin I$_2$ is produced by endothelial cells and probably synergizes with LTB4 to cause edema
4. *Platelet activating factor (PAF)*. A low molecular weight lipid which causes platelet aggregation with release of vasoactive mediators (serotonin) and smooth muscle contraction
5. *Kinins*. Bradykinin (a nonapeptide) and lysyl-bradykinin (a decapeptide) cause increased vascular permeability, decreased blood pressure and contraction of smooth muscle

Mediators which are pro-inflammatory by chemotactic properties
1. *Eosinophil chemotactic factors of anaphylaxis (ECF-A)*. Includes histamine and tetrapeptides from mast cell granules
2. *Neutrophil chemotactic factor of anaphylaxis (IL-8)*. A granule-derived protein of mast cells which attracts and activates neutrophils
3. *Late-phase reactants of anaphylaxis*. Mediators that cause delayed inflammatory cell infiltration
4. *Leukotriene B4 (LTB$_4$)*. Derived from membrane fatty acids, a potent chemotactic factor for PMNs, eosinophils and macrophages, causes adhesion of leukocytes to post capillary venules, degranulation and edema

Mediators which cause tissue destruction
1. *Toxic oxygen and nitrogen radicals*. (e.g., superoxide and nitric oxide). Released from PMNs, macrophages and mast cells.
2. *Acid hydrolases*. From mast cells
3. *Major basic protein*. A very destructive protein from the larger eosinophil granule.

cause anaphylaxis leading to vascular collapse and death if left untreated. Allergic asthma is an important disease which can be triggered by a number of different environmental antigens and is mediated by IgE in its early stages.

Drugs and immunotherapy (desensitization)

Drugs used to treat immediate hypersensitivity act at one of two levels: (i) inhibitors of the production or release of inflammatory mediators. These include nonsteroidal anti-inflammatory drugs (NSAIDs) such as aspirin and indomethicin, synthetic steroids (glucocorticoids) such as dexamethasone and prednisolone, and the inhibitor of histamine release, cromolyn. (ii) Inhibitors of mediator action such as histamine receptor antagonists. Benadryl, dramamine, chlortrimaton and dimetane are representative H1-blocking agents, which are most useful for relief of the sneezing, rhinorrhea (runny nose) and itching eyes associated with hay fever. They are not useful for bronchial asthma or systemic anaphylaxis, where mediators other than histamine play a more important role. Glucocorticoids also inhibit some of the actions of inflammatory mediators. Other drugs such as **epinephrine** and theophyline are used to counteract mediator effects such as low blood pressure and bronchospasm.

Table 2.   Allergens

Pollens	Insect venoms	Microbes	Animals and foods	Drugs
Grass	Bee	Mold	Serum	Penicillin
Timothy	Wasp		Vaccines	Salicylates
Rye	Ant		Nuts	Anesthetics
Ragweed			Seafood	
			Hair	
Tree			Danders	
Plane				
Birch				

Desensitization is used to divert the immune response away from a predominantly Th2 driven IgE antibody response and toward a Th1 driven IgG response. This involves injection or ingestion of allergen in low and increasing amounts. Success has been achieved with only a few allergens e.g. bee venom. An IgG response, which would be driven by Th1 cells, could have two significant effects: (i) Larger amounts of IgG would be produced than IgE and this excess IgG antibody would bind and remove the antigen before it could bind IgE on the mast cells or basophils and trigger degranulation; (ii) IgG would also remove antigen before it could bind to and stimulate Th2 driven IgE producing B cells, thus decreasing the amount of antigen specific IgE produced (*Fig. 3*).

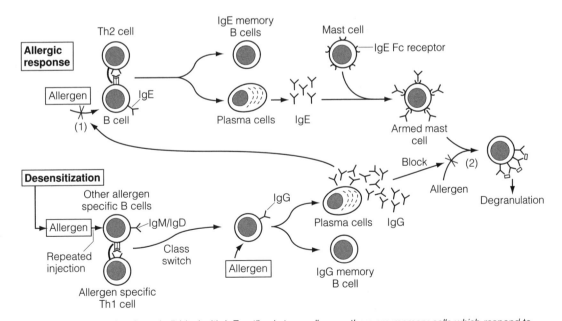

Fig. 3.   Desensitization. In an individual with IgE antibody to an allergen, there are memory cells which respond to allergen by differentiating into plasma cells which produce allergen specific IgE (Topic T2, Fig. 1). This IgE binds to IgE Fc receptors on mast cells which degranulate when allergen is reintroduced and crosslinks IgE on these cells. Repeated injections of allergen is intended to induce an IgG response by stimulating allergen specific B cells which have not yet undergone a class switch. In particular, allergen specific Th1 cells would provide help to these B cells inducing class switch to IgG. This IgG would be produced in larger quantity than IgE and compete effectively for the allergen when it is reintroduced, preventing the allergen from stimulating IgE memory B cells (1) and removing the allergen before it can bind IgE on mast cells (2).

K3 IgG AND IgM-MEDIATED (TYPE II) HYPERSENSITIVITY

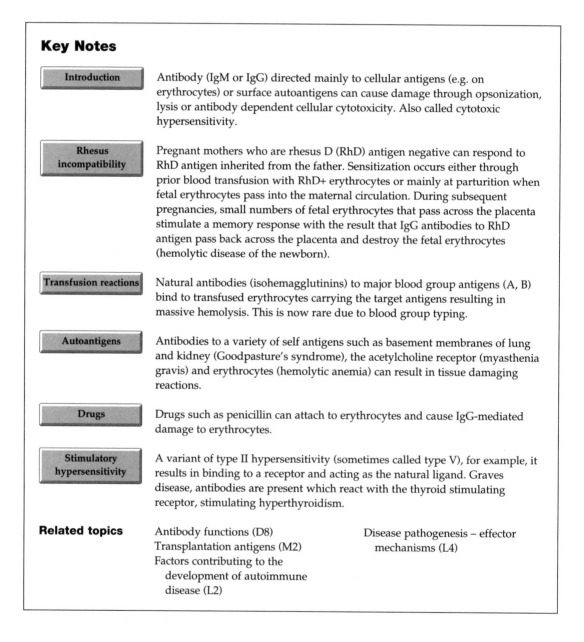

Key Notes

Introduction	Antibody (IgM or IgG) directed mainly to cellular antigens (e.g. on erythrocytes) or surface autoantigens can cause damage through opsonization, lysis or antibody dependent cellular cytotoxicity. Also called cytotoxic hypersensitivity.
Rhesus incompatibility	Pregnant mothers who are rhesus D (RhD) antigen negative can respond to RhD antigen inherited from the father. Sensitization occurs either through prior blood transfusion with RhD+ erythrocytes or mainly at parturition when fetal erythrocytes pass into the maternal circulation. During subsequent pregnancies, small numbers of fetal erythrocytes that pass across the placenta stimulate a memory response with the result that IgG antibodies to RhD antigen pass back across the placenta and destroy the fetal erythrocytes (hemolytic disease of the newborn).
Transfusion reactions	Natural antibodies (isohemagglutinins) to major blood group antigens (A, B) bind to transfused erythrocytes carrying the target antigens resulting in massive hemolysis. This is now rare due to blood group typing.
Autoantigens	Antibodies to a variety of self antigens such as basement membranes of lung and kidney (Goodpasture's syndrome), the acetylcholine receptor (myasthenia gravis) and erythrocytes (hemolytic anemia) can result in tissue damaging reactions.
Drugs	Drugs such as penicillin can attach to erythrocytes and cause IgG-mediated damage to erythrocytes.
Stimulatory hypersensitivity	A variant of type II hypersensitivity (sometimes called type V), for example, it results in binding to a receptor and acting as the natural ligand. Graves disease, antibodies are present which react with the thyroid stimulating receptor, stimulating hyperthyroidism.

Related topics	Antibody functions (D8)	Disease pathogenesis – effector
	Transplantation antigens (M2)	mechanisms (L4)
	Factors contributing to the development of autoimmune disease (L2)	

Introduction   Antibody alone or together with complement can cause hypersensitive reactions. These reactions can be against foreign (often erythrocytes) or autoantigens and usually result in the direct lysis or removal of cells. Type II hypersensitivity is therefore also termed cytotoxic hypersensitivity. Diseases caused by this type of hypersensitivity often involve erythrocytes (anemias) and self cells (auto-immune diseases). Cell death (or lysis) is mediated through normal mechanisms by which antibodies and complement carry out their function including phagocytosis, lysis and antibody dependent cellular cytotoxicity (Topic D8).

Rhesus incompatibility

Rhesus D (RhD) antigen is carried by erythrocytes. Children born to RhD– mothers and RhD+ fathers may express RhD on their erythrocytes. Prior to pregnancy, the mother can become sensitized to RhD antigen through blood transfusion and during pregnancy and especially at birth by the baby's RhD+ erythrocytes coming into contact with the mother's immune system. Some pass across the placenta but most are released into the maternal circulation during placental shedding. Since RhD is not present in the mother, her immune system responds to it as a foreign antigen and makes antibodies (*Fig. 1*). This is usually not a problem during the first pregnancy but in subsequent pregnancies small amounts of erythrocytes passing across the placenta stimulate a memory response leading to specific anti-RhD antibody production. IgG antibodies pass across the placenta and bind to the fetal erythrocytes leading to their opsonization and lysis. This results in hemolytic anemia of the newborn if not prevented. This is often call hemolytic disease of the newborn

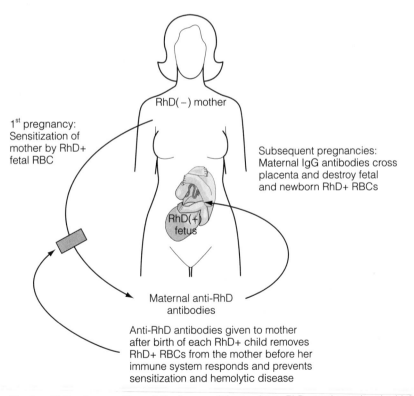

RhD(–) mother

1st pregnancy:
Sensitization of
mother by RhD+
fetal RBC

Subsequent pregnancies:
Maternal IgG antibodies cross
placenta and destroy fetal
and newborn RhD+ RBCs

RhD(+)
fetus

Maternal anti-RhD
antibodies

Anti-RhD antibodies given to mother
after birth of each RhD+ child removes
RhD+ RBCs from the mother before her
immune system responds and prevents
sensitization and hemolytic disease

Fig. 1. RhD antigen and hemolytic disease of the newborn. RhD– mothers who give birth to RhD+ infants become immunized at birth with RhD antigen on fetal red blood cells (RBCs) which pass into the mother's circulation. This results in IgG antibodies to RhD which cross the placenta during subsequent pregnancies and destroy fetal and newborn RhD+ RBCs. This can be prevented by giving the mother anti-RhD antibodies immediately after birth of each RhD+ infant or during pregnancy in order to destroy RhD+ RBCs before they stimulate an active immune response in the mother.

(HDN). Generally, mothers at risk are detected during early stages of pregnancy and monitored thereafter. At termination of each pregnancy with an RhD+ fetus, RhD(–) mothers are given antibodies to RhD which is thought to remove the fetal erythrocytes from the blood stream and suppress the development of a subsequent immune response.

Transfusion reactions

It is common practice to give blood transfusions in cases of severe blood loss. The major blood group antigens A and B are expressed at the surface of erythrocytes and we have natural antibodies (mostly IgM) to these antigens (isohemagglutinins Topic M2). Individuals who are blood group A have antibodies to B antigens, those who are blood group B will have anti-A antibodies and those who are AB will have neither. Those who are blood group O will have both antibodies. It is therefore important to do blood group typing on transfusion donors and recipients. In most cases, this is done accurately but occasionally accidents occur whereby blood is given to a recipient who has the reactive isohemagglutinins. This can result in a transfusion reaction which manifests itself as (a complement mediated) massive intravascular life-threatening hemolysis.

Autoantigens

Antibodies can be made to self antigens when there is breakdown of tolerance to self (Topics M3 and L3). These autoantibodies can cause tissue damaging reactions. In Goodpasture's disease, autoantibodies to the lung and kidney basement membranes cause inflammation and hemorrhage at the site of antibody binding. Antibodies to the acetylcholine receptor cause loss of receptors (*Fig. 2*) reducing conduction of nerve impulses across the neuromuscular junctions (myasthenia gravis). Autoantibodies to erythrocytes result in their lysis and/or removal, leading to autoimmune hemolytic anemia.

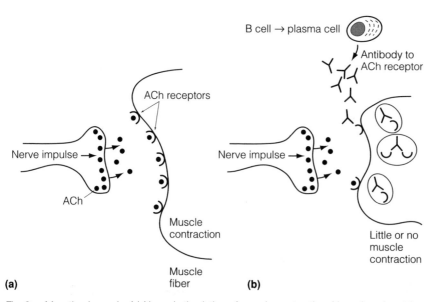

Fig. 2. *Myasthenia gravis. (a) Normal stimulation of muscle contraction. Nerve impulses trigger release of acetylcholine (ACh) from the nerve ending. The ACh then binds to ACh receptors on muscle cells triggering their contraction. (b) Autoantibodies to the ACh receptor bind to these receptors on muscle cells and cause their internalization and degradation so that when ACh is released as the result of a nerve impulse, there are few ACh receptors with which to bind, thus, muscle contraction does not occur or is diminished.*

Drugs

Penicillin, as well as inducing an immediate type hypersensitivity through IgE can also stimulate an IgG response. IgG can then bind to penicillin attached to erythrocytes which induces hemolysis in the presence of complement. This disappears when the drug is removed.

Stimulatory hypersensitivity

Since this relatively newly described type of hypersensitivity is antibody mediated it can be considered as a variant of type II hypersensitivity. In this case, the autoantibodies are directed to hormone receptor molecules and function in a stimulatory fashion, like the natural ligand i.e. the hormone itself. The classical example is Graves' disease where antibodies to the thyroid stimulating receptor result in overactivity of the thyroid (*Fig. 3*).

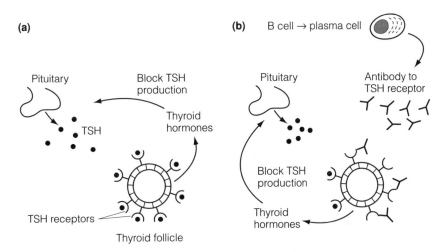

Fig. 3.   Graves' disease. (a) The pituitary makes thyroid stimulating hormone (TSH) which binds to TSH receptors on cells of the thyroid follicle and triggers them to make thyroid hormones. In turn, these thyroid hormones inhibit production of TSH by the pituitary as a form of normal feedback regulation of TSH production by thyroid hormones.
(b) Autoantibodies to TSH receptor bind TSH receptors and trigger the thyroid follicle cells to release thyroid hormones which stop the pituitary from making TSH. However, they have no effect on production of the autoantibody which continues to stimulate thyroid follicle cells to make thyroid hormones, thus causing hyperthyroidism.

K4 IMMUNE-COMPLEX-MEDIATED (TYPE III) HYPERSENSITIVITY

Key Notes

Introduction	Immune complexes can form to foreign serum products e.g. immunoglobulin, as well as microbial and self antigens, either in local sites or systemically, leading to phagocytic and complement mediated damage.
Mechanisms of type III hypersensitivity	Tissue damage is caused mainly by complement activation and release of lytic enzymes from neutrophils. Local damage (Arthus reaction) can be seen in pulmonary disease resulting from inhaled antigen. Systemic antibody complexes with microbial or autoantigens result in immune complex deposition in blood vessels (vasculitis) or in the renal vessels (glomeruli) of the kidneys leading to glomerulonephritis.
Diseases associated with type III hypersensitivity	Pulmonary diseases result from inhalation of bacterial spores (Farmer's lung) or avian serum/fecal proteins (bird fancier's disease). Systemic disease can occur from streptococcal infections (streptococcal nephritis), autoimmune complexes (e.g. systemic lupus erythematosus (SLE)) or drugs (e.g. penicillin) or antisera made in animals.

Related topics	Innate immunity and inflammation (B4)	Antigen/antibody complexes (immune complexes) (D6)
	Antibody classes (D2)	Disease pathogenesis – effector mechanisms (L4)

Introduction

Normally, immune complexes are removed by phagocytic cells and there is no tissue damage. However when there are large amounts of immune complexes and they persist in tissues, they can cause damage which may be localized within tissues (Arthus reaction) or systemic. This type of hypersensitivity can be induced by microbial antigens, autoantigens and foreign serum components.

Mechanisms of type III hypersensitivity

Much of the tissue damage is the result of complement activation leading to neutrophil chemoattraction and release of lytic enzymes by the degranulating neutrophils (Topic B1). Local deposition of immune complexes results in an Arthus reaction (*Fig. 1*). Immune complexes (usually small) can also cause systemic effects such as fever, weakness, vasculitis, arthritis and edema and glomerulonephritis. An example of this is when passive antibodies are given to patients to protect them against microbial toxins such as tetanus toxin (Topic J4). An antibody response can develop (serum sickness) against the horse anti-tetanus toxin and forms immune complexes with them. Serum immune complexes can deposit in blood vessels (vasculitis) or can become trapped in the blood vessels of the kidneys leading to glomerulonephritis.

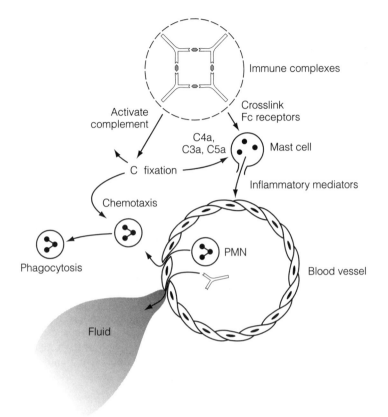

Fig. 1. *The Arthus reaction. Small immune complexes in the skin directly trigger Fc receptors and activate complement resulting essentially in an acute inflammatory response mediated through mast cells. Small immune complexes can also lodge in blood vessels and induce vasculitis or glomerulonephritis in the kidney.*

Diseases associated with type III hypersensitivity

A list of some diseases mediated by type III hypersensitivity is shown in *Table 1*. IgG antibodies complexed with inhaled antigens cause local damage in the airways of the lung (which also includes pneumonitis and alveolitis). Immune complexes made against antigens encountered systemically cause a variety of symptoms and in particular kidney damage through deposition.

Table 1. *Diseases mediated by type III hypersensitivity*

Site of reaction	Antigens	Disease
Localized (inhaled)	Bacterial spores	Farmer's lung
	Fungal spores	
	Pigeon serum/fecal proteins	Bird fancier's disease
Systemic	Microbes including Streptococcus	Streptococcal nephritis
	Hepatitis B	
	Epstein–Barr virus	
	Malaria	
	Autoantigens e.g. DNA	Systemic lupus erythematosus
	Drugs – penicillin, sulphonamides	Drug allergy

K5 DELAYED (TYPE IV) HYPERSENSITIVITY

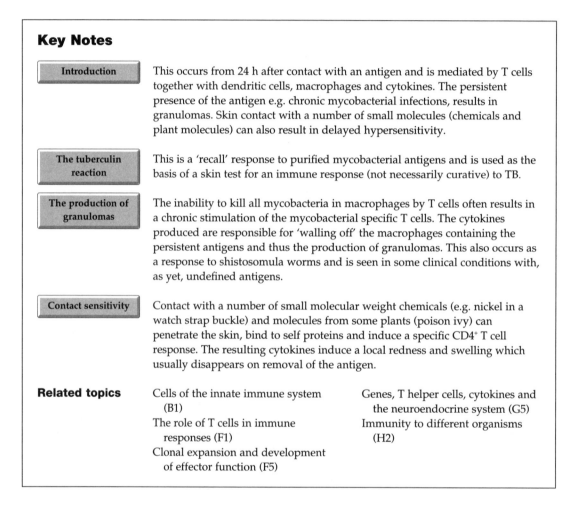

Key Notes

Introduction

This occurs from 24 h after contact with an antigen and is mediated by T cells together with dendritic cells, macrophages and cytokines. The persistent presence of the antigen e.g. chronic mycobacterial infections, results in granulomas. Skin contact with a number of small molecules (chemicals and plant molecules) can also result in delayed hypersensitivity.

The tuberculin reaction

This is a 'recall' response to purified mycobacterial antigens and is used as the basis of a skin test for an immune response (not necessarily curative) to TB.

The production of granulomas

The inability to kill all mycobacteria in macrophages by T cells often results in a chronic stimulation of the mycobacterial specific T cells. The cytokines produced are responsible for 'walling off' the macrophages containing the persistent antigens and thus the production of granulomas. This also occurs as a response to shistosomula worms and is seen in some clinical conditions with, as yet, undefined antigens.

Contact sensitivity

Contact with a number of small molecular weight chemicals (e.g. nickel in a watch strap buckle) and molecules from some plants (poison ivy) can penetrate the skin, bind to self proteins and induce a specific CD4⁺ T cell response. The resulting cytokines induce a local redness and swelling which usually disappears on removal of the antigen.

Related topics

Cells of the innate immune system (B1)

The role of T cells in immune responses (F1)

Clonal expansion and development of effector function (F5)

Genes, T helper cells, cytokines and the neuroendocrine system (G5)

Immunity to different organisms (H2)

Introduction

Unlike type 1 (immediate) hypersensitivity, this hypersensitivity reaction, the only type transferable by cells rather than antibodies, was shown to begin at least 24 h after contact with the eliciting antigen. It was first associated with T cell mediated immune responses to *Mycobacterium tuberculosis* (MTb) and was therefore initially termed 'bacterial hypersensitivity'. Such responses often lead to the production of granulomas some weeks later. This delayed type of hypersensitivity (DTH) now covers a range of T cell mediated responses including those induced by small molecules coming into contact with the skin – contact hypersensitivity. In addition to T cells, the key players in this type of sensitivity are dendritic cells, macrophages and cytokines. This type of hypersensitivity also plays a role in several clinical situations where there is persistence of antigen which the immune system is unable to remove, leading to chronic inflammation.

The tuberculin reaction

Initial experiments by Koch showed that patients with tuberculosis (TB) given subcutaneous injection of mycobacterial antigens derived from MTb, resulted in fever and sickness. This 'tuberculin reaction' is now the basis of a 'recall' test to determine if individuals have T cell mediated reactivity against TB. In this test (Mantoux test) small amounts of the purified protein derivative (PPD) of tuberculin derived from MTb organisms are injected into the skin and the site examined up to 72 h later. A positive skin test shows up as a firm red swelling which is maximal at 48–72 h after injection and is mediated by dendritic cells and an influx of both T cells and macrophages into the site of injection (*Fig. 1*).

The production of granulomas

We now know that CD4$^+$ T cells control intracellular microbial infections such as mycobacteria and some fungi (Topic F5). The problem is that mycobacteria, in addition to some other intracellular infections, have escape mechanisms to prevent their elimination (Topic H3). Thus, the macrophage activation factors produced by CD4$^+$ T cells are not always effective (*Fig. 2*). Antigen therefore persists and leads to the 'chronic' stimulation of CD4$^+$ T cells and continuous production of cytokines. These mediate fusion of the macrophages containing the microbes and fibroblast proliferation, finally resulting in a 'walling off' of the offending microbes in a granuloma. This chronic inflammatory state is seen in both TB and in the tuberculoid type of leprosy caused by *Mycobacterium leprae* (Topic H2). Granulomatous reactions also occur with shistosomula

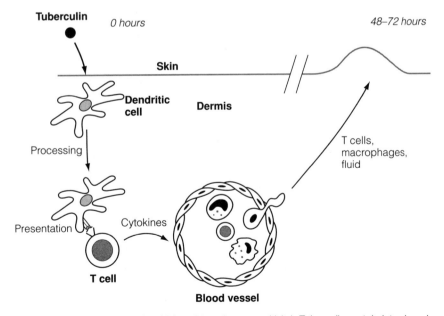

Fig. 1. The tuberculin reaction (delayed-type hypersensitivity). Tuberculin protein introduced into the dermis is processed and presented by dendritic cells to T cells via MHC class II molecules. Cytokines produced by the T cells alter local endothelial cell adhesion molecules allowing monocytes to enter the site of injection and develop into macrophages. T cells and macrophage products result in edema (fluid) and swelling. A positive skin test shows up as a firm red swelling which is maximal at 48–72 h after injection.

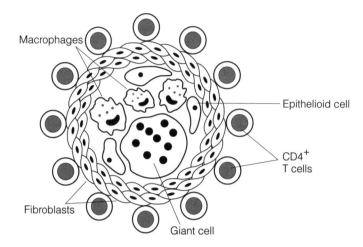

Fig. 2. Granulomas. Immune granulomas are formed in response to chronic stimulation of CD4⁺ T cells by persistent nondegradable antigens including mycobacteria. They consist of epithelioid cells, macrophages and giant cells which are 'walled off' by fibroblasts surrounded by an outer layer of CD4⁺ T cells. Cytokines produced by the different cells all contribute to the granuloma formation which is the immune system's way of isolating the nondegradable microbes from the rest of the body.

infections and in some clinical situations where the antigens have not yet been defined (e.g. sarcoidosis and Crohn's disease). Non-immune granulomas are produced by persistent particles such as asbestos that cannot easily be removed from the body by phagocytosis.

Contact sensitivity

A number of small molecules penetrating the skin can give rise to contact sensitivity, seen clinically as dermatitis. Some chemical agents and plant products shown to produce contact sensitivity are listed in *Table 1*. Classical examples of contact sensitivity include reactions against metal fasteners on watch straps and rashes seen in response to poison oak. Removal of contact with the agent usually results in resolution of the hypersensitivity.

Sensitization against these molecules is thought to be mediated through binding to skin proteins and through the powerful antigen presenting properties of skin dendritic cells, Langerhans cells, which present antigen on MHC class II molecules to CD4⁺ Th1 cells (*Fig. 3*). The subsequent contact sensitivity reaction involves presentation of the antigens to memory CD4⁺ T cells which release cytokines causing vasodilation, traffic into the site of non-specific CD4⁺ T cells and activated macrophages, and localized pustule formation.

Table 1. Agents causing contact sensitivity

Chemicals: nickel, turpentine, some cosmetics, formaldehyde
Plants: poison ivy, poison oak

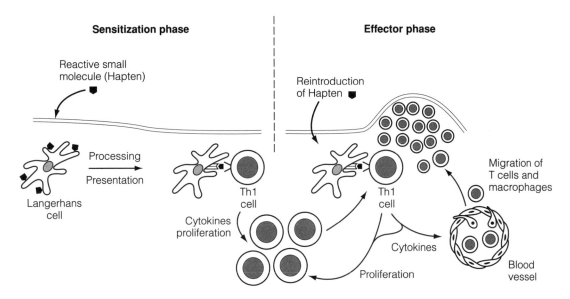

Fig. 3. Contact sensitivity mediated through Langerhans cells. In the sensitization phase, reactive small molecules, haptens (e.g. pentadecacatechol associated with poison ivy), which come in contact with the skin, bind to self proteins (including those on Langerhans cells) and are internalized, processed and presented by Langerhans cells to T cells. These proliferate to form clones of Th1 cells specific for hapten modified self peptide. When hapten is reintroduced, the modified self peptide is again presented on Langerhans cells in MHC class II. Memory T cells eventually find and respond to these antigens by releasing cytokines (e.g. IFNγ) which attract primarily Th1 cells and monocytes to this area and upregulate expression of adhesion molecules on endothelial cells that result in passage of Langerhans cells into the tissues.

L1 THE SPECTRUM AND PREVALENCE OF AUTOIMMUNITY

Key Notes

Autoimmunity and autoimmune disease	Autoimmunity is an acquired immune reactivity to self antigens. Autoimmune diseases occur when autoimmune responses lead to tissue damage.
Spectrum of autoimmune conditions	Autoimmune diseases may be organ specific, e.g. diabetes mellitus where the pancreas is the target organ, or systemic (nonorgan specific), e.g. systemic lupus erythematosus (SLE), where multiple organs may be involved. Pathogenesis associated with these diseases may be mediated primarily by antibody, by T cells or a combination thereof.
Prevalence	Approximately 3.5% of individuals have autoimmune disease, 94% of which are accounted for by Graves' disease/hyperthyroidism, type I diabetes, pernicious anemia, rheumatoid arthritis (RA), thyroiditis, vitiligo, multiple sclerosis (MS) and SLE. Women are more likely than men to develop autoimmune disease.
Related topics	Central and peripheral tolerance (G2) Antigen preparations (I3)

Autoimmunity and autoimmune disease

The immune system has the capacity to mount an immune response to virtually all molecules and/or cells. Although the capacity to respond to self antigen is present in all of us, in most instances such responses result in tolerance or anergy (Section G), indicating that mechanisms must exist to prevent or subdue autoimmune responses. Moreover, autoreactive T and B cells as well as auto-antibodies are found in people who do not have autoimmune diseases, demonstrating that immunological autoreactivity alone is not sufficient for the development of disease. The mechanisms currently thought to prevent/dampen autoimmune responses include inactivation or deletion of autoreactive T and B cells, active suppression by cells or cytokines, idiotype/anti-idiotype interactions, and the immunosuppressive adrenal hormones, the glucocorticoids. When dampening mechanisms fail or are overridden, a response directed against self-antigen can occur, resulting in autoimmune diseases that range from those which are organ specific (diabetes and thyroiditis) to those which are systemic (non-organ specific) such as systemic lupus erythematosus and rheumatoid arthritis.

Several important cofactors in the development of autoimmune disease have been identified and include genetics (e.g. HLA associations), gender, and age. Characteristics of the antigen and how it is 'presented' to the immune system are also important. For example, injection of animals with chemically modified thyroid protein or with normal protein plus Freund's adjuvant (Topic I3) can give rise to severe thyroiditis that is due to immune recognition of normal thyroid proteins. Infection by organisms including Epstein Barr virus (EBV) or mycoplasma can provoke autoantibody production in otherwise normal persons. In addition, certain drugs such as procainamide which is used to treat cardiac arrhythmias, or toxic substances such as mercuric chloride and polyvinyl chloride can induce autoimmune pathology. Moreover, the attack by immune effectors on virus or drug antigens that results in inappropriate tissue damage, may also be considered an autoimmune-like disease (Section K).

Spectrum of autoimmune conditions

That autoimmune diseases involve immune recognition of specific antigens is evidenced by organ-specific diseases including thyroiditis, diabetes mellitus, multiple sclerosis (MS) and inflammatory bowel disease. Antigens shared by multiple tissue sites are apparently involved in systemic autoimmunity in diseases such as SLE, RA, systemic vasculitis and scleroderma. It is also clear that a given individual may develop autoimmune disease of more than one type (e.g. thyroid autoimmune disease is sometimes associated with gastric autoimmunity). Furthermore, the pathogenesis associated with autoimmune disease may be mediated primarily by antibody (e.g. hemolytic anemia), primarily by cellular immunity (e.g. MS) or by a combination of antibody and cell mediated immunity (e.g. RA).

Prevalence

Autoimmune diseases are quite prevalent in the general population, where it is estimated that approximately 3.5% of individuals are afflicted. The most common are Graves' disease/hyperthyroidism, type I diabetes, pernicious anemia, RA, thyroiditis, vitiligo, MS and SLE, which together account for 94% of all cases. Overall, women are 2.7 times more likely than men to develop an autoimmune disease, but the female:male ratio can be as high as 10:1 in SLE (Topic O3).

L2 FACTORS CONTRIBUTING TO THE DEVELOPMENT OF AUTOIMMUNE DISEASE

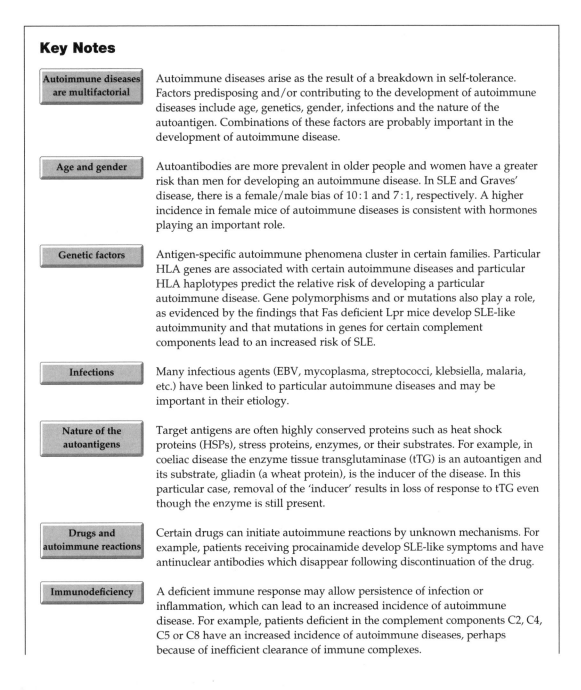

Key Notes

Autoimmune diseases are multifactorial

Autoimmune diseases arise as the result of a breakdown in self-tolerance. Factors predisposing and/or contributing to the development of autoimmune diseases include age, genetics, gender, infections and the nature of the autoantigen. Combinations of these factors are probably important in the development of autoimmune disease.

Age and gender

Autoantibodies are more prevalent in older people and women have a greater risk than men for developing an autoimmune disease. In SLE and Graves' disease, there is a female/male bias of $10:1$ and $7:1$, respectively. A higher incidence in female mice of autoimmune diseases is consistent with hormones playing an important role.

Genetic factors

Antigen-specific autoimmune phenomena cluster in certain families. Particular HLA genes are associated with certain autoimmune diseases and particular HLA haplotypes predict the relative risk of developing a particular autoimmune disease. Gene polymorphisms and or mutations also play a role, as evidenced by the findings that Fas deficient Lpr mice develop SLE-like autoimmunity and that mutations in genes for certain complement components lead to an increased risk of SLE.

Infections

Many infectious agents (EBV, mycoplasma, streptococci, klebsiella, malaria, etc.) have been linked to particular autoimmune diseases and may be important in their etiology.

Nature of the autoantigens

Target antigens are often highly conserved proteins such as heat shock proteins (HSPs), stress proteins, enzymes, or their substrates. For example, in coeliac disease the enzyme tissue transglutaminase (tTG) is an autoantigen and its substrate, gliadin (a wheat protein), is the inducer of the disease. In this particular case, removal of the 'inducer' results in loss of response to tTG even though the enzyme is still present.

Drugs and autoimmune reactions

Certain drugs can initiate autoimmune reactions by unknown mechanisms. For example, patients receiving procainamide develop SLE-like symptoms and have antinuclear antibodies which disappear following discontinuation of the drug.

Immunodeficiency

A deficient immune response may allow persistence of infection or inflammation, which can lead to an increased incidence of autoimmune disease. For example, patients deficient in the complement components C2, C4, C5 or C8 have an increased incidence of autoimmune diseases, perhaps because of inefficient clearance of immune complexes.

Related topics	Genes, T helper cells, cytokines and the neuroendocrine system (G5)	Primary/congenital (inherited) immunodeficiency (J2)

Autoimmune diseases are multifactorial

Autoimmune diseases arise as the result of a breakdown in tolerance to self antigens. Moreover, autoimmune diseases are multifactorial in that their development, in most cases, probably results from combinations of predisposing and/or contributing factors. The factors known to predispose and/or contribute to the development of autoimmune diseases include (*Table 1*): genetics – inheritance of a particular HLA haplotype increases the risk of developing disease; gender – more females than males develop disease; infections – EBV, mycoplasma, streptococci, klebsiella, malaria, etc., have been linked to particular autoimmune diseases; the nature of the autoantigen – highly conserved enzymes and heat shock proteins (HSPs) are often target antigens and may be cross-reactive with microbial antigens; drugs – certain drugs can induce autoimmune-like syndromes; and age – most autoimmune diseases occur in adults.

Table 1. Summary of factors contributing to development of autoimmune diseases

Genetics	Some diseases are HLA associated
Gender	Females generally more prone than males
Infections	Some common infections e.g. EBV, streptococcus, malaria, etc.
Nature of autoantigen	Often conserved antigens e.g. heat shock proteins and enzymes
Drugs	Some drugs e.g. procainamide, hydralazine induce SLE-like symptoms
Age	Higher incidence in aged population

Age and gender

Autoantibodies are more prevalent in older people and animals, perhaps due to less stringent immunoregulation by the aging immune system. Few autoimmune diseases occur in children, the majority being in adults. Women have a greater risk than men for developing an autoimmune disease. In SLE and Graves' disease, there is a female/male bias of 10:1 and 7:1 respectively, whereas ankylosing spondylitis is almost exclusively a male disease. Taken together, these facts suggest that the neuroendocrine system plays an important role in the development of these diseases. This is supported by animal studies where it has been shown that female mice of a particular strain spontaneously develop SLE. This can be prevented by removing their ovaries (estrogen source) or by treating them with testosterone. Similarly, male mice that are more resistant to developing the disease lose this resistance if castrated (Topic O3).

Genetic factors

Antigen-specific autoimmune phenomena cluster in certain families. For example, thyroid-reactive antibodies are much more common in genetically related family members of a person with autoimmune thyroid disease than in the population at large. The role of the MHC (presumably in presenting autoantigenic peptides) is evidenced by the strong association between HLA type and incidence of certain autoimmune diseases. The possession of particular HLA haplotypes predicts the relative risk of developing a particular autoimmune disease (*Table 2*). Polymorphisms and/or mutations of many other genes involved in lymphocyte activation or suppression are also likely to play a

Table 2.   Some autoimmune diseases showing HLA association (Caucasians)

Disease	HLA	Risk*
Ankylosing spondylitis	B27	90
Reiter's disease	B27	36.0
Systemic lupus erythematosus	DR3	15
Myasthenia gravis	DR3	2.5
Juvenile diabetes mellitus (insulin dependent)	DR3/DR4	25
Psoriasis vulgaris	DR4	14
Multiple sclerosis	DR2	5
Rheumatoid arthritis	DR4	4

*Based on a comparison of the incidence of the autoimmune disease in patients with a given HLA type with the incidence of the autoimmune disease in patients without this HLA type.

crucial role. For example, in Lpr autoimmune mice, an autosomal recessive mutation in the Fas apoptosis gene leads to progressive lymphadenopathy and hypergammaglobulinemia, with production of multiple SLE-like autoantibodies. Complement deficiency due to mutations in genes for C2, C4, C5 and C8 results in increased risk of SLE, demonstrating the importance of complement in the clearance of immune complexes.

Infections

Many infectious agents (EBV, mycoplasma, streptococci, klebsiella, malaria, etc.) have been linked to particular autoimmune diseases. Lyme arthritis, for example, is initiated by chronic infection with spirochetes of the genus *Borrelia* (e.g. *Borrelia burgdorferi*) which are transmitted by deer ticks from deer and rodents to people. Some microbial antigens also have structures similar to self-antigens and induce autoimmune responses through 'antigenic mimicry' (see below).

Nature of the autoantigens

Target antigens for autoimmune disease can be cell surface, cytoplasmic, nuclear or secreted molecules (*Table 3*). They are often highly conserved proteins such as HSPs, stress proteins, enzymes or their substrates (*Table 4*). Of importance, the primary immune response to microbial infections includes a strong response to HSPs, followed by a response to a microbe specific component. Since HSPs are highly conserved, a dominant immune response to these antigens may confer on the host an ability to respond generally to other microbial infections. However, microbial and human HSPs have high sequence homology as well. Thus, an immune response to microbial HSP may induce a cross reactive response to human HSP. Target autoantigens are often enzymes (*Table 4*). For example, in coeliac disease the enzyme tissue transglutaminase (tTG) is an autoantigen and its substrate, gliadin (a wheat protein), is the inducer of the disease. Antibodies to both wheat proteins and tTG are found in patients with this disease. However, removal of the wheat protein from the diet leads to the removal of the immune response to tTG as well as to the wheat proteins, although tTG is still present.

Drugs and autoimmune reactions

Certain drugs can initiate autoimmune reactions by unknown mechanisms. For example, antinuclear antibodies appear in the blood of the vast majority of patients receiving prolonged treatment with procainamide for ventricular arrythmias, and nearly 10% develop an SLE-like syndrome which resolves following discontinuation of the drug.

Table 3. Antigens targeted in autoimmune disease.

Organ specific diseases		Nonorgan specific diseases	
Disease	Antigen(s)	Disease	Antigen(s)
Addison's disease	Adrenal cortical cells (ACTH receptor, 17α and 21 hydroxylase)	Ankylosing spondylitis	Vertebral
Autoimmune hemolytic anemia	RBC membrane antigens	Chronic active hepatitis	Nuclei, DNA
Graves' disease	TSH receptor	Multiple sclerosis	Brain/myelin basic protein
Guillain–Barré syndrome	Peripheral nerves (gangliosides)	Rheumatoid arthritis	IgG (rheumatoid factor) connective tissues
Hashimoto's thyroiditis	Thyroid peroxidase thyroglobulin/T4	Scleroderma	Nuclei, elastin, nucleoli, centromeres, topoisomerase 1
Insulin-dependent diabetes mellitus (IDDM)	β cells in the pancreas (GAD, tyrosine phosphatase)	Sjögren's syndrome	Exocrine glands, kidney, liver, thyroid
Pemphigus	Epidermal keratinocytes	Systemic lupus erythematosus	Double stranded DNA, nuclear antigens
Pernicious anemia	Intrinsic factor	Wegener's granulomatosis	Proteinase 3
Polymyositis	Muscle (histidine tRNA synthetase)		
Primary biliary cirrhosis	Pyruvate dehydrogenase		
Several organs affected			
Goodpasture's syndrome	Basement membrane of kidney and lung (type IV collagen)		
Polyendocrine	Multiple endocrine organs (hepatic-cytochrome p450; intestinal-tryptophan hydroxylase)		

Table 4. Enzymes as autoantigens

Enzyme	Disease
Pyruvate dehydrogenase	Primary biliary cirrhosis
Glutamic acid decarboxylase	Insulin dependent diabetes
Myeloperoxidase	Glomerulonephritis
Thyroid peroxidase	Autoimmune thyroiditis
17α and 21 hydroxylase	Addison's disease
Proteinase 3	Wegener's granulomatosis
Tyrosinase	Vitiligo
Transglutaminase	Coeliac disease

Immunodeficiency A deficient immune response may allow persistence of infection or inflammation. This possibility is supported by the observation that immune deficiency syndromes are associated with autoimmune abnormalities. For example, patients deficient in the complement components C2, C4, C5 or C8 have an increased incidence of autoimmune diseases (see Genetic factors). There are also diseases where paradoxically immunodeficiency and autoimmunity coexist. An example of this is in common variable immune deficiency (Topic J2) where autoantibodies to platelets are sometimes found. Autoimmune diseases are also more common in patients with IgA-deficiency (Topic J2).

L3 AUTOIMMUNE DISEASES – MECHANISMS OF DEVELOPMENT

Key Notes

Breakdown of self-tolerance

The mechanisms that lead to autoimmunity are unclear but may include molecular mimicry, defective regulation of the anti-self response through Th1 and Th2 cells, polyclonal activation, modification of self antigens through microbes and drugs, changes in availability of self antigen and dysregulation of the idiotype network.

Molecular mimicry and the T cell bypass

An immune response may be generated against an epitope that is identical, or nearly identical, in both a microbe and host tissue, resulting in attack on host tissue by the same effector mechanisms activated to eliminate the pathogen. For example, a cross-reactive antigen between heart muscle and Group A *Streptococci* predisposes to the development of rheumatic fever as a result of inducing autoantibodies to heart muscle.

Defective regulation mediated via Th cells

Microbial infection induces either Th1 or Th2 cytokines. The Th1 response leads to the production of the pro-inflammatory cytokines, while the Th2 response is associated with anti-inflammatory cytokines and antibody formation. Predominance of Th1 or Th2 responses occurs in some autoimmune diseases and changes in the relative contribution of these subsets (e.g. as seen in pregnancy) can influence disease activity in RA and SLE.

Polyclonal activation via microbial antigens

Some microbes or their products activate lymphocytes independently of their antigenic specificity, i.e. are polyclonal activators, e.g. LPS and EBV. Patients with infectious mononucleosis produce IgM antibodies to several autoantigens including DNA. Since a switch to production of IgG autoantibodies (which requires Th cells) does not occur, T cells are probably not involved or are inhibited in their action.

Modification of cell surfaces by microbes and drugs

Foreign antigens, e.g. viruses and drugs, may become adsorbed onto the surfaces of cells or react chemically with surface antigens in a hapten-like manner to alter their specificity. For example, thrombocytopenia and anemia are relatively common in drug-induced autoimmune disease. Thrombocytopenia is also common in children following viral infections, and may involve association of viral antigens or immune complexes with the surface of platelets.

Availability of normally sequestered self-antigen

Since tolerance induction occurs mainly during embryonic development, antigens which are absent or anatomically separated (sequestered) from the immune system during this period are not recognized as self. Such antigens include the lens proteins of the eye, and molecules associated with the central nervous system, the thyroid and testes.

Dysregulation of the idiotype network	Anti-idiotypic antibodies resulting from an immune response to a hormone could interact with the receptor for the hormone, and thus initiate disease. Animal experiments have verified the existence of this mechanism. Clinical examples include those resulting from development of antibodies to insulin and acetylcholine receptors.
Related topics	Antigens (A4) Central and peripheral tolerance (G2) Regulation by antigen and antibody (G4)
	Genes, T helper cells, cytokines and neuroendocrine system (G5) Pathogen defense strategies (H3)

Breakdown of self-tolerance

The mechanisms that lead to autoimmunity are unclear and involve many factors. In an ideal immune response only foreign antigens activate immune effector mechanisms, the foreign antigens are selectively cleared without damage to the host and immune effector mechanisms are turned off when they are no longer needed. Thus, the immune response may require the orderly interaction of at least four distinct cell types (antigen presenting cells, CTLs, Th cells, and B cells; Topics E3, F2 and F5) that communicate by direct cell to cell contact and through cytokines. Although these interactions are usually well controlled, a defect could result in specific adaptive immune responses to self antigens which cause autoimmune disease. The various mechanisms which may explain breakdown of tolerance to self and how reactions may be initiated to autoantigens include molecular mimicry, defective regulation of the anti-self response through Th1 and Th2 cells, polyclonal activation, modification of self antigens through microbes and drugs, changes in the availability of self antigen and dysregulation of the idiotype network.

Molecular mimicry and the T cell bypass

The adaptive immune response continuously monitors microbial infections and responds accordingly. In some cases, however, a response may be generated against an epitope that is identical, or nearly identical, in both a microbe and host tissue, resulting in attack on host tissue by the same effector mechanisms which are activated to eliminate the pathogen. One example is rheumatic heart disease, which is due to an epitope that is common to heart muscle and Group A *Streptococci* (*Fig. 1*). In this case, previously anergized anti-self B cells (which also crossreact with *Streptococci*) may be reactivated by receiving co-stimulatory signals from microbe-specific T cells. The B cell interacts with the microbial antigen through its antigen receptor and presents microbial peptides to anti-microbial T cells which then provide help and activate the anti-self B cells (*Fig. 2*). Self reactive B cells also become activated if the self antigen forms a complex with a microbial antigen. In this event, the self reactive B cell can endocytose microbial antigens along with the self antigen and present microbial peptides to T cells. The microbe specific T cell in this instance will provide help to the self reactive B cell in the form of costimulatory molecules and cytokines leading to breakdown in tolerance (Topic G1).

Defective regulation mediated via Th cells

The initial response to a microbial infection is usually associated with predominantly either Th1 or Th2 cytokines (Topic G5). The Th1 response leads to the production of the pro-inflammatory cytokines IFNγ, IL2, and TNFα, followed by the release of the anti-inflammatory cytokines TGFβ, IL-4 and IL-10 from Th2 cells. The Th2 response is associated with anti-inflammatory cytokines and

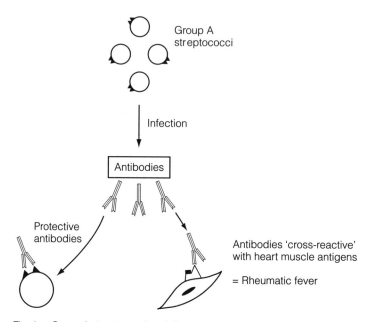

Fig. 1.   Group A streptococci and rheumatic fever. Antibodies to a streptococcal antigen 'cross-react' with heart muscle antigen leading to damage and rheumatic fever. Disease abates when the bacteria are eliminated and antibody production ceases.

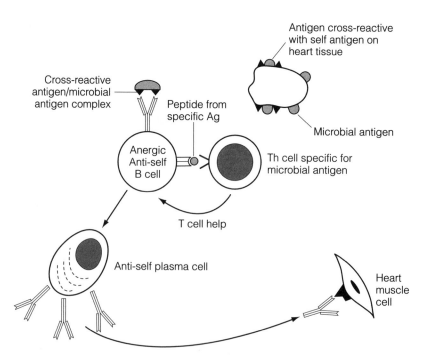

Fig. 2.   Activation of anergic anti-self B cells. The BCR on an anti-self B cell binds to self/microbial Ag complex. The B cell presents the microbial component of the complex to a T cell and receives T cell help for activation (second signal). This is also called the 'T cell bypass' mechanism of autoimmunity since T cell help for self is bypassed by presentation via a nonself antigen.

antibody formation. That polarized Th1 or Th2 responses may be involved in autoimmune pathogenesis is suggested by the observation that during pregnancy, a period when Th2 cytokines predominate, the Th1 autoimmune disease RA is decreased, whereas the Th2 autoimmune disease SLE is exacerbated.

Polyclonal activation via microbial antigens

Some microbes or their products activate lymphocytes independently of their antigenic specificity, i.e. are polyclonal activators. An example of this is endotoxin or lipopolysaccharide (LPS), which is produced mainly by Gram-negative bacteria. Another example involves EBV, which has been linked to autoimmunity in a small subset of infected individuals. Most patients with infectious mononucleosis, which is caused by EBV, develop IgM autoantibodies against several cellular antigens including DNA (*Fig. 3*). Since a switch to production of IgG autoantibodies, which requires Th cells, does not occur, T cells are probably not involved or are inhibited in their action. Moreover, on recovery, when the strong EBV stimulus is removed, autoantibodies disappear. Clearly, multiple factors are important for maintenance of long term tolerance to self, and a defect or impairment of immunoregulation following infection can result in activation and expansion of autoreactive clones.

Modification of cell surfaces by microbes and drugs

Foreign antigens may become adsorbed onto the surfaces of cells or react chemically with surface antigens in a hapten-like manner to alter their immunogenicity. Thrombocytopenia (low platelet levels) and anemia (low red blood cell levels are relatively common examples of drug-induced autoimmune disease. Thrombocytopenia is also common in children following viral infections, and may involve association of viral antigens or virus–antibody immune complexes with the surface of platelets. Similarly, an autoimmune-like situation may result when microbial antigens become actively expressed on the surfaces of infected or transformed cells, especially during viral infection. Although the immune

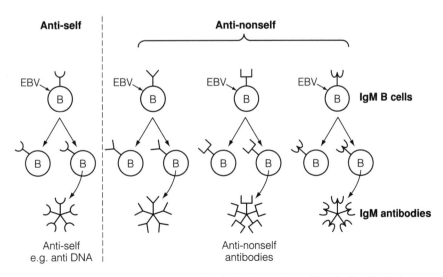

Fig. 3. Autoantibodies produced through polyclonal activation of B cells. B cells of all specificities including self, which have not been eliminated by central tolerance mechanisms, may be polyclonally activated (e.g. by EBV infection) to synthesize and release the antibodies they are programed to produce, perhaps including some autoantibodies. Transient production of the antibodies normally subsides after the microbe is eliminated or controlled.

response that subsequently develops normally results in removal of these infected cells, in some cases the tissue destruction associated with elimination of these antigens may result in immunologically mediated disease which is much more serious than the infection itself. For example, mice infected *in utero* or at birth with lymphocytic choriomeningitis virus (LCMV) become tolerant to the virus and harbor it for life without overt disease symptoms. However, if normal adult mice are exposed to LCMV, the infection is invariably fatal. In X-irradiated or neonatally thymectomized (i.e. immunosuppressed) mice, the viral infection is not lethal. Thus, lethal neurological damage results, not from the virus itself, but from the immune response to LCMV-infected cells.

Availability of normally sequestered self antigen

Since tolerance induction occurs mainly during embryonic development, antigens which are absent or anatomically separated (sequestered) from the immune system during this period are not recognized as self. These antigens are either present in too low amounts to stimulate autoimmunity or are sequestered in immunologically privileged sites. In later life, these antigens may be released as a result of trauma or infection. They may then stimulate lymphocytes that have escaped tolerance, and induce the development of autoimmune disease. Antigens which fit this model include those found in the lens of the eye, central nervous system, thyroid and testes. For example, after vasectomy blocks the release of sperm through spermatic ducts, antibodies to spermatozoa are produced. In addition, trauma to the lens in one eye results in autoantibodies that can damage the nontraumatized eye.

Dysregulation of the idiotype network

Another mechanism by which autoantibodies may arise is through a failure of idiotype/anti-idiotype control (Topics D4 and G4). Anti-idiotypic antibodies resulting from an immune response to a hormone could interact with the receptor for the hormone, and thus initiate disease (*Fig. 4*). Many animal experiments have verified the existence of this mechanism. Possible clinical examples include those resulting from development of antibodies to insulin and acetylcholine receptors (Topic K3).

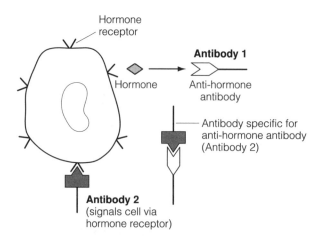

Fig. 4. Antireceptor anti-idiotypic antibody in the development of autoimmune disease. Antibody 1 is directed towards the receptor-binding region of a ligand (e.g. a hormone). Antibody 2 is directed towards the idiotype of antibody 1. Antibody 2 can thus bind the receptor, potentially resulting in autoimmunity.

L4 DISEASE PATHOGENESIS – EFFECTOR MECHANISMS

Key Notes

Tissue damaging reactions in autoimmune diseases	Once autoantibodies have been produced, their mechanisms of tissue destruction are the same as the mechanisms that lead to protective responses – phagocytosis, complement activation and interference with molecular function. Both T and B cells may be involved as well as inflammatory cytokines, immune complexes, phagocytes and complement components. In this case they are considered as hypersensitivity reactions to self antigens. The main difference between anti-microbial and autoimmune responses is that, in autoimmune disease, autoantigen is always present and cannot be removed from the body. Removal of the autoantigen results in eventual loss of autoantibodies.
Autoantibodies can directly mediate cell destruction	Autoantibodies can bind to self cells and, either alone or with complement, cause damage mediated mainly through opsonization via Fc and C3 receptors on phagocytic cells. For example, IgG autoantibodies bind to red blood cells in autoimmune hemolytic anemia (AIHA) or to platelets in immune thrombocytopenic purpura (ITP) and mediate phagocytosis of these self cells.
Autoantibodies can modulate cell function	Antibodies to certain self cell surface molecules can either interfere with or enhance the functional activity of the cell. For example, Abs to the acetylcholine receptor in myasthenia gravis block their effective interaction with acetylcholine. In Graves' disease, Abs to the TSH receptor overstimulate the thyroid.
Autoantibodies can form damaging immune complexes	Circulating immune complexes, whether composed of autologous or foreign antigens, can result in damage to tissue by complement activation and by triggering release of mediators from Fc receptor-bearing cells (type III hypersensitivity). Immune complexes can deposit in the glomeruli, especially in SLE, leading to kidney damage or, in blood vessels, to vasculitis.
Cell mediated immunity in pathogenesis	Although autoantibodies have been most firmly linked to autoimmune disease, it is clear that cell mediated immunity plays an essential part in pathogenesis in some, if not all autoimmune disorders. Inflammatory T cell infiltrates are a hallmark of organ-specific diseases such as diabetes and multiple sclerosis. Their importance is indicated by studies showing that T cells can transfer particular autoimmune diseases.
Related topics	Cells of the innate immune system (B1) Antibody functions (D8) IgM and IgG-mediated (type II) hypersensitivity (K3) Immune-complex mediated (type III) hypersensitivity (K4) Delayed (type IV) hypersensitivity (K5)

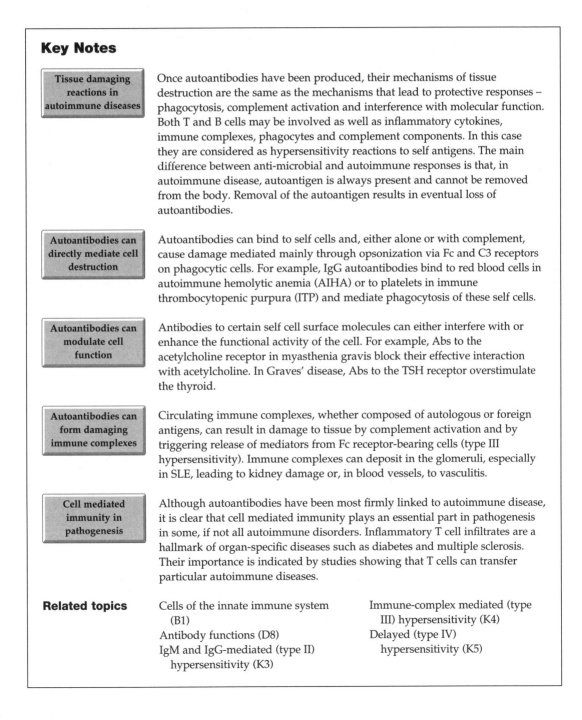

Tissue damaging reactions in autoimmune diseases

The inflammatory processes underlying the tissue damage that occurs in autoimmune disease are complex and may include all of the components of the immune system. The inflammatory infiltrate usually consists of T cells, macrophages, neutrophils, B cells, mast cells and in some instances plasma cells. However, the nature of the primary insult, whether microbial or other, and site of the target tissue may influence the type of cellular infiltrate. For example, increased numbers of mast cells, eosinophils, lymphocytes and plasma cells may be a feature of gastrointestinal associated autoimmune diseases such as coeliac disease and Crohn's disease, whereas, in the pancreas of the diabetic the cellular infiltrate may be mainly mononuclear cells i.e., lymphocytes and macrophages. Some autoimmune diseases such as Goodpasture's syndrome are caused by autoantibodies to lung and kidney basement membranes which leads to renal failure. Immune complexes become deposited in the kidney also leading to kidney failure in SLE (Topic K4). Paradoxically, immunodeficiency is often associated with an increased incidence of autoimmune disease. Thus, the immune system may be an antagonist as well as a protagonist of autoimmunity. Autoimmune diseases are driven by antigen and when this is removed in experimental animals or man the autoimmune response subsides, e.g. removal of the thyroid gland in Hashimoto's thyroiditis removes the source of autoimmune stimulation and autoantibodies are no longer produced.

Autoantibodies can directly mediate cell destruction

Autoantibodies can bind to self cells and either alone or with complement cause damage. This can be mediated through opsonization via Fc receptors or C3 receptors on phagocytic cells. An example of this is IgG autoantibodies binding to red blood cells in autoimmune hemolytic anemia (AIHA), or to platelets in

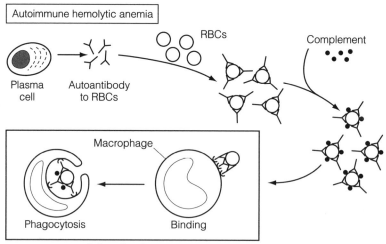

Fig. 1.   Autoantibody mediated removal of erythrocytes (AIHA) or platelets (ITP). In autoimmune hemolytic anemia (AIHA), autoantibody to red blood cells (RBCs) binds to the RBC and as these antibody-coated cells pass through the spleen, liver and lungs, they are recognized and bound by Fc receptors for IgG on macrophages in these organs. The RBCs are phagocytosed by these macrophages and destroyed. Similarly, in idiopathic thrombocytopenia (ITP), which is mediated by autoantibody to platelets, the antibody-coated platelets are removed and destroyed. Complement may also play a role in lysing autoantibody coated RBCs or platelets and/or in opsonizing these self cells for phagocytosis by macrophages.

immune thrombocytopenic purpura (ITP; *Fig. 1*). The Fc mediated mechanism appears to be more important, since successful therapy (e.g. with the immuno-suppressive steroid hormones glucocorticoids or corticosteroids) coincides with decreased Fc receptors on monocytes and macrophages, but not with lower autoantibody titers. Furthermore, the injection of high amounts of nonimmune IgG decreased cell destruction, an effect partly due to blocking of the Fc receptors on the body's phagocytes. Autoantibodies can also bind directly to cells in tissues. For example, in Goodpasture's syndrome, IgG antibodies bind to the basement membranes of kidney and lungs attracting phagocytes, which release enzymes that damage these tissues (frustrated phagocytosis).

Autoantibodies can modulate cell function

Antibodies to certain self cell surface molecules can either interfere with or enhance the functional activity of the cell. For example, myasthenia gravis (MG) is characterized by weakened and easily tired muscles. Serum antibodies directed against muscle, and in particular antibodies to the acetylcholine receptor, play a key role. These antibodies not only block the acetylcholine binding sites, but appear to act by cross-linking the receptor so that it becomes non-functional (Topic K3, *Fig. 2*). This is an example of type II hypersensitivity. The opposite is true in Graves' disease, an autoimmune thyroid disease in which autoantibodies stimulate rather than inhibit receptor function. Both thyroid growth-stimulating immunoglobulin (TGSI: an example of type V hypersensitivity) and thyrotropin binding-inhibitory immunoglobulin (TBII) have been demonstrated. TBII, by binding to receptors for thyroid stimulating hormone (TSH), thyrotropin, stimulates the thyroid gland to make high levels of thyroid hormone resulting in hyperthyroidism. IgG autoantibiodies can cross the placenta and can cause transient hyperthyroidism in the newborns of women who have Graves' disease and MG in the newborns of mothers with MG. It would appear that in MG and Graves' disease, only B-cells specific for a few bodily components are activated. The defect may therefore lie with a very small subset of T or B cells. Since total antibody titer does not correlate well with disease state, antibody class and subclass (e.g. C' binding or nonbinding) may be a crucial consideration.

Autoantibodies can form damaging immune complexes

Circulating immune complexes, whether composed of autologous or foreign antigens, can result in damage to tissue by complement activation and triggering release of mediators from Fc receptor-bearing cells (type III hypersensitivity). Immune complexes may also perturb normal immunoregulation, perhaps through triggering of Fc receptors on lymphocytes. For example, although SLE may involve some target cell-specific autoantibodies (e.g. to erythrocytes), the most life-threatening manifestation of SLE is usually kidney damage, which results from the deposition of soluble immune complexes in the glomeruli. Some immune complexes may deposit in blood vessels leading to vasculitis. Since autoantibodies are produced to many bodily components, there may be a generalized defect in self tolerance similar to the Fas/FasL apoptotic defects seen in certain autoimmune (LPR and GLD) strains of mice. Antibodies to T cells are common as well, and may contribute to progression of the disease.

Cell mediated immunity in pathogenesis

Although autoantibodies have been most firmly linked to autoimmune disease, it is clear that cell mediated immunity plays an essential part in pathogenesis in some, if not all autoimmune disorders. In particular, T cells not only play a helper role in the development of autoimmune disease but also a direct role in tissue inflammation. For example, inflammatory T cell infiltrates are a hallmark of organ-specific diseases such as diabetes and MS, and are also present in skin lesions in SLE. However, a clear understanding of their involvement in auto-immune pathogenesis has been complicated by the MHC restricted nature of T cell recognition and the difficulty in isolating these T cells and in identifying their target antigens. In animal models, using inbred populations, it has been possible to clone autoimmune T cells that are able to transfer the autoimmune disease to other animals. For example, injection of myelin basic protein has been shown to induce experimental allergic encephalomyelitis (EAE) in rats, a disease very like MS in humans. Both encephalogenic and tolerogenic peptides to which T cells bind have been identified and either disease or protection against disease can be transferred to other rats of the same inbred strain with different cloned T cells. In general, clones making Th2 cytokines are protective whereas those making Th1 cytokines elicit disease. Thus, it is clear that T cells play a central role in both pro- and anti-inflammatory aspects of autoimmune disease, and that their MHC restriction, peptide specificity, and Th1/Th2 cytokine profile are important contributors to pathogenesis.

L5 DIAGNOSIS AND TREATMENT OF AUTOIMMUNE DISEASE

Key Notes

Diagnosis

Diagnosis of autoimmune disease is through clinical and laboratory criteria that differ for each disease. Autoantibodies to a variety of autoantigens are detected using tissue sections, immunofluorescence techniques and ELISA. This allows the detection of the IgG Abs to double stranded DNA which are characteristic of SLE, and of rheumatoid factor found in RA patients. Autoantibodies to the acetyl choline receptor or the TSH receptor can be detected by the ELISA.

Replacement therapy

In some cases, critical self antigens are compromised by the autoimmune process and may need to be replaced. In the case of thyroid autoimmunity, the patient is treated with thyroid hormones. In myasthenia gravis, inhibitors of enzymes which break down acetylcholine are given. In diabetes, insulin is given to replace that lost by damage to the islet cells.

Suppression of the autoimmune process

The ideal treatment of an autoimmune disease is to reinstate specific immune tolerance to self antigen. However, more than one autoantigen is often involved and induction of tolerance is very difficult to achieve during an ongoing immune response. Current treatments are aimed at suppressing the autoimmune response. These include nonspecific aspirin-like drugs (nonsteroidal anti-inflammatory drugs; NSAIDs) or glucocorticoids, used to dampen inflammation, and plasmapheresis to remove autoantibodies. Cytotoxic drugs, cyclosporin and MAbs to T or B cells are also used to modulate or eliminate autoreactive lymphocytes. Drugs targeting cytokines (or their receptors) have also demonstrated considerable promise in RA.

Related topics

Monoclonal antibodies (D5)
Antigen/antibody complexes
  (immune complexes) (D6)

Immunoassay (D7)

Diagnosis

Diagnosis of autoimmune diseases is through clinical and laboratory criteria that differ for each disease. In the clinical laboratory, autoantibodies to a variety of autoantigens are detected using tissue sections, immunofluorescence techniques and ELISA (Topic D7). For example, sera containing antinuclear antibodies (ANA), which are characteristic of a number of autoimmune diseases, can be detected on thyroid tissues as can antibodies to thyroid peroxidase which are characteristic of Hashimoto's thyroiditis. Patients with SLE have IgG antibodies to double stranded DNA in their serum, whilst 70% of patients with RA are seropositive for rheumatoid factor – an autoantibody directed to the Fc region of IgG. Autoantibodies to the acetylcholine receptor or the TSH receptor can be detected by ELISA. Antibodies to neutrophil cytoplasmic antigen

(ANCA) are detected by immunofluorescence on normal neutrophils, which if present indicates a diagnosis of Wegener's granulomatosis.

Replacement therapy

In some cases the autoantigen that is being removed either directly by the autoimmune response (e.g. pernicious anemia, autoimmune thyroiditis or indirectly by immune damage (e.g. diabetes) may need to be given back to the patient. This includes platelets in autoimmune thrombocytopenias, thyroid hormones in thyroid autoimmunity, B12 in pernicious anemia and insulin in insulin-dependent diabetes.

Suppression of the autoimmune process

The 'Holy Grail' for the treatment of autoimmune diseases is to reinstate specific immune tolerance to the particular autoantigen. More than one autoantigen is often involved and induction of tolerance is very difficult to achieve during an ongoing immune response (Topic G3). Therefore, current treatment is essentially aimed at reducing specific inhibition of the ongoing inflammatory response (*Table 1*). Nonspecific aspirin-like drugs (nonsteroidal anti-inflammatory drugs; NSAIDs) or glucocorticoids are often used to dampen inflammation. Removal of autoantibodies and immune complexes from the blood and replacement of patient plasma with plasma from normal donors (plasmapheresis) can be useful but has a short-lived effectiveness. Cytotoxic drugs such as those used to treat tumors are used in severe cases of auto-immune disease to eliminate the autoantigen specific T and B cells which are the origin of the disease. Similarly, lymphoid irradiation has been used to treat drug-resistant RA patients with some success. Drugs that more specifically target immune cells include cyclosporin A, which inhibits cytokine release by T cells, and monoclonal antibodies directed to T cells or B cells, which could elim-inate lymphocytes responsible for the disease. However, care has to be taken to avoid elimination of important immune cells leading to secondary immuno-deficiency (Topic J3).

Table 1. Therapy of autoimmune diseases

Current	
Replacement of targeted autoantigen	E.g. thyroid hormone for thyroid autoimmune disease; insulin for type II IDDM.
Nonsteroidal anti-inflammatory drugs (NSAIDs) e.g. aspirin, ibuprofen	Inhibit prostaglandins – RA and others
Corticosteroids e.g. prednisone	Anti-inflammatory
Cytotoxic drugs	
Azathioprine	Inhibits cell division, suppresses T cells
Cyclophosphamide	Blocks cell division, inhibits antibody production
Cyclosporin A	Inhibits T cell cytokine IL-2 production
Experimental/in clinical trials	
Monoclonal antibodies to CD4/CD20	In drug-resistant RA
Inhibitors of TNFα	In drug-resistant RA
Peptides of HSP	IDDM
Antigen given via the oral route to re-establish tolerance	
Myelin basic protein	Treatment of multiple sclerosis
Collagen	Treatment of RA

Drugs targeting cytokines such as inhibitors of IL-1 and monoclonal antibodies to, or soluble receptors for, TNFα have also shown considerable promise in suppressing the inflammatory process in RA and slowing down progression of the disease.

Recent studies have shown that peptide vaccines of self heat shock proteins ameliorate insulin dependent diabetes melitus in a murine model and prevent further damage to the islet cells of the pancreas (Topic L2). This might lead the way to a new approach to treatment of autoimmune diseases in man.

Another approach being developed involves the introduction of antigen via the oral route (mucosal surface) in an attempt to reintroduce specific tolerance (e.g. in RA and MS). There is also experimental evidence that antibodies specific for the autoantibody-producing B cell clones (anti-idiotypic antibodies) may offer effective treatment in the future. Other experimental treatments include targeting the CD40L induced on T cells during cognate interactions with antigen with the idea of removing specific T cell help for autoreactive B cells. This shows promise in re-inducing at least a partial tolerance to the autoantigens.

M1 THE TRANSPLANTATION PROBLEM

Key Notes

Historical perspective	Much of our early knowledge about transplantation rejection was gained during the Second World War when skin grafts were given to treat wounds. Animal experiments led to the first definition of antigens responsible for transplant rejection.
Types of grafts	Transplants are either from one part of the body to another (autografts), to a member of the same species (allografts), or across species (xenografts). Allografts that are commonly used clinically include blood, heart, kidney and liver.
The major problem of rejection	The major transplantation antigens are those of the ABO blood groups and the human leukocyte antigen (HLA) system which are polymorphic, i.e. are coded for by several possible alleles. Antibodies and cell mediated immunity (CMI) are responsible for graft rejection. The likelihood of rejection can be reduced by transplanting within families, tissue typing, and immunosuppression. Bone marrow transplantation can result in graft versus host reactions.
Related topics	Antigens (A4) Transplantation antigens (M2) T cell recognition of antigen (F2)

Historical perspective

Skin grafts were used to treat major wounds acquired during the Second World War, and it was from this experience that the early concept of transplantation rejection was founded. This led to the now widely known fact that transplantation of donor organs/tissues to another individual usually results in rejection, unless histocompatible tissues (based on specific tissue typing) and immunosuppression are used. Early experiments in mice in the 1950s and 60s defined the role of the major histocompatibility molecules in graft rejection. Transplantation is now common medical practice and many different organs/tissues are transplanted (*Table 1*).

Types of grafts

Tissues/organs transplanted from one part of the body to another (autograft) are not rejected since they are self. Transplants of tissue/organs from an individual within the same species are called allografts (e.g. human to human) or

Table 1. Commonly transplanted organs/tissues

Allografts	Autografts
Kidney, pancreas, heart (heart/lung), skin, cornea, bone marrow, liver, blood	Skin, bone marrow

from one species to another are called xenografts (e.g. pig to human). Human transplants are usually allografts but xenografts are now being considered as an alternative due to inadequate supplies of human donor organs/tissues.

The major problem of rejection

That the immune system is responsible for the rejection process has been demonstrated in animal models and in humans. The immune mechanisms used for rejection are the same as those used in immune responses to invading microbes and are essentially adaptive immune responses. The cause of the problem is genetic polymorphism, and in particular that the transplantation antigens are mainly polymorphic gene products, e.g. blood groups and major histocompatibility complex (MHC) molecules, which vary among different individuals within the same species. Rejection can be minimized by using familial donors, tissue typing and immunosuppressive drugs. Bone marrow transplantation given as a source of stem cells can result in graft versus host reactions.

M2 TRANSPLANTATION ANTIGENS

Key Notes

The blood group antigens	The major blood group antigens are those of the ABO system. These carbohydrate antigens are present on erythrocytes and some other tissues. Most individuals have antibodies (isohemagglutinins) which recognize these antigens. Thus, blood group A individuals have antibodies to blood group B, and blood group B individuals antibodies to blood group A. Blood transfused from one group to the other would be rejected.
The major histocompatibility complex antigens	The main tissue transplantation antigens are encoded by the polymorphic MHC locus (HLA in man). The inheritance of two alleles (out of many possible) at six different loci (A, B, C, DP, DQ, DR) means that the chance of all HLA antigens of two individuals being exactly the same is very low (1 in 35 million).
Minor histocompatibility antigens	Minor transplantation antigens include non-ABO blood groups and antigens associated with the sex chromosomes. These are usually 'weaker' than the MHC antigens, and are probably the antigens targeted by the immune system in late onset rejection.
Related topics	Antigens (A4) T cell recognition of antigen (F2)	Genes, T helper cells, cytokines and the neuroendocrine system (G5)

The blood group antigens

The major blood group ABO antigens are mainly present on the surfaces of erythrocytes and the genes encoding them are polymorphic, i.e. there is more than one allele coding for the gene product. This is in contrast to most proteins, e.g. albumin, which are coded for by nonpolymorphic genes or genes which lack allelic variation. The major blood group alleles A and B, code for enzymes which create different sugars on proteins and lipids on the surface of erythrocytes. Blood group O is a null allele and does not add sugars. These alleles are inherited in a simple Mendelian inheritance pattern and are codominantly expressed (i.e. both allelic products are expressed on the erythrocyte surface, *Table 1*). An individual can either be homozygous (the same) or heterozygous (different) for the inherited alleles.

The major problem with transplanting blood is that all of us have antibodies (isohemagglutinins) to these blood group antigens (*Table 1*). The reason for development of these antibodies is unclear, but is probably due to cross-reactivity

Table 1. Blood group antigens and isohemagglutinins

Blood group	A	B	AB	O
Genotype	AA or AO	BB or BO	AB	OO
Isohemagglutinins	Anti-B	Anti-A	None	Anti-A and B

of AB antigens with those of certain ubiquitous microbes (see Topic E3). Transplantation of blood to a recipient who has serum isohemagglutinins can result in a severe transfusion reaction mediated by a type II hypersensitivity reaction (Topic K3).

The major histocompatibility complex antigens

These are the major barrier to transplantation of nucleated cells. As previously described, MHC molecules are expressed on all nucleated cells of the body and their physiological function is to direct T cells to carry out their function. However, like the locus coding for the major blood group antigens and unlike the majority of other gene products, genes coding for MHC molecules are polymorphic. In contrast to the ABO system, each MHC locus can encode for a very large number of different allelic forms and to further increase the complexity, there are six different loci. In humans, this locus is found on chromosome 6 (*Fig. 1*) and encodes HLA, since the antigens were first discovered in humans on leukocytes.

The combinations of the many different allelic forms which are codominantly expressed means that the chances of two individuals having a completely identical set of alleles is extremely remote (1 in 35 million). Thus the different allelic products of the donor organ/tissue will be foreign to the recipient who does not have them and will therefore generate an immune response to them. An example of alleles that might be expressed by donors/recipients is shown in *Table 2* and the

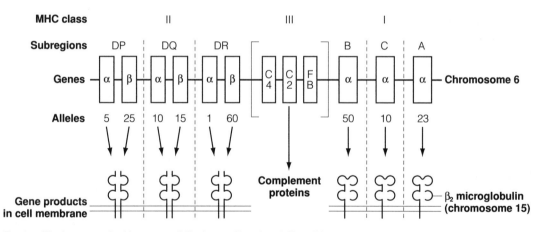

Fig. 1.   *The human major histocompatibility locus. Class I and Class II human leukocyte antigens (HLA) are encoded by three (A, B and C) and six genes (DP, DQ and DR), respectively. Each gene can be coded by many different alleles, the products of which, if different from self, are recognized as transplantation antigens. Thus, there are millions of different combinations of the different allelic products. The class III HLA locus encodes complement proteins.*

Table 2.   *Human leukocyte antigens (HLA) alleles of a hypothetical donor and recipient*

Locus	Donor	Recipient	Alleles to which the recipient's immune system responds
HLA-A	A2/A2	A6/A2	None*
HLA-B	B21/B26	B23/B8	B21, B26
HLA-C	C5/C8	C9/C4	C5, C8
HLA-DR	DR4/DR6	DR8/DR3	DR4, DR6
HLA-DP	DP3/DP1	DP2/DP1	DP3
HLA-DQ	DQ3/DQ3	DQ4/DQ2	DQ3

* The recipient's immune system sees A2/A2 as self.

target of the recipient 's immune system would be the products of the mismatched alleles.

Minor histocompatibility antigens

There are a number of minor transplantation antigens that include non-ABO blood groups and antigens associated with the sex chromosomes. These are usually 'weaker' than the MHC antigens, and are probably the antigens targeted by the immune system in late onset rejection (Topic M3).

M3 REJECTION MECHANISMS

Key Notes

Rejection is an adaptive immune response	Transplants given to recipients that have previously rejected a graft having the same transplantation antigens, are rejected more rapidly. This is due to a specific memory response to these antigens, a property of the adaptive immune system.
Mechanisms of rejection of allografts	The adaptive immune system recognizes the mismatched HLA allelic products expressed on donor tissues and is responsible for rejection. Both antibody and T cell mediated (CMI) rejection occurs depending on the source of tissue for the transplant, e.g. skin, mainly CMI and kidney, antibodies and CMI. The number of HLA mismatches between donor and recipient (i.e. transplantation antigens) usually determines the strength of rejection.
Xenotransplant rejection	Due to the inadequate supply of human donors, animals are being considered as an alternative source of organs/tissues. The pig is deemed appropriate, since the size of many of its internal organs is comparable with that of man. Hyperacute rejection problems have arisen due to the presence in the pig of cell surface sugars to which humans have natural hemagglutinins, similar to those against ABO antigens.
Donor rejection of host tissues	In addition to host rejecting graft tissue, T cells in bone marrow grafts are stimulated by mismatched host HLA leading to a graft versus host reaction. Care to avoid this response is required in using bone marrow as a source of stem cells in cases of anemia, metabolic diseases of the newborn, primary immunodeficiency and some tumors, especially leukemias.

Related topics	The cellular basis of the antibody response (E3)	Prevention of graft rejection (M4)
	The role of T cells in immune responses (F1)	Deficiencies in the immune system (J1)

Rejection is an adaptive immune response

The immune system treats mismatched transplants in the same way as microbes. Thus, if a patient rejects a transplant through transplantation antigens, it will reject a second graft carrying the same or shared transplantation antigens much faster. This 'second set' rejection in due to the sensitization by the first graft and a memory response on subsequent exposure. This is a property of the adaptive immune system.

Mechanisms of rejection of allografts

Graft rejection is mediated by both cell mediated (T cell) and humoral immune mechanisms (antibodies). Furthermore, the number of mismatched alleles also determines the magnitude of the rejection response. The more mismatches, the larger the number of antigens to which an immune response can be made. Thus in Topic M2, *Table 2* above, the recipient's immune response could respond to eight different donor transplantation antigens. Although both T cell mediated responses and antibodies can be generated against the foreign antigens, the rejection of particular types of graft may be preferentially mediated more through antibodies than through T cell mediated immune (CMI) responses and vice versa (*Table 1*). In general, immune responses against transplantation antigens mediated by preformed antibodies result in a rapid rejection (hyperacute).

Allografts can show three main types of rejection patterns. The best studied transplant being the kidney (*Table 2*).

Table 1.   *Main mechanisms of rejection of different kinds of grafts*

Organ/tissue	Mechanism(s)
Blood	Antibodies (isohemagglutinins)
Kidney	Antibodies, CMI (T cell)
Heart	Antibodies, CMI (T cell)
Skin	CMI (T cell)
Bone-marrow	CMI (T cell)
Cornea	Usually accepted unless vascularized, CMI (T cell)

- *Hyperacute rejection* occurs within a few minutes or hours and is believed to be mediated by pre-existing circulating antibody in the recipient to antigens of the donor. Unlike other transplants, the kidney has ABO coded sugar antigens expressed on the endothelial cells of the blood vessels. Thus, if the donor has a different blood group from the recipient, the antibodies will result in a type II hypersensitivity reaction in the kidney graft (Topic K3). Graft recipients might also have some memory responses to HLA through rejection of a previous graft. In addition, multiparous women recipients may have been sensitized to paternal HLA expressed by their child's cells. This could occur during pregnancy and at parturition when small amounts of blood of the newborn may get into the maternal circulation. Prior transfusion with blood containing some leukocytes of a recipient can also result in priming to HLA alleles.
- *Acute rejection* occurs within the first weeks or months following transplantation. The graft shows infiltrates of activated lymphocytes and monocytes. Antibody may be a factor in the process, but the effector mechanism is primarily through cytotoxic T cells or helper/delayed type hypersensitivity T cells (Topic K5) and monocytes/macrophages.
- *Chronic rejection* is the gradual loss of function of the grafted organ occurring over months to years. The lesion often shows infiltration with large numbers of mononuclear cells, predominantly T cells. The mechanism of rejection is not clear but following transplantation, memory (and primary) responses which generate antibody and cellular immunity to HLA may take some time, especially since the patient will be immunosuppressed to improve graft 'take' (see later) and there might be only a limited number of mismatched alleles. Furthermore, minor transplantation antigens may eventually produce a significantly large immune response to result in rejection.

Table 2.   *Kidney graft rejection*

Type of rejection	Time to rejection	Cause
Hyperacute	Within hours	Preformed antibodies (anti-ABO and/or anti-HLA)
Acute	Weeks to months	Cell-mediated (CD8+, CD4+ T cells)
Chronic	Months to years	Cell-mediated (CD8+ T cells), antibodies to tissue antigens

Xenotransplant rejection

The inadequate supply of donor organs/tissues has led to consideration of animals as donors. In particular, the pig appears to be a suitable source of transplantable tissues since the size of many of the internal organs is comparable with that of man. However, a major unforeseen problem is that pig cells have sugars which are not found on human cells and to which humans have serum IgM hemagglutinating antibodies (similar to the ABO isohemagglutinins, *Table 1, Topic M2*). Thus, pig organs will be rejected through a hyperacute mechanism due to preformed hemagglutinins which activate complement resulting in lysis of the grafted cells. Strategies planned to prevent this include:

- Trying to inactivate the gene encoding the glycosyltransferase responsible for the sugar residues.
- Introducing genes into the pig which code for molecules which inhibit the lytic component of complement activation (see Topic D8, G1).

Even if these strategies are successful, there is still the problem of the MHC molecules expressed by pig tissues. The use of nonhuman sources of grafts have additional problems. These include ethical issues and the possibility of transferring unknown viruses that, in the long-term, could enter the germ-line.

Donor rejection of host tissues

Although most transplant rejection is the result of the immune system of the recipient recognizing and responding to the donors' HLA (host versus graft response), in the case of bone marrow transplants there is an additional problem in that the graft (the bone marrow) contains viable active lymphocytes. In particular, T cells may recognize recipient cells as foreign and produce a graft versus host reaction (*Table 3*). More specifically, donor T cells may recognize mismatched HLA alleles and respond to them.

Table 3.   Host versus graft and graft versus host reactions

Host versus graft reaction	Graft versus host reaction
Response to donor HLA by host immune system	Response to recipient HLA by donor T cells

This often results in skin rashes and gastrointestinal problems and may be quite serious. The pathology is probably mediated by inflammatory cytokines released from the donor T cells. In some cases it can be alleviated by cyclosporin A treatment. Bone marrow stem cells are given for a number of clinical conditions to provide functional genes. These conditions include some primary immunodeficiency diseases, anemias, tumors and metabolic diseases (*Table 4*). Other conditions in which bone marrow grafts are being tested are for breast cancer and rheumatoid arthritis following heavy chemotherapy/irradiation to remove the tumor and lymphoid cells, respectively.

Table 4.   Clinical conditions for which bone marrow grafts are given

Anemias	Metabolic diseases	Immunodeficiency diseases	Tumors
Fanconi's anemia	Gaucher's disease	Reticular dysgenesis	Acute lymphoblastic leukemia
	Thalassemias	Severe combined	Acute myeloid leukemia
Aplastic anemia	Osteopetrosis	Chronic granulomatous disease	Acute chronic myeloid leukemia
		Wiskott-Aldrich syndrome	Chronic lymphocytic leukemia

M4 PREVENTION OF GRAFT REJECTION

Key Notes

Familial grafting	Due to the inheritance pattern of the HLA genes, transplantation within families reduces greatly HLA mismatches. Transplants from parents to siblings have at least a 50% match of HLA alleles, whilst sibling to sibling grafts have a 25% chance of having identical HLA alleles.
Tissue typing	Typing of the HLA of both transplant donor and recipient can be done by antibodies or 'typing' cells. Molecular genetic based techniques are also now used by some laboratories.
Cross-matching	Cross-matching is used to test for preformed antibodies in the recipient directed to donor tissues. This is measured by mixing serum from the recipient with blood lymphocytes from the donor.
Immunosuppression	Suppression of the immune system by drugs is usually necessary to aid in maintenance of the graft. The drugs used include corticosteroids, cytotoxic drugs (e.g. azathioprine) and cyclosporin A.
The special case of the 'fetal transplant'	The fetus is an allograft, and yet in most cases it is not rejected due to the body itself suppressing the rejection process. There are probably several mechanisms involved including lack of expression of conventional HLA on the trophoblast, complement inhibitory proteins expressed by the trophoblast and immunosuppressive molecules produced in the placenta.
Related topics	Antibody functions (D8) Rejection mechanisms (M3)

Familial grafting

Transplantation within families significantly reduces allele mismatches because of the inheritance patterns of HLA (*Fig. 1*). In general, there is little crossover within the locus and the whole locus is usually inherited *en bloc*. Thus, if parents donate grafts to their children there is equal to or greater than (due to chance) 50% match of the HLA alleles. If siblings (brothers and sisters) donate to each other there is a one in four chance of a complete match. Thus, if you need a transplant, make sure you come from a family with lots of brothers and sisters! Other tissue antigens that trigger far less vigorous rejection responses (minor histocompatibility antigens) are encoded outside the MHC locus and include male specific antigens. In fact, mismatches of minor transplantation antigens can be important in determining the fate of grafts between HLA matched donor and recipient, especially as it relates to chronic rejection over a longer period of time.

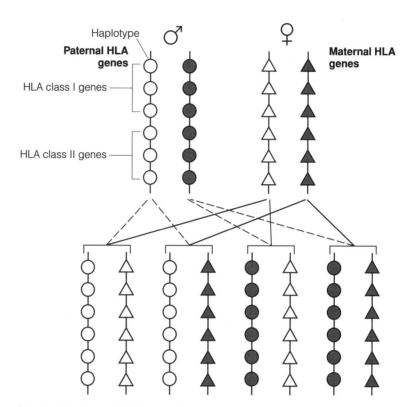

Fig. 1.   Inheritance of HLA genes. Each individual receives one set of HLA genes from each parent (i.e. they receive one haplotype from each parent). Because of their position on the chromosomes, alleles are inherited en bloc. Grafts from parents to siblings and vice versa have at least 50% of matched alleles whilst sibling to sibling grafts have a 1 in 4 chance of a complete match.

Tissue typing

If a familial donor is not available, then the extent of the mismatches between alleles must be determined by tissue typing, in order to best match donor and recipient. In this context, one of the most useful assays involves cytotoxic antibodies (usually mAbs) to individual HLAs. The principal of the antibody method depends on the surface expression of the HLA. Donor and recipient blood for typing are enriched for B cells (they express both class I and II HLA) and specific cytotoxic antibodies are added. Binding of the antibody to a surface HLA in the presence of complement results in the direct killing of the B cells (*Fig. 2*). These can be microscopically scored. Using a panel of antibodies, it is possible to HLA type for the majority of alleles.

Many HLA typing labs are now turning to identification of the HLA genes inherited via molecular genetics based tests that utilize the restriction fragment length polymorphism (RFLP) or polymerase chain reaction (PCR) amplification techniques. These technologies determine the nucleotide sequence of the HLA genes in question and give unequivocal results. Outside its use in tissue typing for transplants, this technology has been particularly important in identifying minor polymorphisms within the HLA-D regions which might be associated with susceptibility to particular kinds of diseases (Topic L2).

Typing can also be done using the 'mixed lymphocyte' reaction also called 'mixed lymphocyte response', which primarily identifies HLA-D class II antigens.

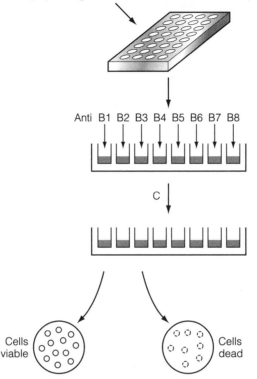

Donor B cells (expressing both MHC I and MHC II molecules)

Anti B1 B2 B3 B4 B5 B6 B7 B8

C

Cells viable

Cells dead

Phenotype for HLA B locus = B3, B8

Fig. 2.   Tissue typing. B cells obtained from the blood of the donor/recipient to be typed are placed in microplates and antibodies to the different MHC allelic products added together with complement. These include antibodies to HLA A, B and C loci and some D antigens. Only antibodies to B1 to B8 are shown here to illustrate the concept. Following incubation at 37°C, lysis (cell death) of the B cells occurs in those wells where antibodies have attached to the B cells. Thus, in this example, lysis of the B cells indicated that the donor was heterozygous for the B locus – B3 and B8.

In this case, 'typing cells' (usually cell lines carrying specific homozygous HLA-D allelic products) are treated with a drug to inhibit their proliferation. They are then mixed with the potential recipient's blood lymphocytes and cultured for 3–5 days. If the recipient's T cells do not carry the typing cell's HLA, they will proliferate in response to 'foreign' HLA since they will not have been eliminated by negative selection in the thymus (Topic G2). By using panels of typing cells, it is possible to determine the HLA type of the donor and recipient.

Matching of HLA for liver transplants does not appear to be of major advantage, probably due to the weak expression of HLA by hepatic cells.

Cross-matching   Cross-matching is used to check that there are no preformed antibodies to donor HLA in the recipient. Blood lymphocytes from the donor are mixed with serum from the recipient (Fig. 3). Anti-donor antibodies are detected by lysis of the cells (mediated by complement) or by using fluorescent staining and flow cytometry. The presence of such antibodies is contraindicatory to the use of the

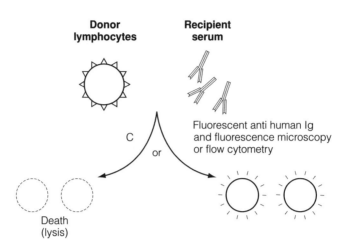

Fig. 3. Cross-matching. Serum from the potential recipient is mixed with donor lymphocytes and is evaluated for lysis (see Fig. 2), in the presence of complement, or stained with fluorescent antibodies to human immunoglobulin (Topic D7) and assayed by fluorescence microscopy or flow cytometry. Dead cells or positive fluorescence signifies the presence of antidonor antibodies which could lead to a hyperacute rejection of the graft. This is contraindicatory to the use of this donor/recipient combination. This assay identifies HLA antibodies in the recipient serum. Cross-matching for blood groups is also carried out for renal transplants.

tissues from that donor. Crossmatching for blood groups is also important for renal transplants (Topic M3).

Immuno-suppression

In the vast majority of cases, there will be some allelic mismatches and some donor minor histocompatibility antigens, therefore the immune system of the recipient has to be suppressed to avoid rejection. The mainstay drug treatment is a mixture of corticosteroids, synthetic cytotoxic drugs and cyclosporin A (a fungal nonapeptide). The mechanisms of immunosuppression by these and other drugs used are shown in *Table 1*. Not surprisingly, a major problem with these drugs is that by inhibiting the immune response against the graft they can also lead to increased susceptibility to infections (see Topic J1). In fact, infection and rejection are the main reasons for the failure of kidney grafts to be main-

Table 1. Drugs used to suppress graft rejection

Drug	Mechanism(s) of immunosuppression
Corticosteroids	
Prednisone	Blocking of migration of neutrophils: Inhibition of IL-1, IL-6 and IL-2 production
Cytotoxics	
Azathioprine	Kills cells at division
Methotrexate	
Cyclophosphamide	
Immunophilins	
Cyclosporin A	Inhibits IL-2 production and/or responses to IL-2
FK506	
Rapamycin	

tained. Other drugs, e.g. anti-lymphocyte antibodies, which kill the recipient's lymphocytes, are also used by some transplant teams.

The special case of the 'fetal transplant' The fetus is a chimera carrying HLA alleles from both parents. It is therefore effectively an allograft in close apposition to maternal tissues. The main potential mechanisms for prevention of rejection are shown (*Fig. 4*) for a recently implanted embryo (day 14), but also play an important role throughout gestation.

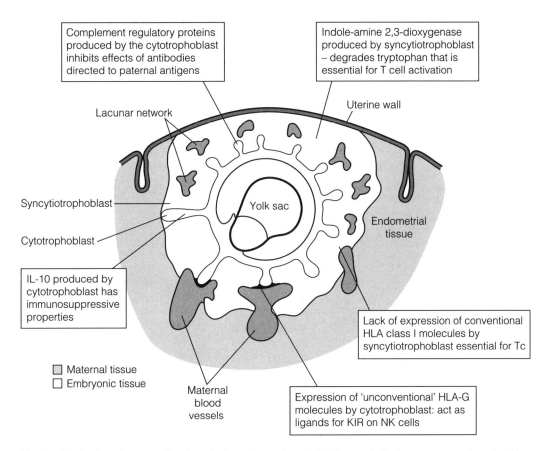

Complement regulatory proteins produced by the cytotrophoblast inhibits effects of antibodies directed to paternal antigens

Indole-amine 2,3-dioxygenase produced by syncytiotrophoblast – degrades tryptophan that is essential for T cell activation

Lacunar network

Uterine wall

Syncytiotrophoblast

Cytotrophoblast

Yolk sac

Endometrial tissue

IL-10 produced by cytotrophoblast has immunosuppressive properties

Lack of expression of conventional HLA class I molecules by syncytiotrophoblast essential for Tc

☐ Maternal tissue
☐ Embryonic tissue

Maternal blood vessels

Expression of 'unconventional' HLA-G molecules by cytotrophoblast: act as ligands for KIR on NK cells

Fig. 4. Mechanisms for preventing the rejection of an embryonic/fetal allograft. During pregnancy, there is a bias towards a Th2 response mediated through estrogen and progesterone, and this is also thought to contribute to the maintenance of the fetal allograft (Topic O3).

N1 ORIGIN AND HOST DEFENSE AGAINST TUMORS

Key Notes

Origin and host defense against tumors	While the etiology of most human tumors is still unknown, it is now clear that radiation as well as a variety of viruses and chemical carcinogens can induce tumors and that immune responses in tumor-bearing patients can develop, or be induced to develop, against antigens associated with these tumors. These responses may be important in tumor regression. Promising therapeutic approaches based on these findings have recently been developed which are efficacious in the treatment of at least some tumors. Vaccines are also likely to become available for therapy of tumors.
Related topics	Cytokine and cellular immunotherapy of tumors (N5) Immunotherapy of tumors with antibodies (N6)

Origin and host defense against tumors

The origin and host response to tumors is currently the focus of extensive basic and clinical research. With regard to origin, a large number of environmental factors have been shown to be carcinogenic and/or mutagenic in animals. Several tumors have, in fact, been associated with exposure to certain substances (asbestos with mesotheliomas in shipyard workers, hydrocarbons with scrotal cancer in chimney sweeps). Viruses are also known to induce tumors in animals. In humans, the Epstein–Barr DNA virus is involved in Burkitt's lymphoma and nasopharyngeal carcinoma, and the hepatitis B virus in liver cancer. The human T cell leukemia virus (HTLV) is involved in certain forms of lymphocytic leukemia and human herpes virus 8 (HHV8) causes Kaposi's sarcoma.

In many instances host immune responses develop against tumors and in some instances may be protective. Based on the development of a clearer understanding of tumor immunology, numerous immunotherapeutic approaches have been explored for the treatment of cancer. Although the results from the use of monoclonal antibodies (mAbs), derivatized mAb, lymphokine-activated killer (LAK) cells, tumor-infiltrating lymphocytes (TILs), cytokines, etc., were initially less promising than hoped, much has been learned about these immunological approaches and how best to use them. In fact, several promising therapeutic approaches have recently been developed which are efficacious in the treatment of at least some tumors. It is very likely that many other effective immunotherapeutic approaches will also soon be available for the treatment of cancer.

N2 TUMOR ANTIGENS

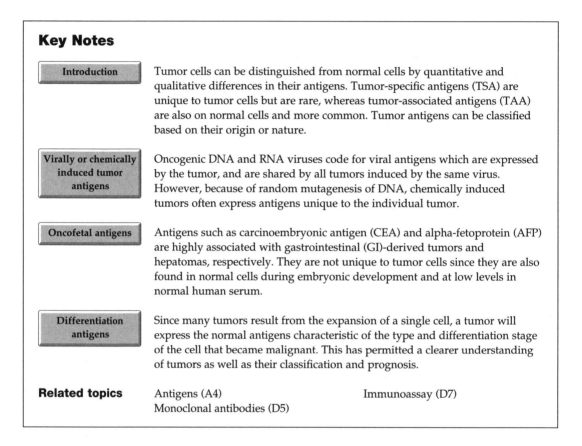

Key Notes

Introduction	Tumor cells can be distinguished from normal cells by quantitative and qualitative differences in their antigens. Tumor-specific antigens (TSA) are unique to tumor cells but are rare, whereas tumor-associated antigens (TAA) are also on normal cells and more common. Tumor antigens can be classified based on their origin or nature.
Virally or chemically induced tumor antigens	Oncogenic DNA and RNA viruses code for viral antigens which are expressed by the tumor, and are shared by all tumors induced by the same virus. However, because of random mutagenesis of DNA, chemically induced tumors often express antigens unique to the individual tumor.
Oncofetal antigens	Antigens such as carcinoembryonic antigen (CEA) and alpha-fetoprotein (AFP) are highly associated with gastrointestinal (GI)-derived tumors and hepatomas, respectively. They are not unique to tumor cells since they are also found in normal cells during embryonic development and at low levels in normal human serum.
Differentiation antigens	Since many tumors result from the expansion of a single cell, a tumor will express the normal antigens characteristic of the type and differentiation stage of the cell that became malignant. This has permitted a clearer understanding of tumors as well as their classification and prognosis.
Related topics	Antigens (A4) Immunoassay (D7) Monoclonal antibodies (D5)

Introduction

A number of properties distinguish tumor from normal cells, including their invasiveness, loss of growth contact inhibition and their lack of response to regulation. In addition, there is considerable evidence for quantitative and qualitative differences in antigens associated with normal vs tumor cells. These antigens can be divided into tumor-specific antigens (TSA), those unique to tumor cells, or tumor-associated antigens (TAA), and those also found on some normal cells. Another classification system is based on the origin or nature of the antigens and includes viral, chemical, oncofetal and differentiation antigens.

Virally or chemically induced tumor antigens

In animal models, oncogenic DNA viruses (*Table 1*) code for both cell surface and nuclear antigens which become expressed by the tumor. RNA tumor viruses induce tumor cell surface antigens which are viral proteins (*Table 1*). Thus, these antigens are shared by all tumors induced by the same virus. On the other hand, because of the random mutagenesis of DNA that occurs, chemically induced tumors express antigens which are unique to the individual tumor.

Table 1.   Virally induced/associated tumors

Tumor viruses	Human tumor
RNA	
Human T cell lymphotrophic virus-1 (HTLV)	Adult T cell leukemia/lymphoma
DNA	
Epstein–Barr (EBV)	B cell and Hodgkins lymphomas, nasopharyngeal carcinoma
Human papillomavirus (HPV)	Cervical carcinomas
Hepatitis B virus (HBV)	Hepatocellular carcinoma
Herpesvirus 8 (HHV8)	Kaposi's sarcoma

Oncofetal antigens

Although highly associated with some tumors, both on their cell surface and in the serum, oncofetal antigens are not unique to tumor cells since they are also found on cells during embryonic development and are found at very low levels in normal human serum (*Table 2*).

Table 2.   Examples of oncofetal antigens

Antigen	MW (kDa)	Nature	Associated tumor
Carcinoembryonic antigen (CEA)	180	Glycoprotein	Gastrointestinal, breast
Alpha-fetoprotein (AFP)	70	Glycoprotein	Hepatomas

Carcinoembryonic antigen (CEA) and alpha-fetoprotein (AFP) are two such antigens. CEA is expressed (both on the cells and in the extracellular fluids) by many gastrointestinal (GI)-derived tumors including colon carcinoma, and pancreatic, liver or gall bladder tumors as well as by breast cancers. It is also expressed by the gut, liver and pancreas of human fetuses (2–6 months). AFP is found in secretions of yolk sac and fetal liver epithelium as well as in the serum of patients with hepatomas (liver tumors). These oncofetal antigens are thus not TSA nor is their presence, even at high concentration, in the serum diagnostic of cancer, because high levels can result from non-neoplastic diseases including chronic inflammation of the bowel or cirrhosis of the liver. However, the quantitation of these molecules in the serum can be used to evaluate the tumor burden and effectiveness of drug treatment.

Differentiation antigens

Some normal cellular antigens are expressed at specific stages of cell differentiation. These differentiation antigens can also be found on tumor cells and can be detected using mAbs (Topic D5). Moreover, since most tumors result from the expansion of a single cell arrested at some point in its differentiation, mAb to differentiation antigens are used to determine the approximate stage of differentiation at which the malignant event occurred. This in turn permits the most appropriate therapy based on a clearer understanding and classification of the malignancy. Using this approach, for example, it has been found that most T cell leukemias are derived from early thymocytes or prothymocytes. Similar approaches have been applied to B cell tumors and other malignant states (*Table 3*).

Table 3. Differentiation antigens on lymphoid and myeloid malignancies*

Acute		Chronic	
Disease	Markers	Disease	Markers
common ALL	CD10 (CALLA), CD19, TdT (n)	B-CLL	CD19, CD20, CD5
null ALL	CD19, TdT (n)	HCL	CD19, CD20, TRAP
Pre-B cell ALL	CD19, IgM (m;cyt)	PLL	CD19, CD20,
T cell ALL	CD7, CD3 (cyt), TdT (n)	Sezary	CD3, CD4
Myeloid leukemia	CD13, CD33, myeloperoxidase	T-CLL	CD3, CD8

*ALL, acute lymphocytic leukemia; CALLA, common ALL antigen; CLL, chronic lymphocytic leukemia; T-CLL, T cell CLL; HCL, Hairy cell leukemia; PLL, pro-lymphocytic leukemia ; TdT, terminal deoxynucleotidyl transferase; n, nuclear; cyt, cytoplasmic; m, membrane; Sezary, *Mycosis fungoides*.

N3 IMMUNE RESPONSES TO TUMORS

Key Notes

Immune surveillance	It is supposed that the immune system surveys constantly for neoplastic cells and destroys them as suggested by the observation of increased incidence of tumors of lymphoid or epithelial cells in immunodeficient animals and humans. NK cells have been proposed to search for and eliminate certain tumors early in their development.
Effector mechanisms	Specific antitumor immunity appears to develop in tumor-bearing patients in much the same way as it does to pathogens or foreign antigens. Both TSA and TAA associated with tumor cells appear to be processed and presented in association with MHC class I molecules, making them potential targets for cytotoxic T cells. NK cells kill tumor cells not expressing MHC class I. Antibody-coated tumor cells can be killed by complement activation, by MØ and PMN-mediated phagocytosis, by ADCC, and/or by induction of apoptosis.
Tumor escape	Mechanisms by which tumor cells may escape killing by the immune system include: (i) induction of tolerance to tumor antigens; (ii) development of tumor cells lacking antigens to which the immune system has responded; (iii) modulation of tumor antigen expression; (iv) tumor suppression of antitumor immunity; (v) poor immunogenicity of the tumor perhaps resulting from lack of expression of MHC class I; (vi) expression of Fas ligand (FasL) on tumors, which may induce apoptosis of effector cells.
Related topics	Cells of the innate immune system (B1) Central and peripheral tolerance (G2)
	The cellular basis of the antibody response (E3) Deficiencies in the immune system (J1)
	Clonal expansion and development of effector function (F5)

Immune surveillance

It is supposed, but difficult to prove, that the immune system surveys constantly for neoplastic antigens associated with a newly developing tumor and destroys the cells bearing them. Evidence supportive of this possibility comes from the observation of increased tumor incidence in immunodeficient animals or humans. However, congenitally athymic mice do not have high tumor rates, suggesting that the T cell system may not be involved in surveillance for most tumors. Moreover, congenitally immunodeficient and immunosuppressed patients have high rates of tumors only of lymphoid or epithelial cells. Thus, a less-specific tumor surveillance system, perhaps NK cells, may search for and eliminate certain types of tumor cells early in their development. The best evidence for a surveillance mechanism involving T cells comes from experimental mouse models with virus-induced tumors but here the response is essentially directed to viral antigens and not tumor antigens.

Effector mechanisms

If a tumor evades the surveillance system, it might then be recognized by the specific immune systems. In models of chemically and virally induced tumors, the tumor-associated antigens are immunogenic and trigger specific cellular and antibody responses against the tumor. This immunity may be protective and can be passively transferred with immune cells. In tumor-bearing patients as well, it is possible to demonstrate antitumor antibody, which may mediate some tumor cell lysis.

It is likely that antitumor immune responses develop in tumor-bearing patients in much the same way as they do to pathogens or foreign antigens. Thus, antitumor antibodies and T cells are generated and, along with more non-specific immune defense mechanisms, play a role in tumor immunity. More specifically, it is likely that both TSA and TAA are associated with tumor cells and, after their intracellular synthesis, are processed and presented in association with MHC class I molecules, making them potential targets for cytotoxic T cells. Overall, the potential effector mechanisms which may be involved in human tumor cell lysis *in vivo* are the same as those used in microbial immunity (*Table 1*).

Table 1.   Potential tumor immune effector mechanisms

Killing by specific cytotoxic T cells recognizing TAA or TSA peptides associated with MHC class I

Antibody induction of apoptosis

Killing mediated by antibody and complement

Antibody-dependent cellular cytotoxicity (ADCC) mediated by MØ, PMNS or lymphocytes with Fc receptors

Phagocytosis by activated macrophages

Killing by natural killer (NK) cells. These cells have surface Fc receptors for IgG (FcγRIII). They are activated for antitumor activity by IFNγ and/or IL-2 and kill antibody coated tumor cells. Cells lacking, or with decreased expression of, MHC class I molecules are particularly susceptible to NK cell killing.

Tumor escape

If tumors possess immunogenic antigens which eventually stimulate specific immune responses, how do they escape rejection? The various possibilities which may explain tumor cell escape from the immune system include:

- *Tolerance to tumor antigens.* This might happen if the antigen is a TAA and thus also associated with normal cells and/or if the antigen is presented in a form or under conditions such that T cells are rendered unresponsive to it.
- *Selection for tumor-antigen-negative variants.* If antigens associated with tumor cells are able to elicit strong effective immune responses, tumor cells bearing these antigens would be rapidly eliminated, and only those tumor cells lacking, or with decreased amounts of, these antigens would survive.
- *Modulation of tumor antigen expression.* Binding of antibody to antigens on the surface of tumor cells may result in rapid internalization of antigen and its loss from the cell surface, permitting the tumor cell to escape temporarily from further detection by antibody and thus from FcR-bearing effector cells.
- *The tumor may immunosuppress the patient.* Tumors may release molecules such as TGFβ or IL-10 which have immunosuppressive properties (see Topic B2).
- *The tumor may have low immunogenicity.* Tumor cells having little or no MHC

class I on their surface are able to avoid recognition by cytolytic T cells. Although these tumor cells are more susceptible to NK cells, NK cells do not have memory and thus there may be insufficient expansion of these cells to deal with a large tumor burden.

- *Tumor cells sometimes express Fas ligand (FasL)*. When FasL on the tumor interacts with Fas on T cells, T cell apoptosis may result (see Topic F5).

N4 IMMUNODIAGNOSIS

Key Notes

Classification	MAbs to antigens associated with a particular differentiation state can sometimes be used to classify the origin of the tumor and its stage in normal cell differentiation. This information permits prediction of the likelihood of success of current therapy.
Monitoring	MAbs can sometimes be used to determine the rate of change of TAA (oncofetal antigens, PSA, CA-125, CA-19-9) within the serum of a patient as a measure of tumor progression and duration of remission. Using cytological analysis, mAbs to certain TAA (e.g. cytokeratin, MUC-1) can be used to search for micrometastases.
Imaging	Radioconjugated mAbs specific for an appropriate TAA can sometimes be used to locate and image metastases in a tumor-bearing patient.
Related topics	Hemopoiesis – development of blood cells (A5) Monoclonal antibodies (D5) Immunoassay (D7)

Classification

Numerous mAbs have been developed against tumor cells. Thus far, few of these antibodies are absolutely tumor specific. Therefore, binding of mAbs to tissues from a patient will not necessarily indicate the presence or location of a tumor. However, because tumors often appear to be monoclonal in origin (develop from a single cell that has undergone a malignant event) and to have characteristics of the cell of origin, mAbs to antigens associated with a particular differentiation state can be used to classify the origin of the tumor and the stage in normal cell differentiation most similar to that of the tumor cell (Topic N2). One of the most prominent uses of this approach is in the subgrouping of leukemias (*Fig. 1*).

In particular, mAbs have permitted the definition of a large number of markers associated with lymphoid and myeloid cell populations, and with different stages of their differentiation. Information obtained using panels of such mAb permits classification of some types of tumors, and as a result, it is possible to develop patterns of tumor cell progression and responsiveness to therapy for tumors subclassified in this way. Thus, it becomes possible to predict, for a particular tumor subtype, whether or not current therapy will be effective, and if it is not, the need to pursue a different therapeutic approach (*Table 1*).

Monitoring

MAbs to TAA can sometimes be used to monitor the progression of tumor growth in a patient. Oncofetal antigens, because of their presence in serum, are useful for this purpose. That is, because they are normally only present at very low levels in normal human serum, the presence of large amounts of CEA and AFP may indicate a gastrointestinal or liver tumor, respectively. However, since

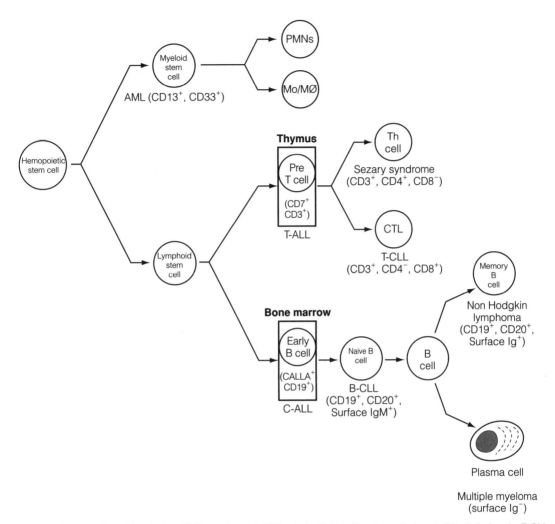

Fig. 1. Subgrouping of leukemias. AML, acute myeloid leukemia; T-ALL, thymic acute lymphoblastic leukemia; T-CLL, T-cell chronic lymphocytic leukemia; c-ALL, common acute lymphoblastic leukemia; B-CLL, B-cell chronic lymphocytic leukemia. Each myeloid or lymphoid tumor expresses a set of markers (molecules) typical of normal myeloid or lymphoid cells at a particular stage of their differentiation.

Table 1. Acute lymphocytic leukemias (ALLs)

Name	% of ALLs	Markers	Prognosis
Common ALL (CALLA)	60%	CD10, CD19	
Pre- B cell ALL	20%	CD19, IgM (cyt)	POOR
T cell ALL	20%	CD7, CD3	

ALL, acute lymphocytic leukemia; cyt, cytoplasmic.

conditions other than tumors elevate the level of these molecules in the serum, their levels are most useful in tumor-bearing patients whose serum level of the oncofetal protein is known. Relapses or duration of remission can be followed by monitoring the rate of change of the amount of oncofetal antigen in the serum (*Fig. 2*).

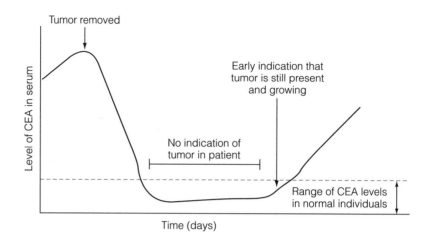

Fig. 2.   Monitoring serum levels of CEA in a cancer patient with a CEA expressing tumor.

In addition, quantitation of other TAA are used to monitor tumor presence and growth in patients with other tumor types. The serum levels of the mucins CA-125 and CA-19-9 (both high-molecular-weight proteoglycans) in a patient with ovarian cancer are useful in following the status and progression of this tumor. Prostate-specific antigen (PSA) is similarly useful in prostate cancer.

Using cytological analysis, mAbs to certain TAA (e.g. cytokeratin) can be used to search for micrometastases in bone marrow or lymph node. Similarly, another mucin, MUC-1, is expressed on breast carcinomas in a pattern different from that on normal breast epithelium.

Imaging

By linking a radioisotope (e.g. [131]I) to a mAb specific for an appropriate TAA (e.g. CEA), and intravenously injecting this construct into a tumor-bearing patient, it is possible to image tumor metastases using scintigraphy.

N5 CYTOKINE AND CELLULAR IMMUNOTHERAPY OF TUMORS

Key Notes

Immunostimulation and cytokines	Nonspecific immunostimulants induce cytokine-producing immune responses that activate effector cells, but have limited ability to mediate tumor cell lysis. Cytokines are critical to the development of immunity, but to be effective in tumor therapy, they will probably need to be used in conjunction with specific immunotherapy.
Lymphokine-activated killer (LAK) cells	Lymphocytes from a tumor-bearing patient are cultured in IL-2 to expand and activate cytotoxic LAK cells, primarily NK cells. They are then infused into the patient with or without more IL-2.
Tumor-infiltrating lymphocytes (TILs)	TILs are CD8$^+$ T cells isolated from patient tumor samples, some of which react with tumor antigens. After expansion and activation with IL-2, these cells are infused into the patient with or without more IL-2, with the goal that they will home to tumor cell sites and kill tumor cells. As with LAK therapy there is significant toxicity if high doses of IL-2 are used.
Macrophage-activated killer (MAK) cells	Monocytes isolated from peripheral blood of tumor-bearing patients are cultured *in vitro* with cytokines which activate these cells for enhanced cytotoxicity before reinjection into the patient.
Related topics	Cells of the innate immune system (B1) Clonal expansion and development of effector function (F5) Molecules of the innate immune system (B2)

Immuno-stimulation and cytokines

Initially, immunotherapy in humans utilized nonspecific immunostimulants such as BCG and *C. parvum*, which resulted in some tumor cell killing but overall did little to reduce the tumor cell burden. These results probably reflect the development of strong immune responses against antigens associated with these microbes, including production of cytokines capable of activating immune effector cells. The resulting activated cells (e.g. macrophages) then mediated increased tumor cell lysis. When recombinant cytokines became available, they were tried, but again with limited success. Thus, although cytokines are critical to the development of specific immune responses, when used alone they primarily enhance nonspecific activation of immune cells (Topic B2). To be effective antitumor agents they will probably need to be used in concert with induction of more specific immune responses to the tumor.

Lymphokine-activated killer (LAK) cells

This approach involves expansion and activation of cytotoxic cells outside the body, which are then reinjected (*Fig. 1*), and is based on the fact that most tumor-bearing patients have lymphocytes reactive to their tumor.

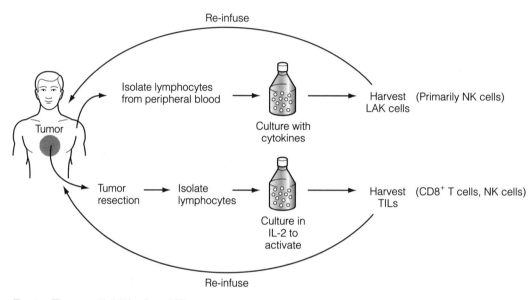

Fig. 1.   Therapy with LAK cells and TILs.

Peripheral blood lymphocytes from a tumor-bearing patient are cultured in IL-2 to expand and activate cytotoxic LAK cells. These are primarily NK cells and thus do not have the specificity of T cells, but rather react with and kill tumor cells which express little or no cell surface MHC class I molecules (*Table 1*). LAK cells are then infused back into the patient with or without more IL-2. Although some tumor regression occurs with this approach, significant toxicity is evident if high doses of IL-2 are used.

Table 1.   Natural killer (NK) cells

1. Activated for anti-tumor activity by IFNγ and/or IL-2
2. Specificity:
    Have cell surface receptors for the Fc portion of Ig (FcγRIII)
    Have cell surface receptors for certain self molecules
3. Mediate killing of:
    Antibody-coated, virus-infected or tumor cells
    Virus-infected or tumor cells with little or no MHC class I

Tumor-infiltrating lymphocytes (TILs)

As with LAK cells, TILs are obtained from tumor-bearing patients, expanded and activated with IL-2 (*Fig. 1*). In particular, TILs are lymphocytes isolated from patient tumor samples that are primarily CD8⁺ T cells, at least some of which are thought to be specific for tumor antigens. They are also infused back into the patient with or without more IL-2. TIL therapy induces tumor regression in some patients and especially in patients with renal cell carcinoma.

Again, there is significant toxicity if high doses of IL-2 are used to maintain the active status of the TIL cells *in vivo*.

Macrophage-activated killer (MAK) cells

Another immunotherapeutic approach involves the use of cytokines and activated macrophages. Monocytes are isolated from peripheral blood of tumor-bearing patients and cultured *in vitro* with cytokines (e.g. IFNγ) which activate these cells for enhanced cytotoxicity before reinjection into the patient. Although these cells are highly cytotoxic and phagocytic, they are relatively nonspecific, and may require co-injection with antibody to TAAs to be most effective.

N6 IMMUNOTHERAPY OF TUMORS WITH ANTIBODIES

Key Notes

Specificity of mAbs to tumors	The vast majority of mAbs prepared against human tumors are not truly tumor specific. The TSAs which have been identified include: (i) idiotypes of antibody on a B cell tumor; and (ii) a mutant form of epidermal growth factor receptor (EGF-R) which has a deletion of an extracellular domain. Additional TSAs are now being identified as a result of analysis of translocations associated with tumor development.
Tumor therapy with antibodies alone	MAbs kill tumor cells by apoptosis or through complement activation, ADCC or phagocytosis. Several humanized mAbs have demonstrated efficacy including mAbs to: (i) HER2/neu for treatment of breast cancer; and (ii) CD20 for therapy of B cell tumors. Thus, mAbs may be useful if they are human or humanized, react with an antigen highly expressed on the tumor, are used to treat minimal disease and are used in patients whose immune system is fully functional.
Tumor therapy with immunotoxins (ITs)	ITs are mAbs to TAA that are linked to a toxin or radioisotope. MAbs coupled to toxin are internalized where they inhibit critical cellular processes. Radioisotope-coupled mAbs mediate killing by DNA damage from decay and release of high-energy particles.
Tumor therapy with bispecific antibodies (BsAbs)	BsAbs are engineered molecules which have two different covalently linked specificities, one against a TAA, the other to a trigger molecule on a killer cell. *In vivo*, BsAbs bind to immune effector cells, arming them to seek out and kill tumor cells.
Purging of bone marrow for analogous transplants	The high doses of chemotherapy or irradiation necessary to cure some patients of their tumor are toxic to hemopoietic stem cells. Thus, bone marrow transplants are sometimes used in which stem cell-containing blood or bone marrow is taken from the patient, after which the patient is treated with high doses of chemotherapy or irradiation. The patient is then rescued by infusion of their own stem cells that have been purged of contaminating tumor cells using mAbs to antigens associated with the tumor.
Related topics	Hemopoiesis – development of blood cells (A5) Monoclonal antibodies (D5) Allotypes and idiotypes (D4) The transplantation problem (M1)

Specificity of mAbs to tumors

Considerable effort has been expended on the development of mAbs to TSA, since it was thought that only mAbs specific for tumor cells would be useful in the diagnosis and treatment of tumors. However, few if any mAbs prepared against human tumors have been found to be truly tumor specific. Examples of antigens which could be considered to be TSA include:

- The idiotype of the antibody on a B cell tumor (e.g. CLL). The first successful use of an mAb in tumor therapy involved treatment of a patient with anti-idiotype antibody prepared specifically against the patient's tumor. DNA coding for idiotypes is currently being explored as a potential way to immunize patients against their own B cell tumor (Topic N7). This approach could also be used to treat T cell tumors based on their expression of a unique binding site.
- A mutant form of the epidermal growth factor receptor (EGF-R) which has a deletion of an extracellular domain. That this molecule is antigenic and uniquely expressed on tumors may be the basis for an antibody-based therapeutic agent or for a vaccine to induce a CTL response.
- As information becomes available on the mutations and translocations associated with various tumors, unique gene products are being identified that serve as TSAs.

Tumor therapy with antibodies alone

Although mAbs can cause tumor cell lysis through complement activation, by targeting NK cells, Mo, and/or MØ ADCC or phagocytosis, or by inducing apoptosis, the use of mAbs to treat human tumors has had, until recently, little success. To some extent these failures probably resulted from: (i) the lack of specificity of the mAb utilized; (ii) the presence of soluble forms of the antigen in the serum that effectively interfered with the interaction of antibody with the tumor cell; (iii) modulation and loss of the antibody–antigen complexes from the tumor cell surface before antibody-mediated killing could occur; (iv) outgrowth of (selection for) tumor cells not expressing the antigen; and (v) the use of mouse mAbs, which do not interface well with human effector molecules (complement) and cells (NK cells, macrophages, PMNs), and being foreign, induced a human anti-mouse antibody (HAMA) response that eventually compromised the effectiveness of the mAb.

Nonetheless, the clearer appreciation that developed on how to use mAbs more effectively in cancer therapy has resulted in a renaissance in antibody therapy (*Fig. 1*).

Many trials are currently ongoing with human or humanized mAbs (Topic D5). In addition, several mAbs have been approved by the US FDA for treatment of different cancers (*Table 1*), including a mAb to HER2/neu (Herceptin) which has been approved for treatment of breast cancer and a mAb to CD20 (Rituximab) a molecule expressed on B cells and B cell tumors. This anti-CD20 mAb may also be of significant utility in the treatment of antibody-mediated autoimmune diseases. Other mAbs still in clinical trials are also demonstrating efficacy as indicated by tumor regression in some patients. Thus, there is growing optimism that mAbs

Table 1. Monoclonal antibodies approved for cancer therapy

Name (date approved)	Specificity	Tumor
Herceptin (98)	HER2/neu	Breast
Rituximab (97)	CD20	B cell lymphoma
Campath (01)	CD52 (on B and T cells)	B cell CLL
Mylotarg (00) mAb-toxin	CD33	AML
Zevelin (02) mAb-radionuclide	CD20	B cell lymphoma

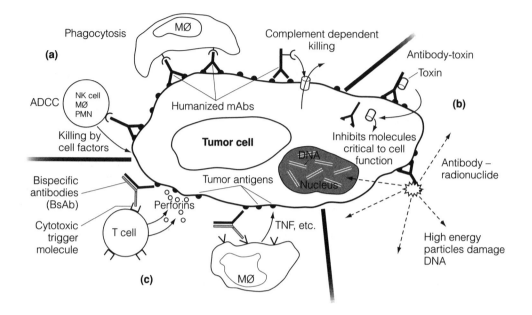

(d) Purging of tumor cells from bone marrow before autologous transplantation

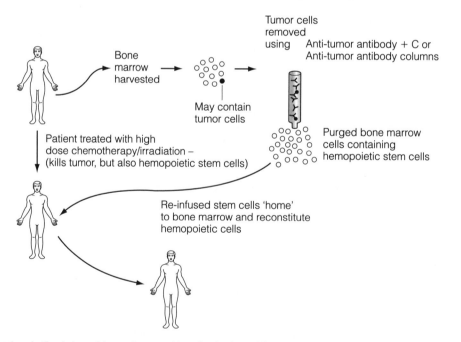

Fig. 1.   Antibody-based tumor therapy. (a) antibody alone; (b) antibody toxin/radionuclides constructions; (c) bispecific antibodies; (d) purging of tumor cells from bone-marrow or stem cell populations.

will be very useful tumor therapeutic agents, especially if: a) they are human or humanized to permit long-term use; b) the antigen to which they react is expressed at a high level on the tumor; c) the mAb is used to treat minimal disease; and d) the patient's immune system is fully functional.

Tumor therapy with immunotoxins (ITs)

Many studies, including clinical trials, have used mAbs to which toxins or radioisotopes have been coupled (*Fig. 1*). Thus, when injected into a patient, ITs would not need to activate patient effector mechanisms. Rather, ITs would seek out and bind to tumor cell antigens, and mediate their own lethal hit. Toxins such as ricin are very potent inhibitors of critical intracellular processes, with a single molecule able to kill a cell. It is essential, however, that the targeting mAbs react with a TAA that is internalized on binding of IT. Mylotarg, an IT in which a humanized mAb to CD33 has been conjugated to the toxin calicheam-icin, has been approved for treatment of patients with acute myeloid leukemia.

Radioisotope-coupled mAbs mediate killing by DNA damage from decay and release of high-energy particles. This kind of IT will kill bystander cells (those nearby) which may result in killing of normal cells, but also of adjacent tumor cells which do not express the targeted antigen. The development of useful ITs has taken more time than initially anticipated due to toxic side effects, but many of the problems have been solved and some ITs are now in late-stage clinical trials. The same anti-CD20 mAb which has been approved for therapy of B cell lymphoma has also been coupled to a radionuclide, yttrium, and the resulting immunotoxin (Zevelin) has been approved for therapy of B cell lymphoma.

Tumor therapy with bispecific antibodies (BsAbs)

Directing or redirecting immune effector cells is also being explored as a way to enhance the ability of a patient's own immune system to reject their tumor. BsAbs, consisting of the binding sites of two different covalently linked mAbs, have been engineered as anti-tumor therapeutics. One specificity of this BsAb is to a TAA (e.g. HER2/neu), the other to a trigger molecule on a killer cell (e.g. CD64 on macrophages). When injected into a tumor-bearing patient, the BsAb binds to the immune effector cell thereby arming it to seek out, and kill, tumor cells. Several BsAbs have shown considerable promise and one is now in late-stage clinical trials for therapy of ovarian cancer.

Purging of bone marrow for autologous transplants

Much of cancer therapy involves the use of cytotoxic drugs and/or irradiation, both of which primarily target dividing cells. Although effective for many patients, a significant number are not cured and eventually succumb to their tumor, partly because the amount of chemotherapy or irradiation a patient can receive is limited by the toxicity of these agents to normal cells and especially hemopoietic stem cells (cells that give rise to platelets, PMNs, lymphocytes, etc.). In order to be able to increase the dosage of chemotherapy or irradiation, bone marrow transplants are sometimes used in conjunction with chemother-apy and irradiation. In particular, stem-cell-containing blood or bone marrow is first taken from the cancer patient. The patient is then treated with doses of chemotherapy or irradiation high enough to kill all tumor cells, but doses likely to kill all hemopoietic stem cells as well. The patient is then 'rescued' by infusion of their own stem cells which repopulate the bone marrow (Topic E1). Autologous marrow is commonly given because donor marrow of identical MHC types is not often available (Topic M2). However, because tumor cells may contaminate the stem cell populations harvested before therapy, mAbs to antigens associated with the tumor are used to purge the marrow so that these cells are not returned to the patient to re-establish the tumor. This approach has been successfully used in the treatment of some tumors, including myeloid leukemia.

N7 TUMOR VACCINES

Key Notes

Prophylactic vs therapeutic vaccines	The development of vaccines for treatment of cancer is a very active area of research. Prophylactic vaccines induce immunity to viruses associated with tumor development; other approaches are designed to enhance/induce effective immunity in tumor-bearing patients.
Immunization with tumors and tumor antigens	Killed or irradiated patient tumor cells or appropriate TAAs and their peptides are being tested for induction of patient anti-tumor immunity to antigens that are primarily tumor associated. Immunizing with DNA or peptide for the TAA may induce a stronger CTL response.
Immunization with transfected tumors	Transfecting tumor cells with co-stimulatory molecules enhances their immunogenicity and ability to induce a CTL response. Tumor cells transfected with cytokine genes attract, expand and activate immune cells reactive to tumor antigens.
Immunization with APCs loaded with TAA	Since immature dendritic cells (DC) are best able to ingest antigen and mature DCs are best at presenting antigen, considerable effort is directed at determining optimal conditions for loading and maturing DCs *ex vivo* so they induce strong CTL anti-tumor responses when re-introduced into the patient.
Related topics	Clonal expansion and development of effector function (F5) Antigen preparations (I3)
	Vaccines to pathogens and tumors (I4)

Prophylactic vs therapeutic vaccines

Numerous approaches are being used to develop vaccines for use in the treatment of cancer. Prophylactic approaches focus on the use of vaccines that induce immunity to viruses known to be associated with the development of a tumor. Hepatitis B vaccines would prevent infection by this virus and reduce the incidence of liver cancer. Human papilloma virus (HPV) vaccines would prevent the development of cervical carcinoma. Vaccines developed against specific viral proteins of HPV are currently in clinical trials. In contrast, most other tumor vaccine approaches are designed to enhance or induce effective tumor immunity in patients who have already developed cancer.

Immunization with tumors and tumor antigens

A variety of approaches have been explored for inducing or enhancing a patient's immunity to their tumor. These include injecting killed or irradiated tumor cells from the patient, an approach which has had little success. The identification of appropriate TAAs (those expressed at low levels on normal cells and high levels on tumors), and their potentially immunogenic peptides has resulted in their use in vaccines to focus the patient's immune system to respond to antigens that are primarily tumor associated. As with immunization using whole cells, these antigens would most likely induce a T helper cell rather than a more desirable CTL response, as they would enter APCs by the exogenous pathway and be presented on MHC class II molecules (Topic F2). However, it is now clear that the APC-presenting antigen to the CTL needs first to be conditioned by interaction with a T helper cell before it can effectively induce a CTL response (Topic F6). Moreover, antigens entering by the exogenous pathway may in some instances be presented on MHC class I molecules and initiate a CTL response.

Still another approach that is being very actively pursued involves immunizing with DNA encoding the TAA or peptide, either alone or in an appropriate expression vector. This DNA introduced into a cell would be integrated, expressed, and translated into proteins in the cytosol, some of which would be degraded to peptides for loading onto MHC class I molecules and thus the potential induction of a CTL response.

Immunization with transfected tumors

Since most kinds of tumor cells do not express the co-stimulatory molecules (e.g., B7.1, B7.2) that are important to the induction of an immune response, studies have been carried out to determine if transfecting tumor cells with these molecules would enhance their immunogenicity. In fact, B7-transfected tumor cells induced a strong CTL response against the tumor. Furthermore, these CTLs were sometimes able to lyse parent tumor cells not expressing B7, because once activated, CTLs do not need the B7 co-stimulatory signals to kill.

Another approach involves transfecting tumor cells from a patient with a cytokine gene, as certain cytokines expressed by the tumor may attract, expand and activate cells of the immune system and induce or enhance immunity to tumor antigens. In experimental models, tumor cells transfected with cytokine genes (e.g., IL-2, IFNγ, GM-CSF) are able to induce immunity to the tumor resulting in its regression or rejection. IL-2 may, for example, enhance the development of cytotoxic cells to TAAs from their precursors (e.g. in melanoma).

Immunization with APCs loaded with TAA

A very active area of tumor vaccine research at the present time involves loading of patient dendritic cells *in vitro* with TAA and re-injection of these cells into the patient. This approach has the benefit that potential APCs can be isolated from a patient's peripheral blood and manipulated such that their antigen-presenting capabilities are optimal. In particular, monocytes readily obtained from the peripheral blood of a patient can be induced with cytokines to differentiate into immature dendritic cells (*Fig. 1*). Since immature DCs are best able to ingest antigen and mature DCs are best at presenting antigen, loading of monocyte-derived immature DCs followed by cytokine-induced differentiation of these cells to mature DCs is more readily accomplished *in vitro* than *in vivo*. These mature, loaded APCs are then reintroduced into the patient, fully able to stimulate T cells. Many research groups are currently trying to define the optimal conditions for obtaining immature DCs, for loading and maturing them, and for their reintroduction into the patient.

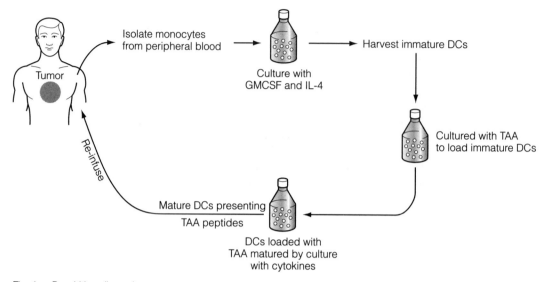

Fig. 1.   Dendritic cell vaccines.

01 OVERVIEW

Key Note

Overview	Gender-associated differences in immunological function have been recognized for some time. Females have marginally higher levels of serum IgG and IgM, a better primary and secondary response to infectious agents and an increased frequency of autoimmune diseases compared to males. Sex hormones have important effects on the immune system. Estrogens are associated with increased B cell synthesis of immunoglobulins while testosterone is associated with suppression of B cell activity. The anatomical distribution of lymphoid tissue is the same in both sexes with the exception of the reproductive tracts. In the female, highly organized lymphoid tissue is distributed throughout the reproductive tract and appears to be influenced by hormones associated with menstruation and pregnancy.
Related topics	Mucosa-associated lymphoid tissues (C3) The cellular basis of the antibody response (E3)
	Antibody classes (D2) Antibody responses in different tissues (E4)

Overview

Before the advent of antibiotics there was an increase in prevalence of infectious disease (morbidity) and mortality in male children compared to females and while the mortality has decreased, morbidity is still greater in male children. In recent years a better understanding of the effect of gender on the immune system has thrown some light on the basis of these findings. For example, there is a tendency for levels of serum IgG and IgM antibodies to be higher throughout life in females compared with males. This could contribute to the decreased susceptibility to infection and general trend in heightened immune response to microbial infections compared to males (*Table 1*).

Both increased primary and secondary responses to microbial infections such as *E. coli*, *Brucella*, measles, rubella and hepatitis B have also been reported. Perhaps as a consequence of their tendency to heightened immune response, females have a much higher frequency of autoimmune diseases pre- and post-puberty compared to their male counterparts. These autoimmune diseases include juvenile arthritis, Hashimoto's thyroiditis, systemic lupus erythematosus (SLE), primary biliary cirrhosis and rheumatoid arthritis (Topic L2). In

Table 1. *Gender-associated immunological differences*

	Female	Male
Susceptibility to infection	<	>
Immune response to infection	>	<
Frequency of autoimmune disease	High	Low

certain strains of mice (New Zealand Black), female mice are much more susceptible to the human equivalent of SLE than their male counterparts. Furthermore, male mice that have had an orchidectomy (removal of the testes) develop the same incidence as females, whilst ovariectomy (removal of the ovaries) has a protective effect in females. This provides strong evidence for the role of sex hormones on the adverse immune response in autoimmune diseases. Indeed, experimental evidence suggests that sex hormones in females modulate the immune system at all stages of life from prenatal to post menopause. In addition, they have been shown to have pivotal and different immunological functions in the developmental phase of the immune system and in its functional activity. In experimental systems it has been shown that estrogens are associated with increased B cell synthesis of immunoglobulins whilst testosterone is associated with suppression of B cell activity. Sex hormones appear to have major influences on immune cell types and function during the menstrual cycle and pregnancy. During cycle, NK cells increase in numbers in the late secretory phase compared to the late proliferative phase and in pregnancy there is an increase in the numbers of γδ T cells. The anatomical distribution of lymphoid tissue is the same in both sexes with the exception of the reproductive tracts. In the female highly organized lymphoid tissue is distributed throughout the reproductive tract and appears to be influenced by hormones associated with menstruation and pregnancy. The male, in contrast, has only occasional lymphocytes distributed throughout his reproductive tract. The lymphoid tissue associated with the reproductive tracts is part of the mucosa-associated immune system (Topic C3).

02 IMMUNE CELLS AND MOLECULES ASSOCIATED WITH THE REPRODUCTIVE TRACTS

Key Notes

The female reproductive tract

The female reproductive tract contains all of the cells associated with an appropriate immune response. These are distributed throughout the reproductive tract in the vagina, cervix, endometrium and in the epithelial layers of the fallopian tubes. Protective antibodies of both IgA and IgG classes are found in the lumen of the tract.

Immunological changes during the menstrual cycle

There are both numeric and functional changes in NK cells and T cells in the endometrium during the menstrual cycle. These changes are thought to be related to the marked fluctuations in estradiol and progesterone during the cycle.

Immune-associated changes during pregnancy

Pregnancy can be considered an immune privileged state. This immune privilege permits acceptance of the fetal allograft and is thought to be under the influence of pregnancy-associated hormonal regulation. Immunological changes include a shift towards a Th2-type cytokine profile.

The role of the lactating breast in immune defense

Plasma cells associated with the acini of the lactating breast are responsible for the production and secretion of IgA into colostrum and breast milk that is important for protection of the newborn.

The male reproductive tract

The lower male reproductive tract (penile urethra) resembles other mucosal sites in that it has abundant CD4$^+$ and CD8$^+$ T lymphocytes in the lamina propria (although CD8 T cells predominate). Macrophages are also frequent and dendritic cells restricted to the distal tip of the urethra. Occasional lymphocytes, mainly CD8$^+$ T cells, are found among the epithelial cells in the vas deferens and epididymis. IgA antibodies derived from plasma cells in the urethra and prostate glands are found in the seminal fluid.

Related topics

Cells of the innate immune system (B1)

Molecules of the innate immune system (B2)

Lymphocytes (C1)

Mucosa-associated lymphoid tissues (C3)

Antibody classes (D2)

Antibody functions (D8)

Antibody responses in different tissues (E4)

The female reproductive tract

Localization of immune cells in the tract

The female reproductive tract (FRT) is composed of vagina, cervix, uterus (containing endometrium), ovaries and fallopian tubes (*Fig. 1*). The vagina and

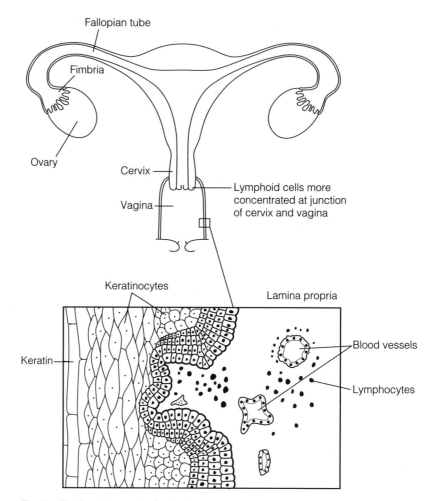

Fig. 1.   The female reproductive tract.

the outer portion of the cervix contain a highly vascularized mucosal layer and can act as a portal for microbial infection. The mucosal layer is an important barrier against infection. It contains immunologically reactive tissues that can mount local responses to foreign antigens in the same way as other mucosal surfaces. Active sites of mucosal immunity (Topic C3) include the cervix and vagina, although IgA plasma cells have been found in the fallopian tubes, endometrium, as well as in the cervix and vagina. Plasma cells, CD4$^+$ and CD8$^+$ lymphocytes, and MHC class II positive dendritic cells are distributed throughout the lower reproductive tract in both epithelial and sub-epithelial layers of the cervix and the vagina. Unlike the ileum of the gastrointestinal tract, no epithelial M cells have been found in the FRT for efficient transport of antigens into the subepithelial layers (Topic C3). The majority of lymphocytes appear to be located at the junction of the cervix and vagina. The cells in the epithelial layer of the cervix are mainly CD8$^+$ T cells and those in the subepithelial layer are mainly CD4$^+$ T cells. Most of the cells associated with the immune response in the female reproductive tract are summarized in *Table 1*.

Table 1.　Cells of the immune system associated with the female reproductive tract

NK cells	Endometrium
CD4, CD8 T cells	Vagina, cervix, endometrium, fallopian tubes
γδ T cells	Endometrium
B cells	Endometrium
Plasma cells	Vagina, cervix, endometrium, fallopian tubes
Macrophages	Vagina, cervix, endometrium
Dendritic cells	Vagina, cervix

Immunity in the FRT

IgG and IgA are both normally found in secretions of the cervix and vagina. IgA is derived locally from IgA plasma cells while IgG is thought to be mainly derived from the serum, although some local IgG production does take place. IgA is transported across the mucosal surfaces of the tract via poly Ig receptors on specialized epithelial cells (Topic E4). It is less certain how IgG is transported, although it is likely that there are IgG Fc receptors on specialized epithelial cells that can carry out this activity. Interestingly, the levels of IgG are usually higher than those of IgA in the non-pregnant female reproductive tract but vary during cycle. This is unusual at mucosal sites, e.g. intestine, where mostly secretory IgA is found in the secretions (Topic D2). The FRT, like other mucosal surfaces, is constantly open to the outside world and therefore direct exposure to pathogens (Topic C3). Vaginal immunization gives rise to both IgA and IgG responses to the immunizing antigen in both the vagina and cervix, confirming the ability of the lower reproductive tract to respond to foreign antigens. Independent of immunization, post-menopausal women tend to have higher concentrations of IgA and IgG in the cervix than non-immunized pre-menopausal women. Since the vagina is an efficient site for immunization, it could be expected that sexually active women would mount potent responses to sperm antigens and other proteins associated with the male ejaculate. For the most part, however, this appears not to be the case, as females are unresponsive to sperm antigens perhaps as the result of tolerance induction (Topics G2 and G3). In addition, the high concentrations of prostaglandins (which have potent immunosuppressive properties) in seminal fluid may inhibit immune responses. Antibodies to sperm antigens are produced in some women and this can lead to infertility.

Immunological changes during the menstrual cycle

As described earlier, NK cells, CD4$^+$ T cells, CD8$^+$ T cells, B cells and macrophages are distributed throughout the endometrium. The number of NK cells increases from the late proliferative phase (LP) and is maximal at the late secretory phase (LS) at which time it constitutes the largest number of lymphocytes. *Figure 2* shows the different phases of the cycle.

　　T cell numbers appear to remain relatively unchanged during the cycle, although the ratio of CD8 to CD4 T cells is lower at the LS phase compared to the LP phase. Between the LP phase and LS phase of the menstrual cycle, NK cells increase from 20% to 80%, whereas T cells decrease from 50% to less than 10%. In contrast, a group of potential regulatory cells, NKT cells, are increased in the late secretory phase of the menstrual cycle and are unusual in that they have NK cell markers as well as CD3 but not CD4 or CD8 (Topic C1). No classical MHC class II positive dendritic cells are present in the uterus. Changes in cell populations are summarized in *Table 2*. Organized lymphoid aggregates are also found in the

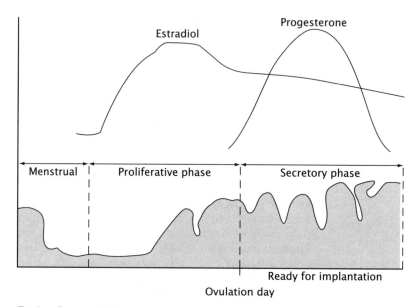

Fig. 2.   *Endometrial thickening during the menstrual cycle.*

Table 2.   *Changes in lymphocyte populations during the menstrual cycle*

	Late proliferative phase	Late secretory phase
NK cells	20%	80%
T cells	50%	<10%
NKT cells	lower	higher

endometrium. They have a core of B cells surrounded by more numerous T cells and an outer halo of monocytes/macrophages. The T cells in these lymphoid aggregates are mainly CD8⁺. The number and size of the aggregates increase during the menstrual cycle and their absence in post-menopausal women suggests that they are hormonally influenced. The function of these aggregates is at present unknown. The phagocytic activity of mononuclear cells decreases during the early phase of the cycle compared to the later phase, whereas T cell responses to *Candida* antigens are reduced during the secretory phase. Interestingly, this appears to be the time of increased susceptibility to *Candida albicans* infections. Taken together, the marked fluctuations in estradiol or progesterone during the menstrual cycle may influence not only the accumulation of different populations of immune cells but also their response to microbial antigens.

Immune-associated changes during pregnancy

Following implantation of the blastocyst, there is an increase in estradiol and progesterone, the latter being essential for maintaining the pregnant state. This prepares the uterus for reception and development of the fertilized ovum and induces changes in the endometrium resulting in a modified mucosa (decidua) (*Fig. 3*). Changes occur in immune cell populations in the endometrium and in the overall immune system presumably to provide an 'immune privileged state' for the maintenance of the fetal 'transplant' (Topic M4). During the first trimester of pregnancy, endometrial NK cells account for between 60–80% of

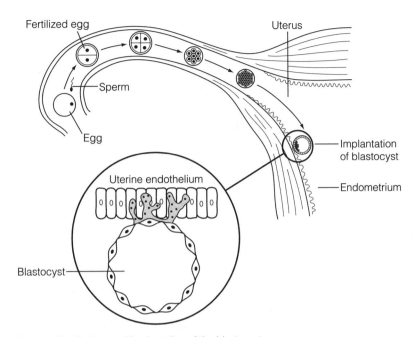

Fig. 3. Fertilization and implantation of the blastocyst.

the immune cells and these rapidly decrease after the second trimester. The remainder of the immune cell population consists of approximately 12% CD3⁺ T cells of which CD4⁺ and CD8⁺ are expressed in equal numbers, γδ T cells, NKT cells and a small percentage of B cells.

During the early phases of pregnancy, Th2 lymphocytes are the dominant T lymphocyte subset in the decidua. Th2-type cytokines, such as IL-4, IL-6, induce the release of human choriogonadotrophin (HCG) from trophoblasts, which in turn stimulates the production of progesterone from the corpus luteum. The decidua (part of the placenta) itself secretes IL-6, IL-10, IL-13 and TGFβ and diminishes the secretion of Th1-type cytokines. Moreover, trophoblasts are a source of IL-4 and IL-10. Thus Th2-type T cells and placenta-derived Th2 cytokines may contribute to the maintenance of pregnancy by modulating the immune (e.g. Th1 cell function: Topic G5) and endocrine systems. Interestingly, in animal models of pregnancy, Th1-type cytokines such as IFNγ have been shown to be associated with spontaneous abortion.

The role of the lactating breast in immune defense

Hormonal changes during pregnancy prepare the female breast for the supply of milk to ensure the healthy development of the newborn child. The importance of breast feeding in the prevention of respiratory and gastrointestinal infections has been emphasized by the World Health Organization and they have predicted that increasing breast feeding by 40% would reduce respiratory and gastrointestinal death by approximately 50% worldwide in children under the age of 18 months.

Localization of immune cells in the lactating breast
The female breast is composed of fatty and connective tissue, milk ducts and lobules (see *Fig. 4*). The lobules contain the specialized epithelial cells for

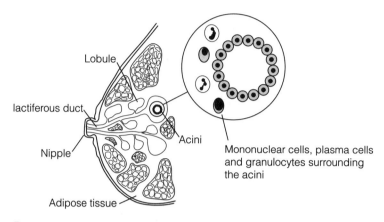

Lobule

lactiferous duct

Nipple

Acini

Adipose tissue

Mononuclear cells, plasma cells
and granulocytes surrounding
the acini

Fig. 4.   The lactating breast.

producing milk and are surrounded by stroma or lamina propria containing capillaries, lymphatics, mononuclear cells and granulocytes. The initial secretions from the breast (colostrum) contain between 10^6 and 10^7 leukocytes/ml and reduce to between 10^4 and 10^5/ml in mature milk. Colostrum and breast milk also contain a variety of cytokine and growth factors (*Table 3*). It is presently unclear how these factors and cells contribute to protection in the hostile environment of the infants' intestine.

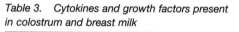

*Table 3.   Cytokines and growth factors present
in colostrum and breast milk*

- TGF-β
- EGF
- Colony-stimulating factor
- IL-1
- IL-6
- TNF-α

Antibodies in colostrum and breast milk

The lactating breast is an important site of mucosal immunity. In humans, approximately 80% of plasma cells in the lactating breast contain IgA. This immunoglobulin, in addition to other factors such as cytokines, growth and nutritional factors provide help to the newborn in thriving and preventing infection. **Secretory IgA** is produced by plasma cells derived from B cells that originally homed to the breast under hormonal influences from other mucosal surfaces such as the respiratory or gastrointestinal tracts – major portals of microbial entry (Topic C3). Lymphocytes entering the breast tissue contain homing molecules to allow them to enter mucosal tissue (Topic C4). Like secretion across the intestinal wall, IgA dimers are bound by the polymeric immunoglobulin receptors located on the basolateral surface membranes of mammary gland epithelial cells. The antibody receptor complex is then internalized and transported to the apical surface of the cell. Since these secretory IgA antibodies are derived from B cells that have originated from other mucosal surfaces such as the respiratory or gastrointestinal tracts, they usually have specificity against microbial antigens found in these tissues. The concentration of IgA is greatest in colostrum, the initial secretion from the breast. These levels fall rapidly postpartum in the breast milk to the equivalent of serum IgA concentrations. While IgA in the serum is mainly IgA1 (85%) compared to IgA2 (15%), breast IgA contains more IgA2 than IgA1 and is similar to intestinal IgA (Topic D2). The importance of IgA2 in the secretions may be related to its increased resistance to degradation by proteases produced by microbial pathogens (*Pseudomonas* sp., *Neisseria* sp., *Haemophilus influenzae* and *Streptococcus pneumoniae*, etc.) found in the mucosa. The mechanisms by which ingested IgA functions to protect against infection presumably involve blocking of attachment and entry of microbes (Topic D8). This passive IgA-mediated immunity is especially important immediately after birth because, as described previously, production of IgA by the infant only begins after birth (Topic C5). Many of the IgA antibodies found in breast milk are also directed against antigens derived from the mother's diet. Thus, in addition to protecting against microbial infection these antibodies may also protect against absorption of certain food antigens in early development. Small amounts of IgM and even smaller amounts of IgG are also found in breast milk. The mechanism of transport of these immunoglobulins across the breast epithelial cells is unclear.

The male reproductive tract

The penile urethra is the first point of contact of microbes entering the lower male reproductive tract (*Fig. 5*). It resembles other mucosal sites in that there are abundant CD4$^+$ and CD8$^+$ T lymphocytes in the lamina propria and epithelium (although CD8$^+$ T cells predominate). These cells are mainly of the memory phenotype (CD45RO), and many of them carry mucosa-associated homing molecules (Topic C4). Macrophages are also frequent within the lamina propria but dendritic cells are restricted to the distal tip of the urethra where they are intraepithelial in location. IgA plasma cells are also found in the lamina propria and home there from other mucosal surfaces. As in the gut, epithelial cells with poly Ig receptors transport the IgA into the lumen. IgA plasma cells are also found in the prostate gland and the secreted IgA derived from both these sites is found in the seminal fluid.

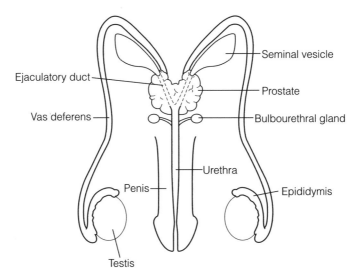

Fig. 5. The male reproductive tract.

Only occasional lymphocytes, mainly CD8 cells, and macrophages are found further up the reproductive tract amongst the epithelial cells in the vas deferens and epididymis. Thus, the urethral mucosal tissue is an extremely important site of immunological protection against ascending microbial infections.

03 FUNCTIONAL EFFECTS OF SEX HORMONES ON THE IMMUNE SYSTEM

Key Notes

Effects of estrogen and progesterone on immune function	In experimental systems, the hormones estrogen and progesterone have effects on immune function both *in vivo* and *in vitro*. Estrogens are associated with increased immunoglobulin synthesis and progesterone with a shift from Th1- to Th2-type cytokine production.
The effect of testosterone on immune function	Testosterone would appear to have a contrary effect to estrogens on some immunological functions in that it has been shown to inhibit immunoglobulin synthesis by B cells and is associated with protection against some autoimmune diseases.
Gender-associated autoimmunity: the role of sex hormones	Most autoimmune diseases are found with higher frequency in females than in males. This would suggest that sex hormones may play a pivotal role in the development and/or maintenance of these diseases.
Related topics	B cell activation (E2) Genes, T helper cells, cytokines and the neuroendocrine system (G5)	Factors contributing to the development of autoimmune disease (L2)

Effects of estrogen and progesterone on immune function

Estrogen and progesterone are the main female sex hormones. Estrogen is the term used collectively to denote a group of steroid hormones, which includes estradiol, estriol and estrone. Estradiol is produced by the ovaries and progesterone is produced by the corpus luteum and the uterine endometrium. Experimental studies *in vitro* and *in vivo* have shown several diverse effects of estrogen (and progesterone) on the immune system (*Table 1*). NK cells, monocytes/macrophages and T and B cells all have cell surface estrogen receptors. B cell immunoglobulin production is enhanced in the presence of estrogen. This is probably due to the direct effect of estrogen on B cells and/or plasma cells, as well as to enhancement of a Th2 cytokine response. Consistent with this finding, the anti-estrogen drug Tamoxifen causes an increase in the production of IL-2 and IFNγ in animal models, while reducing the levels of the Th2-associated cytokine IL-10. Similar effects are seen with progesterone suggesting that both of these hormones can regulate immune responses (Topic G5). That estrogens can directly activate some lymphocyte populations is indicated by their ability to stimulate lymphocyte proliferation *in vitro* and influence the expression of lymphocyte surface molecules. Estradiol has also been shown to suppress the cytotoxic activity of NK cells and downregulate IFNγ production. In experi-

Table 1.   Effects of estrogen on the immune system

Enhances immunoglobulin synthesis
Induces Th2 type responses*
Decreases NK cell cytotoxicity*
Downregulates IFNγ production
Prevents Fas-dependent apoptosis of CD4 Th2 cells

*Progesterone also has these effects.

mental models, estrogen has been shown to influence development of T and B cells. Thymic stromal cells and immature thymocytes express estrogen receptors and their absence in knockout mice results in decreased thymic size. Estrogen also inhibits the synthesis of thymosin α1, a thymic hormone, produced by thymic epithelial cells. Since thymosin α1 has a role in the maintenance of thymic homeostasis, the inhibition of this hormone may have a role in involution of the thymus.

In addition to preparing the uterine endometrium for implantation, progesterone has some effects on immune cells similar to those of estrogens (*Table 1*). Thus, the decreased NK cell function and biased Th2 response throughout pregnancy mediated by these two hormones is likely to reduce the potential 'rejection' of the fetal allograft mediated through a Th1-type mechanism (Topic M4).

The effect of testosterone on immune function

Testosterone is the main male-associated sex hormone and is produced mainly by the testes. Receptors for testosterone appear to have a similar distribution to estrogen receptors on cells associated with the immune system. The effects of testosterone on the immune system can be similar to those of estrogens but can also be different and even opposite. Testosterone, like estrogen, has a profound effect on thymic development leading to regression. In animal models, removal of the testes (orchidectomy) or removal of the ovaries (oophorectomy), causes thymic enlargement (hypertrophy) after birth. The mechanisms whereby testosterone and estrogen cause the thymus to regress are not fully understood but would appear to involve the thymocytes and thymic epithelial cells both of which have receptors for estrogen and testosterone.

Testosterone has also been shown to induce CD4$^+$ T cells to produce IL-10 (*Table 2*). This would tend to suppress Th1 cell responses leading to decreased cell-mediated immunity. Unlike the effects of estrogen, *in vitro* B cell differentiation to mitogens (Topic E2) is inhibited and not enhanced by testosterone. In addition, one of the mechanisms by which lymphocytes are regulated is through Fas-mediated cell death through apoptosis (Topic G2). Testosterone promotes, while estrogen prevents, Fas-dependent apoptosis of Th2 cells by reducing the expression of the apoptosis-suppressing mitochondrial proteins. Interestingly, there is now evidence that lymphocytes can produce small amounts of testosterone but the significance of this is currently unclear.

Table 2.   Effect of testosterone on the immune system

Induces IL-10 from CD4 cells
Inhibits B cell responses to mitogens
Promotes Fas-dependent apoptosis of CD4 Th2 cells

Gender-associated autoimmunity: the role of sex hormones

Apart from anatomical differences giving rise to increased frequencies of urinary tract infections in the female, the major gender-associated diseases are those caused by autoimmunity. Autoimmune diseases are disproportionately more common in females than in males (*Table 3*) with few exceptions. For example, ankylosing spondylitis is mainly a male autoimmune disease. The observation that autoimmune diseases are more frequently found in females than males and occur more frequently post puberty suggests a major immunological role for sex hormones in these conditions. Moreover, post-menopausal women have less clinical disease activity than their pre-menopausal counterparts. This may be as a result of the changing hormone profiles seen in women post menopause where estrogen levels are reduced and it has been shown that both IL-2 and IFNγ levels are increased compared to women in the pre-menopausal state. Hormone replacement therapy has been shown to reverse this decreased clinical disease activity in post-menopausal women. Clinical activity in SLE is also known to cycle with menses. Moreover, pregnancy can ameliorate certain autoimmune diseases. For example in RA, symptoms of the disease are markedly reduced during pregnancy. This is further support for the concept that hormones altered during pregnancy can have a major influence on the immune system.

Table 3.   Incidence of autoimmune diseases in females compared with males

Hashimoto's disease	30-1
Sjögren's syndrome	9-1
Systemic lupus erythematosus	9-1
Primary biliary cirrhosis	9-1
Antiphospholipid syndrome	9-1
Chronic active hepatitis	8-1
Mixed connective tissue disease	8-1
Graves disease	6-1
Rheumatoid arthritis	3-1
Scleroderma	3-1
Type 1 diabetes	2-1
Multiple sclerosis	2-1
Myasthenia gravis	2-1
Coeliac disease	2-1

In animal models of diabetes such as the non-obese diabetic (NOD) mouse or the BB rat, diabetes develops spontaneously but the severity of the disease is much more common in the female of the species. This severity can be reduced by gonadectomy (removal of reproductive organs) in female mice or treatment with testosterone. Sjögren's syndrome, which is primarily a female autoimmune disease, is also found in hypogonadal males. In mouse models of Sjögren's syndrome, treatment with testosterone delays disease progression. Taken together the greater predisposition of autoimmune diseases in females would appear to be related to the effects of the different sex hormones on the autoimmune response.

P1 OVERVIEW

Key Note

Overview	It is now clear that as humans age defects in both innate and adaptive immune systems occur and the overall effectiveness of their immune system decreases (termed *immunosenescence*). T cell function is reduced, the affinity of antibodies decreases and the response to vaccination is diminished. In addition, there are changes in neural and endocrine networks that influence immune responsiveness. Overall, infections are more common with an increase in morbidity and mortality, and there is an increased predisposition to malignancies.
Related topics	Cells of the innate immune system (B1) The role of T cells in immune responses (F1)
	Lymphocytes (C1) Genes, T helper cells, cytokines and the neuroendocrine system (G5)
	Antibody structure (D1)

Overview

A decline in immune competence is well recognized in the elderly. Aged people show a decline in many aspects of protective immunity including a tendency to produce lower-affinity antibodies, a failure to generate long-lasting immunity to vaccination and a loss of delayed-type hypersensitivity to antigens previously encountered in life (*Table 1*). Bacterial and viral diseases such as tuberculosis and herpes zoster (shingles), respectively, are found much more frequently in the elderly compared to young adults. Septicemia (infectious microbes in the bloodstream) is also more common in the elderly. Pneumonia is more prevalent and more often fatal and other viral and bacterial infections are more common in older people leading to an increase in morbidity and mortality. This decline in immune competence is not solely a result of a defective immune system, as it is also a result of changes in the endocrine and nervous systems, as well as nutritional and other factors including the general state of health of the older individual.

Table 1. Microbial infections associated with aging

Tuberculosis	Shingles
Pneumonia	Influenza
Urinary tract infections	Cytomegalovirus (CMV)

Malignancies are seen much more frequently in older people and while many of these may be related to inappropriate DNA translational events, a defective immune system may also be responsible since there is an association between immune deficiency and increased malignancy (Topic J3).

Defects in all compartments of the immune system have been reported in the elderly. While studies are often contradictory, reliable data indicate that defects develop in T and B cell immunity as well as in the phagocytic component of immunity. Increased NK cell numbers and decreased γδ T cell function are also a feature of aging (Topic B1). IL-6 and IL-10 production by monocytes is increased with aging as well as the pro-inflammatory cytokines IL-1β and TNFα. MHC molecules are expressed at lower density on a variety of cells and fewer T cells expressing CD28, important for T cell signaling, are found in the elderly (Topic F1). Antibody responses are usually of lower affinity and auto-antibodies are found much more frequently. Hemopoiesis is impaired with fewer progenitor cells produced. Thymic involution is well established in the elderly with fewer T cells entering the vascular pool and hence secondary lymphoid organs. AICD and apoptosis are increased. Age-related changes in hormonal and neurotransmitter function may also have an impact on immune function and may determine morbidity, mortality and longevity.

P2 DEVELOPMENTAL CHANGES IN PRIMARY LYMPHOID TISSUE AND LYMPHOCYTES WITH AGE

Key Notes

Hemopoiesis and aging	With increasing age, the number of progenitor cells produced decreases. This is seen in the bone marrow and in the thymus, organs that give rise to the specialized cells of the immune system.
Thymic involution and aging	One of the major immunological events associated with aging is the involution of the thymus. This begins after puberty and continues to senescence and decreases the thymic output of mature T cells.
AICD and apoptosis in aging	There is an increase in the expression of Fas (CD95) and FasL (CD95L) on T cells in the elderly. Increased levels of soluble FasL (sCD95L) are also found in the serum of aged individuals. This may lead to an increase in activation-induced cell death (AICD) and apoptosis and may explain the lower numbers of lymphocytes seen in the elderly.
Related topics	Hemopoiesis – development of blood cells (A5) Shaping of the T cell repertoire (F3)
	Lymphoid organs and tissues (C2) Central and peripheral tolerance (G2)

Hemopoiesis and aging

Hemopoiesis (blood cell and platelet development) is maintained during aging although at a reduced level. The proliferative capacity of cells of the bone marrow peaks during middle age and decreases thereafter. This is associated with a decrease in colony-stimulating factors (Topic B2), a decrease in the number of progenitor cells produced and an increase in apoptosis. There is a decreased capacity to deal with severe bleeding in the elderly, suggesting a decline in the function of bone marrow stem cells. This may be a result of diminished numbers of stem cells produced or micro-environmental changes in hormones, stromal cells or cytokines responsible for stem cell growth and differentiation. These changes probably also contribute to immunosenescence in that there would be fewer progenitor cells committed to the maturation processes of the immune system leading to fewer naïve lymphocytes entering the vascular pool and secondary lymphoid tissues. Even though there are fewer progenitor cells in the marrow, hemopoiesis has been achieved with progenitor cells from aged individuals in autograft treatments for multiple myeloma and other malignant blood disorders.

Thymic involution and aging

One of the most obvious effects of aging on the immune system is the involution of the thymus. This begins in adolescence and progresses to near total atrophy in the elderly where lymphoid tissue is replaced by fat. There is an approximate 3% decrease per year in the size of the thymus until middle age and an approximate 1% decrease per year thereafter (*Fig. 1*). As a result of this, the number of T cells entering the vascular pool and secondary lymphoid organs and tissues decrease with age. Data from studies on the rearrangement of genes encoding the T cell receptor have suggested that there is continuing thymic function in the elderly and that adult memory T cells in the periphery have undergone many replications.

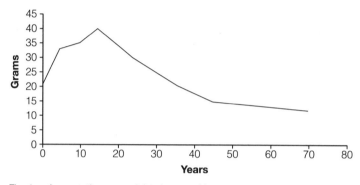

Fig. 1.   Average thymus weight change with age.

That changes occur in the thymus during aging is also indicated by observations on the recovery of CD4+ T cells following chemotherapy or therapy with anti-CD4 antibodies. The CD4+ T cells return to normal levels faster in younger individuals than adults and are mainly of the naïve phenotype (CD45RA) compared with those with a memory phenotype (CD45R0) in the elderly.

Thymic atrophy is probably under the control of many factors including T cell cytokines, thymic hormones and products of both the nervous and endocrine systems. Thymic involution is thought to result in the failure of the thymic microenvironment to support lymphopoiesis. Significant cytokine changes occur in the thymus during aging, including increases in IL-6 and macrophage colony-stimulating factor (M-CSF), and decreases in IL-2, IL-10 and IL-13. Other important thymic cytokines such as IL-7 and IL-15 remain stable during the aging process. Thymic status may also be under the control of signals from the nervous and endocrine systems. There is an age-associated increase in acetylcholinesterase-positive structures in the human thymus. In rodent models, older mice have increased noradrenergic sympathetic nerves and a 15-fold increase in the concentration of noradrenaline. The significance of this finding is presently unclear but does point to a role for the nervous system in thymic function especially in old age.

AICD and apoptosis in aging

The number of cells expressing Fas (CD95) and Fas ligand (CD95L) are increased in the elderly. In contrast, there is a decreased expression of CD95 in those of advanced age (>90).

Moreover, the amount of soluble CD95L is increased in older individuals compared to young. There is also an increased expression of CD95L on both

CD4$^+$ and CD8$^+$ T cells in the aged, and a strong correlation between the levels of CD95L on these cells and activation-induced cell death (apoptosis: Topic F5). In the elderly Fas-mediated apoptosis is increased in both 'memory' and 'naïve' T cells, although it is observed much more frequently in the 'memory' subset, and is associated with a reduced level of the anti-apoptotic mitochondrial proteins. Furthermore, lymphocytes in the elderly are more susceptible to TNFα-induced apoptosis than those in newborn blood. These findings suggest that AICD and apoptosis may contribute to immunosenescence by reducing the numbers of lymphocytes (*Table 1*).

Table 1. Factors that influence immunosenescence

- Hemopoietic failure
- Thymic involution
- Endocrine senescence
- Neural senescence
- Apoptosis

P3 EFFECTS OF AGING ON INNATE IMMUNITY

Key Notes

Aging and innate immunity	Macrophages, neutrophils and NK cells are the major components of the innate immune system. They function immediately after birth and continue to do so throughout life although some changes occur with aging.
Aging and neutrophils	Functional phagocytic defects occur in neutrophils of aged individuals. This leads to an inability to combat certain microbial infections, e.g., those caused by *Staphylococcus aureus*.
Aging and monocyte/MØ function	Monocytes/macrophages from aged individuals show changes compared to those of young adults. These changes include increased cytokine production and diminished phagocytic activity.
Aging and NK cells	NK cell numbers and function are essentially intact in the aged although some cytokines may be reduced.
Related topics	Cells of the innate immune system (B1) Molecules of the innate immune system (B2)

Aging and innate immunity

Macrophages, neutrophils and NK cells are the major components of the innate immune system. Innate immunity functions immediately after birth and although its activity persists throughout life, some functional changes occur with aging. While many innate pattern recognition receptors (PRR) for bacterial components are not affected by aging, the activity of other important components of innate immunity do change. In particular, the generation of superoxide by neutrophils and monocytes during phagocytosis tends to decrease. In contrast to innate immunity, adaptive immunity is not completely mature at birth, but peaks at puberty and declines thereafter (*Fig. 1*).

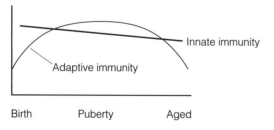

Birth   Puberty   Aged

Fig. 1. Changes in innate and adaptive immunity over time.

Aging and neutrophils

Changes in neutrophil function occur in the elderly, including reduced superoxide production in response to staphylococcal infections and reduced ability to respond to survival factors such as GM-CSF, G-CSF (Topic B2). There is also a marked reduction with aging in the expression of CD16 (an IgG/antigen complex receptor) by these cells (Topic B1). Taken together these factors may contribute to the inability of elderly patients to deal effectively with microbial infections and in particular with staphylococcal infections.

Aging and monocyte/MØ function

Monocytes from older adults frequently show signs of activation and secrete increased levels of IL-6 and IL-10 compared to monocytes from young adults. In the elderly, macrophages produce less superoxide, a molecule associated with intracellular killing (Topic B1). Accessory cell function is critical for T cell activation. This is achieved by presenting antigens through class I and class II HLA antigens. HLA class I molecules (Topic M2) are less well transcribed (as measured by levels of mRNA) in monocytes from the elderly compared to those from younger controls, and may give rise to less-efficient antigen presentation and poorer immune responses, especially those involving cytotoxic $CD8^+$ T cells (Topic F5).

Monocytes express the molecule CD14 (Topic B1) that is involved in activation via LPS and is therefore important in protection against Gram-negative bacteria. The percentages of monocytes bearing CD14 decrease with age and there is an increase in the number of monocytes expressing low-density CD14. Compared with the monocytes expressing the higher density of CD14, they have increased production of IL-6, IL-10 and decreased cytotoxicity. LPS-stimulated monocytes from the elderly produce less C-CSF, GM-CSF, IL-8, TNFα and IL-1 but normal levels of IL-12 (Topic B2). Taken together these data suggest that an inappropriate microenvironment for antigen presentation and T cell proliferation could contribute to poorer responses made against Gram-negative bacteria in the aged (*Table 1*).

Table 1.   Changes in monocyte function in the aged

Decreased CD14 expression
Decreased cytotoxicity
Decreased superoxide production

Aging and NK cells

Studies on peripheral blood NK cells indicate that their numbers generally increase in the elderly and that they appear to function normally. However, NK cells in the elderly only release 25% of the IFNγ released by NK cells from young adults on a cell-to-cell basis. In mouse models of aging, similar results are found for peripheral blood NK cells, although NK cells from spleen and lymph nodes of older animals have a profound loss of NK function. Whether this is true in humans has yet to be ascertained.

P4 THE EFFECTS OF AGING ON T CELL IMMUNITY

Key Notes

T cell phenotypes in the elderly

In aged individuals memory T cells are increased while naïve T cells are reduced in number. While there is evidence for increased T cell activation in the memory T cell population, total T cell numbers tend to be reduced with a loss of both CD4⁺ and CD8⁺ T cells.

T cell receptor usage in the aged

T cell receptor diversity is reduced in the aged. Reduced T cell receptor expression is associated more with CD8⁺ T cells than with CD4⁺ T cells.

T cell responses to mitogens and antigens

T cell responses to mitogens and antigens are reduced in the aged. This reduction is related to a number of intrinsic and extrinsic defects including defects in antigen presentation, signaling and cytokine expression.

Related topics

The role of T cells in immune responses (F1)

T cell recognition of antigen (F2)
T cell activation (F4)

T cell phenotypes in the elderly

Total T cell numbers are lower by approximately 30% in the aged (>60 years) compared to young adults (<35 years). Moreover, the composition of T cells is also different. Most T cells in young adults resemble 'naïve' (CD45RA⁺) cells, and in newborn blood nearly 100% are naive. In contrast, there are more primed or 'memory' T cells (CD45RO) and less 'naïve' cells in the elderly. Furthermore, these memory T cells appear to be more activated, based on the increased number of these cells that express CD25 and HLA-DR. Even so, there tend to be fewer CD3⁺ T cells as well as a decrease in the expression of CD3. This decrease is of both CD4⁺ T cells and CD8⁺ T cells, although the CD4/CD8 ratio does not differ significantly with age.

CD28 is critical as a 'second signal' for both CD4⁺ and CD8⁺ T cell activation (Topic F5). The number of CD28⁺ T cells and the density of its expression generally decreases in the elderly. Since centenarians have higher numbers of CD8⁺ T cells expressing CD28 than in the average elderly individual, it is possible that prolonged survival could be associated with number of CD28⁺ T cells. In addition, because T cells undergoing excessive replication, such as that seen in Crohn's disease, show a decrease in CD28 expression, the decreased expression of CD28 on cells from aging individuals may also be the result of excessive T cell replication (replication senescence; *Table 1*).

T cell receptor usage in the aged

T cell repertoire changes are also associated with aging. Although the CD4⁺ T cell population remains polyclonal during aging, the CD8⁺ population more frequently develops clonal expansions thus skewing the repertoire in favor of the TCRαβ chains (Topic F3) represented by the expansions. However, these

Table 1.   Major T cell changes associated with aging

- Reduced T cell numbers
- Increase in memory T cells (CD45RO)
- Decrease in naïve T cells (CD40RA)
- Decrease in proliferative responses to mitogens and antigens
- Decrease in DTH
- Decreased expression of CD3, CD154 and CD28
- Increased expression of CD25 and HLA-DR

expansions do not seem to be associated with childhood illnesses or vaccination in these individuals in earlier life. The ability to be successfully vaccinated against influenza in the aged is also related to the wider repertoire of different TCRs to which they make a response. Thus, in those elderly who are unresponsive to influenza vaccination, there is a marked restriction of the TCR-Vβ usage by their CD8⁺ cells. A restricted TCR repertoire in some individuals could therefore contribute to impaired immune responses to microbes in the aged. CD8⁺ T cells are also important in maintaining immune surveillance against tumors and thus a restriction in available TCR repertoires could help explain the increased incidences of malignancies that are seen in the elderly (Topic J3).

T cell responses to mitogens and antigens

In the elderly, T cell proliferation in response to PHA, anti-CD3 or IL-2 is diminished. This reduced proliferation may be a result of an intrinsic defect in T cells, defective accessory cell function, or inappropriate signaling through cell surface receptors. Resting T cells require signaling through the TCR **and** co-stimulatory molecules such as CD28 (by B7). The lack or inefficiency of this second signal may lead to apoptosis or anergy. In the elderly it has been shown that T cells expressing CD28 are reduced and CD154 and CD3 expression are also downregulated in both naïve and memory cells. Such age-associated changes in the expression of these co-stimulatory molecules could have profound effects on the immune response leading to immunosenescence.

There is also a defect at the level of signaling (Topic F4). Defective phosphorylation of tyrosine residues mediated by lck and ZAP70 in CD4⁺ T cells of the elderly, suggests that T cell activation via the T cell receptor is impaired (see *Fig. 4*, Topic F4).

Most studies on cytokine secretion in the elderly are equivocal, although it is generally agreed that IL-2 secretion is reduced. Similarly, IL-2 receptor expression is also decreased on elderly T cells. As IL-2 is important for lymphocyte expansion, a deficit in IL-2 or its receptor could lead to a loss of the stimulatory effect of this cytokine and thus poor proliferative responses to an antigen.

P5 THE EFFECTS OF AGING ON HUMORAL IMMUNITY

Key Note

The effect of aging on humoral immunity	In the elderly there is a reduction in the number of both B1 and B2 cells. Hypermutation is decreased and there is a tendency toward an increase in autoantibodies and toward a failure to produce high-affinity antibodies.
Related topics	Antibody structure (D1) T cell activation (F4) B cell activation (E2)

The effect of aging on humoral immunity

Several alterations in the B cell compartment are associated with aging, including a reduction in the total number of B cells, and of both the B1 and B2 subsets (Topic C1). Although the amount of antibody in the circulation does not appear to decrease significantly (*Table 1*), there are changes in the quality of the antibody response, including:

- A decrease in antibody affinities.
- A diminished ability to produce antibodies to vaccines (e.g. influenza) and to novel antigens.
- A change in the isotype of antibody responses. For example, in the young, antibody responses to influenza vaccine are primarily of the IgG1 subclass, whereas in the elderly they are of the IgG3 subclass.
- Hypermutation associated with increased antibody diversity appears to be impaired.
- An increase in autoantibody production especially rheumatoid factor, antidsDNA, antihistones and anticardiolipin antibodies (Section L). Although found more frequently, these autoantibodies seem to be of low specificity and of unknown pathological significance.

Some of these events may be related to dysfunctional T cell help and in particular to defective co-stimulation. Thus, these changes could result from deficient T cell signaling through B7-CD28 and/or CD40L–CD40 interactions.

Table 1. *Normal ranges for serum immunoglobulin concentrations in European Caucasians in different age groups*

	IgG		IgA		IgM	
	Males	Females	Males	Females	Males	Females
20–35 yrs	6.7–12.5	6.8–12.6	0.8–2.6	0.7–2.4	0.6–1.6	0.7–2.0
40–45 yrs	6.7–12.4	6.8–12.7	1.0–3.2	0.8–2.7	0.6–1.6	0.7–2.0
60–75 yrs	6.7–12.5	6.8–12.6	1.0–3.0	0.8–2.6	0.5–1.5	0.6–1.7

The restriction in antibody repertoire may also be related to a failure of development of precursor B cells in the bone marrow.

It is also interesting that there is some evidence for a decrease in IgE-mediated allergies with age and an increase in salivary IgG and IgA levels, perhaps reflecting changes in mucosal immunity. Moreover, gastrointestinal immunosenescence is associated with deficits in differentiation and homing of IgA plasmablasts to the lamina propria and the initiation and regulation of local antibody production.

P6 IMMUNOSENESCENCE AND MORBIDITY, MORTALITY AND LONGEVITY

Key Notes

Immunosenescence and disease	Tuberculosis, pneumonia, urinary tract infections and septicemia (bacteria in the bloodstream) are much more common in the elderly. Infections with influenza, rhinovirus and cytomegalovirus (CMV) are much more frequent and morbidity and mortality greater. This is related to a number of factors including immunosenescence.
Immune response genes and aging	Immune response genes (especially HLA genes) are important in helping the immune system respond effectively to microbial infections. Different HLA haplotypes may confer greater mortality or longevity.
Immunosenescence and the nervous and endocrine systems	Immunosenescence is complicated by senescence of the endocrine and nervous systems. This is shown not only as a decline in immune function but also by changes associated with aging of the neural and endocrine systems and their combined interactions.
Related topics	T cell recognition of antigen (F2) Immunity to different organisms (H2)

Immuno-senescence and disease

The incidence of microbial disease and malignancies are increased in the elderly compared to the young. Tuberculosis, pneumonia, urinary tract infections and septicemia (bacteria in the bloodstream) are much more common. Morbidity associated with gastroenteritis caused by *Salmonella* and other enteric bacteria such as *E. coli 0157* is greater. Infections with influenza, rhinovirus and CMV are much more frequent and morbidity and mortality greater. There is a ten-fold increase in the incidence of TB in the elderly. In some studies the major cause of death in individuals >80 years is infections.

Deficiencies in any component of the immune system can lead to a predisposition to infections. However, it appears that defects in NK cell numbers and function are related to death due to infections: NK activity is well preserved in centenarians. Shingles is a good indicator of immunosenescence and suggests decreased functional activity in both the T cell and NK cell compartments. Decreased T cell function can readily be shown by DTH tests to recall antigens (Topic J4). However, other factors such as nutritional status, stress, gender and previous vaccination history must be considered. Individuals who are malnourished are prone to vaccination failure. Autoantibodies are increased in the elderly although not necessarily associated with pathology (Topic P5). In fact

SLE becomes milder in patients as they age, as does primary Sjögrens syndrome. Immunosenescence may have some benefits in some clinical situations. Acute graft rejection to kidney, heart or liver is less in the elderly and the incidence of asthma and specific IgE responses to allergens decreases.

Immune response genes and aging

The immune response genes that encode the HLA molecules involved in presenting microbial antigenic peptides to T cells are the HLA class I and class II genes (Topic G5). The cellular expression of these genes is decreased in the elderly compared to younger controls. This may give rise to less-efficient antigen presentation and poorer immune responses. There is also an increase in the presence of soluble class I MHC molecules in the elderly, the significance of which is unclear.

Certainly, the number and kind of the different HLA types inherited determine to a significant degree the nature, extent and effectiveness of an individual's immune response. Thus, although there are no changes in these genes during aging, longevity or lack thereof, is to some extent influenced by these genes. For example, some HLA haplotypes are frequently associated with autoimmunity, e.g. HLA-DR3 – diabetes and HLA-DR4 – rheumatoid arthritis (Topic L1). In contrast, the inheritance of some IR genes is associated with longevity in some populations. However, immune response (IR) genes alone probably do not dictate mortality or longevity. Rather, it is likely that a combination of factors, including exercise, diet, stress, environment and other genetic components such as those associated with increased synthesis of pro- or anti-inflammatory cytokines will determine morbidity, mortality and longevity.

Immuno-senescence and the nervous and endocrine systems

The immune, endocrine and nervous systems influence each other through cytokines, hormones and neurotransmitters. During aging, changes occur in all areas of these interactive systems. Some pro-inflammatory cytokines such as IL-1 and TNFα are frequently increased and can affect the HPA axis. There is a loss of dehydroepiandrosterone (DHEA), dehydroepiandrosterone sulfate (DHEAS), progesterone and aldosterone. Growth hormone, melatonin and the sex hormones estrogen and testosterone are all reduced. It is not clear if these hormones influence immunosenescence, although some circumstantial evidence suggests that they do. For example, cortisol, a stress-related hormone, is increased in aging and is a powerful anti-inflammatory. Estrogen stimulates immune function and testosterone is inhibitory. In mouse models, melatonin improves the DTH response, prevents thymic involution and increases antibody responses.

Supplementation of DHEA and DHEAS, which are reduced in the elderly, results in enhanced lymphocyte mitogenic responses and in the number and activity of NK cells, but there is no improvement in antibody responses to 'flu' vaccines. Leptin is another hormone that is known to affect the pro- and anti-inflammatory cytokine response. While commonly associated with obesity, increased leptin levels are known to affect the Th1/Th2 balance by increasing the proinflammatory cytokine response. Leptin levels are increased by estrogen and decreased by testosterone. Since these hormones decrease with age, changes in leptin levels may contribute to the T cell cytokine status.

The autonomic nervous system also changes during aging. The sympathetic response is increased, although there is a decrease in sympathetic innervation; these events are accompanied by an increase in noradrenaline (norepinephrine) in the circulation. Cortisol and noradrenaline are thought to induce a Th2 type response. Cortisol increases immunoglobulin production and IL-4, IL-5 and IL-10 secretion, whereas noradrenaline inhibits IL-2, IL-12 and IFNγ synthesis, although stimulating IL-6 and IL-10 (*Fig. 1*). Moreover cortisol increases noradrenaline production from sympathetic nerve terminals. The expression of dopamine D3 receptors on lymphocytes is also rapidly reduced during aging. Dopamine induces T cell adherence to fibronectin, which is important in T cell trafficking. Taken together these findings show the interplay between the nervous, endocrine and immune system and the associated changes during senescence (*Table 1*).

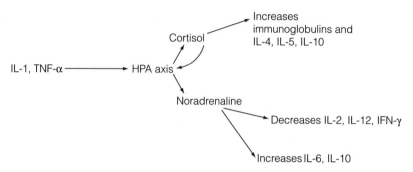

Fig. 1.   Interplay between the immune, endocrine and nervous systems.

Table 1.   Hormonal changes associated with aging

• Cortisol	Increased
• Noradrenaline (norepinephrine)	Increased
• Melatonin	Decreased
• DHEA, DHEAS	Decreased
• Growth hormone	Decreased
• Estrogen	Decreased
• Testosterone	Decreased

FURTHER READING

A large number of textbooks in immunology are now available which are good reference books for those interested in more detail. In addition, specific detailed information can often be obtained through the WEB and through specialist journal databases, including Medline, PubMed etc.

General textbooks

Abbas, A.K. and Lichtman, A.H. (2003) *Cellular and Molecular Immunology*, 4th edn., W.B. Saunders Company, Philadelphia, USA.

Janeway, C.A., Travers, P., Walport, M. and Shlomchik, M. (2001) *Immunobiology*, 5th edn., Garland Publishing, London, UK.

Kuby, J., Goldsby, R., Kindt, T.J. and Osbourne, B.A. (2002) *Immunology*, 5th edn., W.H. Freeman, Oxford, UK.

Playfair, J.H.L. and Lydyard, P.M. (2000) *Medical Immunology for Students*, 2nd edn. Churchill Livingstone, Edinburgh, UK.

Roitt, I.M., Brostoff, J. and Male, D. (eds.) (2001) *Immunology*, 6th edn., Mosby, London, UK.

Roitt, I.M. and Delves, P. J. (2001) *Essential Immunology*, 10th edn., Blackwell Scientific, Oxford, UK.

Sharon, J. (1998) *Basic Immunology*, William and Wilkins, Baltimore, USA.

MULTIPLE CHOICE QUESTIONS

The following pages contain multiple choice questions for self assessment. They are presented in the style of the US Medical Boards part 1 but are used universally in examinations. The questions are based on the material presented in the corresponding Sections into which they are grouped. Answers to these questions can be found on page 313. To make the most effective use of these questions do not try to answer them immediately after reading or reviewing the material on which they are based. Rather, let the knowledge settle overnight and then try the questions. Choose the single best answer.

A–E

1. Tears contain ...

A   IgA
B   IgG.
C   lysozyme.
D   all of the above.

2. Macrophages ...

A   circulate in the blood stream.
B   produce nitric oxide.
C   have receptors for IgM.
D   are the first leukocytes to arrive at the site of a skin infection.
E   are the main immune cells for dealing with viruses.

3. Phagocytosis ...

A   is carried by cells of the adaptive immune system.
B   is restricted to macrophages.
C   is important in bacterial infections.
D   is a process that does not involve energy.
E   results in division of the cell.

4. Molecules directly involved in NK cell mediated killing include ...

A   muramyl dipeptide.
B   granzyme A and B
C   complement.
D   IFNγ.
E   superoxide.

5. Opsonins include ...

A   perforin.
B   magainins.
C   C9.
D   IFNγ.
E   C3b

6. Dendritic cells are characterized by ...

A   the presence of major basic proteins.
B   expression of CD3.
C   expression of IgM molecules.
D   their ability to release histamine.
E   their interface between the innate and adaptive immune systems.

7. Both mast cells and basophils ...

A   are phagocytic
B   circulate in the blood stream.
C   are found primarily in lymph nodes.
D   have receptors for IgM antibodies.
E   release histamine.

8. Activation of the alternate pathway involves ...

A   C1.
B   C3.
C   C2.
D   C4.

9.   **Control of the activated complement components results from ...**

A   agglutination.
B   immune adherence.
C   instability and inactivation of some of these components.
D   mobility of phagocytes.

10.   **All of the following are true about acute phase proteins EXCEPT ...**

A   they include C-reactive protein.
B   they include complement proteins.
C   they are mainly produced in the liver.
D   they function to limit tissue damage.
E   they are not induced by cytokines.

11.   **Complement inhibitory proteins include the following EXCEPT ...**

A   decay accelerating factor (DAF).
B   CD59 (protectin).
C   membrane cofactor protein (MCP).
D   ICAM-1.

12.   **B cells are distinguished from T cells by the presence of ...**

A   CD3.
B   CD4.
C   CD8.
D   surface Ig.
E   Class I MHC antigen.

13.   **Lymphocytes of the mucosal immune system ...**

A   are normally primed in the lamina propria of the intestine.
B   home mainly to mucosal sites and not systemic lymphoid organs.
C   make up less than 10% of the lymphoid tissues in the body.
D   mainly produce IgG antibodies.
E   are only of the T cell type.

14.   **Newborns ...**

A   receive IgM antibodies from the mother through placental transfer.
B   have virtually a full complement of maternal IgG antibodies.
C   have very few lymphocytes in their circulation.
D   respond to antigens as well as adults.
E   receive maternal B cells.

15.   **Rearrangement of VH genes begins during ...**

A   the pre-B cell stage.
B   the pro-B cell stage.
C   maturation of B cells into plasma cells.
D   development of dendritic cells.
E   thymus development.

16.   **All of the following are true about the development of blood cells EXCEPT ...**

A   cytokines are required
B   IL-7 is involved in T cell development.
C   M-CSF is required for granulocyte development.
D   B cell development takes place mainly in the bone-marrow.

17.   **Allotypes are ...**

A   antigenic determinants which segregate within a species.
B   critical to the function of the antibody combining site.
C   involved in specificity.
D   involved in memory.

18.   **IgE ...**

A   is bound together by J chain.
B   binds to mast cells through its Fab region.
C   differs from IgG antibody because of its different H chains.
D   is present in high concentration in serum.

19.   Ig heavy chains are ...

A   encoded by a Constant region exon, Variable exon, Diversity exon, and Joining exon.
B   not glycosylated
C   not important to binding of antigen.
D   expressed by T cells.

20.   The Fab portion of Ig ...

A   binds to an Fc receptor.
B   contains the J chain.
C   contains the idiotype of the Ig.
D   mediates biological effector functions of Ab molecules (e.g. complement fixation).

21.   Cells destined to become IgA producing plasma cells do not ...

A   migrate from mucosal areas on stimulation with antigen.
B   home to any mucosal area
C   produce secretory component.
D   produce J chain.

22.   IgA ...

A   is present in milk and saliva
B   is involved in hay fever.
C   activates complement by the classical pathway.
D   crosses the placenta

23.   Antibody dependent cell mediated cytotoxicity (ADCC) ...

A   is carried out by B cells.
B   is the main mechanism for killing intracellular microbes.
C   involves Fc receptors on the effector cells.
D   is primarily mediated by IgE antibody.

24.   The Fc region of antibody ...

A   contains both heavy and light chains.
B   is required for antigen binding.
C   is not a requirement for placental transmission.
D   is not important for triggering of IgE mediated hypersensitivity.
E   generally confers biological activity on the various molecules.

25.   Human IgM ...

A   crosses the placenta
B   consists of 3 subunits linked together by a J chain.
C   protects mucosal surfaces.
D   is largely restricted to the circulation.
E   is the antibody produced by high affinity plasma cells.

26.   Immunoglobulin light chains ...

A   are joined to heavy chains by peptide bonds.
B   can be present as both κ and λ chains as part of a single Ig molecule.
C   are not found in every major immunoglobulin class.
D   all have the same amino acid composition.
E   are present in the Fab fragment of IgG.

27.   The fixation of complement by an antigen-antibody reaction can lead to ...

A   formation of a factor chemotactic for mononuclear cells.
B   enhanced phagocytosis.
C   activation of T cells.
D   increased synthesis of antibody.

28.   Both interleukin 1 and 2 ...

A   are produced by the same cell.
B   require complement for their biological activity.
C   act on T cells.
D   trigger histamine release.

29.   Tumor necrosis factor ...

A   decreases macrophage effector functions.
B   increases expression of adhesion
    molecules on endothelial cells.
C   decreases vascular permeability.
D   decreases blood flow.

**30.   Cytokines that directly elevate body
        temperature include ...**

A   IL-10.
B   TGFβ
C   IL-4.
D   IL-5.
E   IL-6.

31.   A B cell can express on its cell surface ...

A   membrane IgM and IgD at the same time.
B   both types of light chain.
C   secretory component.
D   IgG that can bind several different
    unrelated antigens.

**32.   All of the following are true about
        receptors of the innate immune system,
        EXCEPT that they ...**

A   include those of the Toll family.
B   recognize molecular patterns associated
    with groups of microbes.
C   include CD14 and scavenger receptors.
D   include MHC molecules.
E   do not include Igα and Igβ.

**33.   On the B cell surface, receptors for
        antigen are associated with ...**

A   CD3γ chains.
B   Igα and Igβ.
C   MHC class II molecules.
D   MHC class I molecules.
E   Toll receptors.

34.   Direct causes of inflammation include ...

A   TGFβ.
B   histaminase.
C   ICAM-1.
D   VCAM.
E   LPS.

**35.   Which of the following is a known
        inhibitor of inflammation ...**

A   TNFα.
B   nerve growth factor.
C   protein C.
D   neuropeptide Y.
E   reactive oxygen species.

36.   Clonal selection ...

A   necessitates that proteins are
    multideterminant.
B   requires that each antigen reactive cell
    have multiple specificities.
C   involves binding of Ab Fc regions to mast
    cells.
D   explains specificity and memory in
    immunity.

**37.   Stimulation of B cells to proliferate and
        differentiate requires ...**

A   B cell immunoglobulin binding of peptide
    in association with T cell MHC class II.
B   binding of CD40 on B cells by its ligand
    on T cells.
C   IFNγ.
D   B cell surface antibody binding to C3b.

**38.   Type 1 thymus-independent antigens
        characteristically are ...**

A   small peptides.
B   bacterial proteins.
C   viral nucleic acids.
D   bacterial polysaccharides.
E   haptens.

39. Among the steps of maturation of a pre-B cell to a plasma cell, the only one that does not require antigen is ...

A   affinity maturation.
B   development of memory.
C   clonal selection or tolerance.
D   recombination of the V, D, J gene loci.
E   tolerance.

40. Reaction between an IgG anti-albumin monoclonal antibody and albumin might result in ...

A   precipitation.
B   lattice formation.
C   agglutination.
D   complex formation.

41. ELISA assay ...

A   results in cell lysis.
B   uses a radiolabeled second antibody.
C   involves addition of substrate which is converted to a colored end-product.
D   requires sensitized red blood cells.

42. Monoclonal antibodies produced by hybridoma technology ...

A   are usually of human origin.
B   are each the result of immortalization of a single monocyte.
C   usually have specificity predetermined by prior immunization.
D   are prepared by fusion of T lymphocytes and myeloma cells.

F–I

43. Helper T cells are distinguished from cytotoxic T cells by the presence of ...

A   CD2.
B   CD4.
C   CD3.
D   IL-2 receptor.
E   Class II MHC antigen.

44. T-cells in lymph nodes ...

A   occur predominantly in the medullary region.
B   are only of the cytotoxic type.
C   are phagocytic
D   are absent in Di-George syndrome.
E   express surface immunoglobulin.

45. IFNγ ...

A   is produced by all nucleated cells of the body.
B   induces Th2 responses.
C   can activate macrophages.
D   was discovered because of its effect on tumors.

46. Viral replication within cells is inhibited by ...

A   IL-13.
B   IL-1.
C   IFNα
D   TNFα
E   IL-4.

47. Cytotoxic T cells generally recognize antigen in association with ...

A   class II MHC determinants.
B   class I MHC determinants.
C   class III MHC determinants.
D   HLA-DR determinants.

48. The T cell antigen receptor ...

A   recognizes epitopes on linear peptides associated with MHC determinants.
B   has Ig light chains.
C   is made up of a heavy chain and $\beta2$ microglobulin.
D   recognizes conformational epitopes on the native antigen.

49. **TCR gene rearrangement ...**

A takes place primarily in the bone marrow.
B is antigen independent.
C involves immunoglobulin.
D requires costimulation by antigen presenting cells.

50. **The class I MHC processing pathway primarily ...**

A processes antigens that are present in the cytosol.
B processes antigens from the extracellular environment.
C generates peptides, complexes them with class I MHC molecules for presentation to helper T cells.
D generates peptides, complexes them with class I MHC molecules for presentation to NK cells.

51. **The endogenous pathway of antigen presentation involves ...**

A mostly peptides derived from extracellular pathogens.
B presentation of antigen on MHC class II molecules.
C presentation of antigen to cytolytic T cells.
D presentation of antigen to Th1 cells.
E presentation of antigen to B cells.

52. **Potent chemotactic factors (chemotaxins) for neutrophils include ...**

A C-reactive protein.
B C3b.
C arachidonic acid.
D LTB4.
E IFNα.

53. **All of the following are true about class switching of antibodies EXCEPT that ...**

A particular Th subsets are required.
B it occurs in germinal centers of lymph nodes.
C cytokines are required.
D it occurs in patients with Di George syndrome.
E it does not occur in patients with a genetic defect in CD40L.

54. **The following are required for, or are sequelae of clonal selection EXCEPT ...**

A recognition of antigen by specific antigen receptors on lymphocytes.
B proliferation of cells triggered by specific antigens.
C activation of T lymphocytes by superantigens.
D generation of T cell dependent B cell memory responses.

55. **T cells do not ...**

A make IL-2.
B respond to IL-4.
C respond to IL-2.
D mediate their functions solely by cell to cell contact.

56. **Th1 cells do not ...**

A express CD4.
B produce IFNγ.
C activate macrophages.
D bind soluble antigen.

57. **CD8 positive cells ...**

A can be classified into Th1 and Th2 subgroups based on their biological function.
B do not produce IFNγ.
C can recognize and kill virus infected cells.
D can bind free virus.
E do not require direct cell to cell contact with their targets for killing.

58. CTL ...

A do not mediate cytotoxicity of other T cells infected with virus.

B mediate killing by insertion of perforin into the membrane of the target cell.

C do not need to recognize MHC antigens on the target cell to kill.

D recognize antigens with MHC class II antigens.

E normally help B cells to make antibodies.

59. Superantigens ...

A activate large numbers of T cells by directly binding to the TCRβ chain and class II MHC

B are high molecular weight antigens that can trigger T cell proliferation in the absence of antigen presenting cells.

C can activate all B cells by binding to IgM.

D can only trigger CD8+ T cells.

60. Molecules involved in lymphocyte activation include all of the following EXCEPT ...

A CD3.

B CD79b.

C CD14.

D lck.

E CD28.

61. Stimulation of antigen-specific T cells by appropriately presented antigen alone results in ...

A induction of cytotoxicity.

B production of IL-2 but not other cytokines.

C activation resulting in cell division.

D anergy.

62. The stage in B-cell development at which tolerance can be most easily induced is ...

A memory B.

B pre-B.

C immature B.

D mature B.

E plasma cell.

63. Mechanisms whereby peripheral tolerance may be maintained include all of the following EXCEPT ...

A the absence of co-stimulation by CD80 or CD86.

B treatment with glucocorticoids.

C failure of cytokine signalling.

D apoptosis of activated T cells induced by Fas ligand on other cells.

E the absence of co-stimulation by CD154.

64. Properties of antigen that may influence its role in the induction of tolerance include ...

A its nature.

B its route of administration.

C the dose of antigen.

D maturity of the immune system.

E all of the above.

65. The process involved in allowing T cells to survive in the thymus is ...

A positive selection.

B negative selection.

C apoptosis.

D necrosis.

E complement inactivation.

66. **All of the following are true of the tolerant state EXCEPT ...**

A   its induction is dependent on the immunologic maturity of the individual.
B   it is observed when CD28-B7 interactions are blocked.
C   it is generally dependent on the presence of antigen.
D   its maintenance does not involve activation induced cell death (AICD).

67. **Central tolerance takes place in ...**

A   lymph nodes.
B   thymus.
C   spleen.
D   liver.
E   pancreas.

68. **One reason why different individuals can mount T cell responses to specific peptides and others cannot is because ...**

A   they lack the expression of class I or class II MHC molecules on specific cell types.
B   the peptides that can be presented by the MHC molecules that a person inherited are limited.
C   of an imbalance in the CD4/CD8 T cell ratio.
D   of mutations in the constant region of MHC class I genes.

69. **The main cytokine responsible for immunosuppressing Th1 responses is ...**

A   IL-1.
B   IL-2.
C   IL-4.
D   IL-10.
E   TNFα

70. **Which of the following cell types (or their products) is least effective against extracellular bacterial pathogens?**

A   B cells.
B   cytotoxic T cells.
C   helper T cells.
D   neutrophils.
E   macrophages.

71. **Complement components facilitate immunity to extracellular pathogens by all of the following mechanisms EXCEPT ...**

A   opsonizing the pathogen.
B   mediating the chemotaxis of inflammatory cells to the site of infection.
C   increasing vascular permeability to increase access to the site of infection.
D   binding to T cells inducing their activation.

72. **Extensive cooperation between phagocytes and lymphocytes is essential *in vivo* for ...**

A   elimination of inert carbon particles (e.g. a splinter).
B   elimination of non-encapsulated bacteria (e.g. *S. epidermidis*, a normal skin bacterium).
C   NK cell killing of tumor cells.
D   elimination of encapsulated bacteria (e.g. pneumococci).

73. **A tetanus booster shot results in the increased production of ...**

A   tetanus-specific NK cells.
B   T cells that recognize tetanus toxoid but not tetanus toxin.
C   antibodies which neutralize tetanus toxin.
D   T-cells which kill *Clostridium tetani*.

74. For adjuvants to be effective, they need to do all of the following EXCEPT ...

A prolong antigen exposure.
B enhance release of TGFβ.
C induce high affinity responses.
D increase quantitative response.

75. DNA vaccines can be effective if they ...

A can be engineered to contain DNA motifs that have an adjuvant effect.
B encode expression of antigen.
C encode expression of appropriate cytokines.
D all of the above.

76. Polysaccharides are rarely effective vaccines by themselves because they ...

A have repeating B cell epitopes.
B lack classical T cell epitopes.
C only induce CTL responses.
D are usually the same in people and bacteria.

77. Vaccines may fail to induce a protective response because they induce ...

A humoral immunity when cell mediated immunity is needed.
B IgM but not IgG or IgA.
C production of IL-4 when IFNγ is needed.
D all of the above.
E items A and B only.

78. An antibody to CD40 would be expected to enhance vaccine effectiveness by ...

A blocking CD40 signalling on dendritic cells.
B activating CD40 signalling on dendritic cells.
C linking dendritic cell CD40 to lymphocyte CD154 (CD40 ligand).
D inducing dendritic cell apoptosis.
E none of the above.

J–L

79. An anti-idiotypic antibody was infused into a patient with autoimmune hemolytic anemia. This treatment improved the anemia for 2 days, followed by recurrence of the anemia. The improvement was most likely related to binding of anti-idiotypic antibody to ...

A the B-cells making the autoantibody.
B plasma cells making the autoantibody.
C autoantibody specific T helper cells.
D circulating serum autoantibody alone.

80. The presence of 70% CD3 positive lymphocytes in the peripheral circulation of a patient indicates that the patient has normal ...

A humoral immunity.
B cellular immunity.
C numbers of B lymphocytes.
D numbers of T lymphocytes.

81. HIV infects all of the following EXCEPT ...

A monocytes.
B T cells.
C macrophages.
D B cells.

82. The receptor through which HIV infects is ...

A CD2.
B CD3.
C CD4.
D CD5.

83. Immunoglobulin deficiency can be detected by ...

A   flow cytometry.
B   DTH skin test.
C   mixed lymphocyte response (MLR).
D   serum protein electrophoresis.

84. Cell-mediated immune responses are ...

A   enhanced by depletion of complement.
B   suppressed by cortisone.
C   enhanced by depletion of T cells.
D   suppressed by antihistamine.
E   enhanced by depletion of macrophages.

85. Treatments for immunodeficiency would not include ...

A   antibiotics.
B   bone marrow transplantation.
C   interleukins.
D   anti-CD4 antibody.

86. Immediate hypersensitivity usually involves ...

A   mast cells.
B   antibodies to mast cells.
C   platelets.
D   IgG.

87. Mast cell products mediate some of the symptoms of immediate hypersensitivity by increasing ...

A   IgE receptors.
B   secretion of IgE.
C   capillary leakage.
D   secretion of IgG.

88. Therapy for immediate hypersensitivity includes injection of antigen (allergen) to ...

A   induce wheal and flare.
B   increase T cells making IL-4.
C   cause anaphylaxis.
D   increase T cells making IFNγ.

89. Slow-reacting substance of anaphylaxis (SRS-A) constricts airways and arteries and increases bronchial mucus production. The chemical nature of SRS-A is ...

A   histamine.
B   leukotrienes.
C   prostaglandin D2.
D   thromboxane.
E   chondroitin sulfates.

90. The predominant antigen presenting cell in contact hypersensitivity (e.g. poison ivy) is the ...

A   T lymphocyte.
B   B lymphocyte.
C   basophil.
D   Langerhans cell.
E   NK cell.

91. The cutaneous response of delayed hypersensitivity ...

A   can be passively transferred by antibody.
B   shows erythema (redness) and induration 1–2 days after injection of the antigen.
C   depends upon the attachment of IgE antibody to mast cells.
D   is mediated by B lymphocytes.

92. Anti-RhD antibody ...

A   is not given to RhD negative mothers after birth of an RhD positive infant.
B   does not react with RhD antigens on RBC.
C   does not block the development of active immunity to RhD antigen.
D   is obtained from RhD negative women.

93. Inflammation resulting from
     IgG–antigen complexes ...

A   requires IgM to activate complement.
B   involves complement activation.
C   produces the rash of poison ivy.
D   requires T cells.

94. Immune complex disease ...

A   requires cytotoxic T cells.
B   requires neutrophils.
C   usually involves IgE.
D   usually involves IgA.

95. Serum sickness occurs only ...

A   when anti-basement-membrane antibodies
     are present.
B   in cases of extreme excess of antibody.
C   when IgE antibody is produced.
D   when soluble immune complexes are
     formed.
E   in the absence of neutrophils.

96. Both immune complex disease and
     delayed type hypersensitivity involve ...

A   phagocytic cells.
B   IgG or IgM antibodies.
C   NK lymphocytes.
D   B cells.

97. Hemolytic disease of the newborn due
     to RhD incompatibility depends upon
     the ...

A   mother possessing RhD antigens not
     present on the baby's red cells.
B   inability of the baby to react against the
     mother's red cells.
C   transplacental passage of IgM anti-RhD
     antibodies.
D   transplacental passage of IgG anti-RhD
     antibodies.
E   production of cytotoxic antibodies by the
     baby.

98. Delayed hypersensitivity as typified by
     the Mantoux reaction to tuberculin is
     mediated by ...

A   lymphocytes.
B   polymorphonuclear cells.
C   anaphylactic antibodies.
D   complement binding antibodies.
E   antigen–antibody complexes.

99. Complement receptors on red blood cells
     and Fc receptors on platelets probably
     facilitate ...

A   immune phagocytosis of immune
     complexes by red blood cells and
     platelets.
B   immune pinocytosis of immune
     complexes by red blood cells and
     platelets.
C   the synthesis of gamma interferon by the
     platelet.
D   the elimination of immune complexes by
     phagocytic cells.

100. The broad spectrum of autoantibody
     formation in patients with systemic
     lupus erythematosus is probably
     indicative of ...

A   excess production of macrophages.
B   failed regulation of a multi-specific B-cell
     clone.
C   the presence of many auto-reactive B-cell
     clones.
D   heterozygosity at the HLA B locus.

101. The clinical disease most likely to
     involve a reaction to a hapten in its
     etiology is ...

A   systemic lupus erythematosus after
     treatment with glucocorticoids.
B   hemolytic anemia after treatment with
     penicillin.
C   juvenile diabetes after treatment with
     insulin.
D   rejection of kidney graft after treatment
     with cyclosporin.

102. IgG antibodies against 'self' proteins ...

A   are only found in patients with tumors.
B   are only produced in the spleen.
C   can cross the placenta.
D   are more common in men.

103. Goodpasture's disease involving lesions in the kidney and in lung alveoli is caused by ...

A   deposition of soluble antigen–antibody complexes.
B   cell mediated hypersensitivity to kidney antigens.
C   IgE antibodies to proximal tubules.
D   antibodies to basement membranes.
E   non-specific reactions due to a high level of serum IgG.

M–P

104. Tumors induced by chemical carcinogens ...

A   express unique TSA.
B   express TSA that are the same for all tumors induced by the same carcinogen.
C   do not usually express MHC antigens.
D   can be treated by immunosuppression.

105. Host antibody against a tumor would most likely be directed against ...

A   MHC class II antigens.
B   viral antigens.
C   differentiation antigens.
D   MHC class I antigens.

106. Tumor immune surveillance may be mediated by ...

A   mast cells.
B   neutrophils.
C   Langerhans cells
D   NK cells.

107. The HLA typing in a paternity case is as follows:

mother:	A8	B3	C2	DR10
	A23	B8	C4	DR5

potential father #1: A2,3; B8,27; C2,11; DR3,9
child: A3,23; B8,27; C2,4; DR5,10

Based on this information potential father #1 should ...

A   be convinced that the child is his because a crossover generating a recombinant maternal haplotype explains the only discrepancy.
B   sue the hospital for mixing up newborns because the child cannot belong to either him or the mother.
C   review his knowledge of immunogenetics and determine his haplotypes from his previous children's HLA types because without this information he cannot be sure if he is the father of this latest child.
D   determine the HLA type of potential father #2.

108. Graft survival can be enhanced *without* generalized immunosuppression by ...

A   matching for HLA antigen.
B   anti-thymocyte globulin.
C   cyclosporin A therapy.
D   steroids or cytotoxic drugs.

109. The mixed lymphocyte reaction ...

A   can be used to determine if two individuals have HLA-D differences.
B   if carried out with the cells of identical twins, would show a marked increase in proliferation because the cells are antigenically compatible.
C   is carried out with the cells from both individuals treated with mitomycin C or X-ray to eliminate extraneous proliferation.
D   is assayed by measuring cell lysis.

110. **Immunosuppression is not induced by ...**

A   antihistamines.
B   removal of lymphoid tissue.
C   use of anti-lymphocyte antibodies.
D   cytotoxic drugs.

111. **Bone marrow engraftment is a unique type of organ transplantation because ...**

A   MHC differences are not recognized.
B   minor histocompatibility differences are the only antigenic differences that can lead to rejection.
C   graft versus host disease may occur.
D   immunosuppression is never required.

112. **A major transfusion reaction may occur if the recipient ...**

A   has antibodies to transfused cells.
B   has T cells reactive to blood group antigens.
C   is RhD compatible.
D   is AB positive.

113. **The most acute form of graft rejection (termed hyperacute rejection) results from ...**

A   occlusion of blood vessels by proliferating endothelial cells.
B   killing of grafted tissue by cytotoxic T cells.
C   occlusion of blood vessels as a result of coagulation.
D   attack by natural killer cells.

114. **In some instances, a graft made between two unrelated donors, who are perfectly matched at HLA-A, B, C, and D, is still rejected. The possible cause of this rejection is ...**

A   β2-microglobulin differences.
B   mismatching of immunoglobulin allotypes.
C   prior sensitization to major histocompatibility antigens.
D   minor histocompatibility differences.

115. **The immune effector system responsible for acute graft rejection is ...**

A   cytotoxic T lymphocytes.
B   mast cells.
C   activated macrophages.
D   complement.

116. **An HLA haplotype is ...**

A   the total set of MHC alleles present on each chromosome.
B   a specific segment of the MHC locus.
C   genes outside the MHC locus that contribute to rejection.
D   one allele of HLA-B.

117. **Graft rejection ...**

A   occurs between identical twins.
B   rarely involves T lymphocytes.
C   can be accelerated by a previous graft from the same donor.
D   can be prevented by immunostimulation.
E   is mainly prevented by matching at the HLA A, B or C loci.

118. The antigenic component of a vaccine for melanoma is a 20 amino acid peptide. This peptide ...

A   could induce both T cell tolerance and T cell activation.

B   would be expected to work for most people.

C   would be expected to work for a subset of people.

D   items A and C only.

119. Major histocompatibility antigens are not ...

A   linked with a number of autoimmune diseases.

B   important for interactions between T and B cells during an immune response.

C   the only antigens which result in graft rejection.

D   important for graft versus host reactions.

120. HLA disease association ...

A   means that the particular HLA antigen or haplotype involved causes the disease.

B   may in some instances be useful in diagnosis.

C   means that every person with that HLA type will contract the disease.

D   may suggest that genes near the MHC locus code for T cell antigen receptors specific for self antigens.

121. The major immunoglobulin class found in colostrum is ...

A   IgG.

B   IgA.

C   IgM.

D   IgE.

E   IgD.

122. B cells found in the lactating breast are likely to have homed from the ...

A   Spleen.

B   Bone marrow.

C   Liver.

D   Gastrointestinal tract.

E   Thymus.

123. NK cells are more numerous during ...

A   Early secretory phase of the menstrual cycle.

B   Late secretory phase of the menstrual cycle.

C   Early proliferative phase of the menstrual cycle.

D   Late proliferative phase of the menstrual cycle.

124. The major T cell change associated with aging is ...

A   Increased numbers of CD4 cells.

B   Increased numbers of CD8 cells.

C   Increased numbers of memory T cells.

D   Increased numbers of B cells.

125. Which of the following is associated with aging ...

A   Increase in antibody affinity.

B   Decrease in antibody affinity.

C   Increased response to vaccination.

D   Increased response to novel antigens.

ANSWERS

1.	D	43.	B	85.	D
2.	B	44.	D	86.	A
3.	C	45.	C	87.	C
4.	B	46.	C	88.	D
5.	E	47.	B	89.	B
6.	E	48.	A	90.	D
7.	E	49.	B	91.	B
8.	B	50.	A	92.	D
9.	C	51.	C	93.	B
10.	E	52.	D	94.	B
11.	D	53.	D	95.	D
12.	D	54.	C	96.	A
13.	B	55.	D	97.	D
14.	B	56.	D	98.	A
15.	B	57.	C	99.	D
16.	C	58.	B	100.	C
17.	A	59.	A	101.	B
18.	C	60.	C	102.	C
19.	A	61.	D	103.	D
20.	C	62.	C	104.	A
21.	C	63.	B	105.	B
22.	A	64.	E	106.	D
23.	C	65.	A	107.	D
24.	E	66.	D	108.	A
25.	D	67.	B	109.	A
26.	E	68.	B	110.	A
27.	B	69.	D	111.	C
28.	C	70.	B	112.	A
29.	B	71.	D	113.	C
30.	E	72.	D	114.	D
31.	A	73.	C	115.	A
32.	D	74.	B	116.	A
33.	B	75.	D	117.	C
34.	E	76.	B	118.	D
35.	C	77.	D	119.	C
36.	D	78.	B	120.	B
37.	B	79.	D	121.	B
38.	D	80.	D	122.	D
39.	D	81.	D	123.	B
40.	D	82.	C	124.	C
41.	C	83.	D	125.	B
42.	C	84.	B		

Appendix I SELECTED CD MOLECULES

CD	Cell distribution	Function
1a,b,c	thymocytes, Langerhans cells, DCs, B cells (CD1c)	MHC-class I like molecule; presents lipid antigens
2	T cells, NK cells	also called LFA2; adhesion, binds to CD58 (LFA3)
3	All T cells	signalling molecules associated with TCR
4	T cell subset	binds to MHC II; activation; co-receptor for HIV
5	T and B cells	binds to CD72; negative regulation of B cells
8	T cell subset	binds to MHC I; co-receptor for activation
10	T and B cell progenitors	also called CALLA; metalloproteinase
11a	leukocytes	subunit of LFA-1; associated with CD18; adhesion
11b	myeloid and NK cells	also called Mac-1, CR-3; adhesion; binds to CD50, 54, 102
11c	myeloid cells	also called CR-4; adhesion; binds to CD54, C3bi
11d	leukocytes	associated with CD18; adhesion; binds to CD50
14	myeloid cells	binds LPS/LPS binding protein complex; activation
15	G, M	CHO on cell surfaces; binds to CD62E/L/P
16	NK cells, G, M subset	low affinity FcR for IgG (FcγRIII); act and phagocytosis
18	leukocytes	Integrin; β2 subunit associates with CD11a, b, c, d
19	B cells	part of the BCR; complexes with CD21; involved in activation
20	B cells	ion channel?; involved in activation
21	B cells, FDC	also called CR2; complement receptor
22	resting B cells	binds to sialo-conjugates (BL-CAM); act; negative regulation
23	B cells, act M, eos, FDC, Pt	low affinity FcR for IgE (FcεRII)
25	act T, B cells and act M	also called TAC ; IL2 receptor α chain
27	thy, T, NK act B cells	binds CD70; co-stimulator for T and B cell activation
28	T cells, act B cells	binds to B7.1 (CD80) and B7.2 (CD86); co-stimulatory for T cells
29	leukocytes	binds to FN, collagen
30	act T, B and NK cells, M	binds CD30L; involved in activation
31	M, Pt, G, T cell subset, End	also called PECAM-1; binds to endothelial cells
32	Mac, G, B, Eos	FcR for IgG (FcγRII)
33	myeloid progenitors, M	binds sialoconjugates
34	hemopoietic precursors	also called My 10; binds CD62L
35	G, M, B, some T/NK, eryth	also called CR1, C3b/4bR; complement receptor; binds C3b, C3bi, C34b;
40	B, DC, Mac	binds to T cell CD40L (CD154); co-stimulatory for B/class switching; cytokine production by MAC and DCs.
45	leukocytes	also called LCA; phosphatase; 2 main isoforms – RA and RO
45RA	leukocytes	on T cells RA is associated with naïve cells
45RO	leukocytes	on T cells RO is associated with antigen experienced (memory) cells
46	leukocytes	also called membrane co-factor protein (MCP); complement inhibition; binds to C3b and 4b to permit degradation by Factor 1
49	broad distribution	multiple families: integrins associated with CD29; bind coll and lam (VLA-1,2), coll and FN (VLA-3, VLA-5) and V-CAM-1 (VLA-4) and lam (VLA-6)
50	broad distribution	also called ICAM-3; binds integrins CD11a/CD18 (LFA-1)
52	thymocytes, T,B cells (not PC), M,G	also called CAMPATH-1; molecule not characterized
54	broad distribution	also called I-CAM-1; binds LFA-1 and Mac-1; receptor for rhinovirus
55	broad distribution	also called Decay Accelerating Factor (DAF); inhibits complement; binds C3b and disassembles C3/C5 convertase

CD	Cell distribution	Function
56	NK cells, act T cells	also called N-CAM, NKH1
58	broad distribution	also called LFA-3; binds to CD2
59	broad distribution	also called protectin; inhibits complement; blocks assembly of the membrane attack complex
62E	End	also called ELAM-1 and E-Selectin; binds sialyl-Lewis^x
62L	B, T, M, NK cells	also called LAM-1, L-Selectin, LECAM-1; binds CD34
62P	Pt, megakaryocytes, End	also called P-selectin; binds CD162 on lymphocytes, M and N
64	M, Mac, act G	high affinity FcR for IgG (FcγRI)
71	all proliferating cells	transferrin receptor
72	B cells	binds to CD5; involved in activation
79a	B cell	Igα chain; signalling molecule for BCR
79b	B cells	Igβ chain; signalling molecule for BCR
80	B cells, Mac, DC	also called B7-1; co-stimulator for CD28/CTLA-4
86	act B cells, Mac, DC	also called B7-2; co-stimulator for CD28/CTLA-4
89	M, Mac, G	FcR for IgA (FcαR)
95	broad distribution	also called FasL; binds to Fas and involved in induction of apoptosis
106	End	also called VCAM-1; ligand for VLA-4
152	act T cells	also called CTLA-4; binds to CD80, CD86
154	act CD4+T cells	also called CD40L; binds to CD40 on B cells and DC
158a	NK cells, T cell subset	Killer Inhibitory Receptor (KIR)
178	act T cells, other cells	also called FasL; binds to CD95

CD (Cluster of differentiation) antigens are defined by groups of monoclonal antibodies that recognize leukocyte-derived molecules with a common molecular mass and cellular distribution. A series of workshops are organized frequently to define different CDs. Abbreviations: **act**, activated; **B**, B cell; **BCR**, B cell receptor; **CHO**, carbohydrate; **coll**, collagen; **CR**, complement receptor; **DAF**, decay accelerating factor; **DC**, dendritic cells; **End**, endothelial cells; **Eo**, eosinophil; **EPC**, epithelial cell; **Eryth.** erythrocytes; **FcR**, Fc receptor; **FIB**, fibrinogen; **FN**, fibronectin; **G**, granulocyte; **HIV**, human immuno-deficiency virus; **ICAM**, intercellular adhesion molecule; **LAM**, Leukocyte Adhesion Molecule; **Lam**, laminin; **LCA,** leukocyte common antigen; **LFA**, leukocyte function antigen; **VLA**, very late antigen; **LPS**, lipopolysaccharide; **MHC**, major histocompatibility complex; **M**, monocyte; **Mac**, macrophage; **N**, neutrophils; **NK**, natural killer cell; **Pt**, platelet; **T**, T cell; **Thy**, thymocytes; **MCP**, membrane cofactor protein; **VN**, vitronectin; **VCAM**, vascular cell adhesion molecule

Appendix II THE PRINCIPAL CYTOKINES

Cytokine	Main source	Action
IL1α and β	Mac, Epc	activates T cells and Mac; fever
IL2	T cells	T cell growth factor, causes T cell proliferation
IL3	T cells	growth of many cell types
IL4	T cells, mast cells	B cell activation; class switch to IgE; suppresses Th1 cells
IL5	T cells, mast cells	B cell growth factor; eosinophil growth
IL6	T cells, Mac, End	T and B cell growth, production of APP
IL8	T cells	chemokine; attracts PMNs and monocytes
IL9	T cells	mast cell growth factor
IL10	T cells, Mac, EBV ACT B cells	inhibits Mac function and production of other cytokines
IL11	BM stromal cells	involved in hemopoiesis
IL12	APC, Mac, B cells	activates NK cells; induces Th1 cells
IL13	T cells	B cell growth factor; suppresses Th1 and Mac inflammatory cytokines
IFNα	most nucleated cells	antiviral; enhances MHC class I expression
IFNβ	most cells, especially fibroblasts	antiviral; enhances MHC class I expression
IFNγ	T cells, NK cells	enhances MHC class II expression; activates Mac; induces IgG class switching; suppresses Th2 cells
TGFβ	T cells, monocytes	inhibits cell growth; anti-inflammatory; induces IgA secretion
TNFα	Mac, T cells	pro-inflammatory; causes shock and endothelial activation
TNFβ (LT)	T cells, B cells	cytotoxic; activates endothelial cells
G-CSF	monocytes, fibroblasts	induces granulocyte growth
GM-CSF	Mac, T cells	induces differentiation of myelomonocytic lineage especially dendritic cells
M-CSF	BM stromal cells	stem cell factor (SCF-1); induces monocyte growth and differentiation

ACT, activated; **APC**, antigen presenting cells; **APP**, acute phase proteins; **BM**, bone marrow; **EBV**, Epstein Barr virus; **End**, endothelial cells; **endo**, endothelial; **Epc**, epithelial cells; **G-CSF**, granulocyte colony stimulating factor; **GM-CSF**, granulocyte monocyte colony stimulating factor; **IFN**, interferon; **IL**, interleukin; **LT**, lymphotoxin; **M-CSF**, monocyte colony stimulating factor; **Mac**, macrophages; **SCF**, stem cell factor; **TGF**, transforming growth factor; **TNF**, tumor necrosis factor

GLOSSARY

Active/passive immunization. Active immunization requires that the immune system of the host participate in the protective immune response against a microbe (e.g. following vaccination), whereas passive immunization results when 'preformed' antibodies made in another person or animal are injected into the host.

Acute phase proteins. Found in the blood soon after the onset of an infection, they limit damage caused by the organism and implement repair; mainly produced by the liver, they include CRP, mannose binding lectin, etc.

ADCC. Antibody dependent cellular cytotoxicity; cytotoxicity mediated by effector cells bound to antibodies attached to surface antigen of target organisms, e.g. parasites or tumour cells.

Adhesion molecules. Cell surface molecules that are involved in cell–cell interactions, e.g. ICAM-1.

Adjuvant. A substance included with an antigen that potentiates (non-specifically) an immune response (e.g. alum in human vaccines).

Affinity. The binding strength of a single receptor to its ligand (e.g. one antibody binding site binding to one antigenic determinant).

Allograft. A transplant made between genetically different individuals within the same species.

Allotype. The product of an allele detectable as foreign by another member of the same species (e.g. MHC antigens, blood groups, IgG).

Allelic exclusion. In a heterozygous individual only one of the two allelic forms are expressed as proteins; relates to antibody variable region genes where only one antibody receptor can be expressed by a single B cell.

Anergy. A state of tolerance involving non-responsiveness to antigen rather than cell deletion.

Antigen. a substance that induces an antibody or a T cell response. Generally used for any molecule that binds specifically to an antibody or T cell receptor.

Antigenic determinant (see also epitope). The portion of an antigen recognized and bound by antibody (3–5 amino acids in size) or the T cell receptor (8–20 amino acids in size). Thus, even the smallest protein would have numerous determinants.

Antigen presentation. The display of peptide fragments bound to MHC molecules on the cell surface, necessary for recognition by T cells.

Antigen processing. Enzymatic degradation of proteins into peptides to be associated with MHC molecules for T cell recognition.

Apoptosis (programmed cell death). Cell death occurring under physiological conditions that is controlled by the dying cell itself (i.e. 'cell suicide'); does not normally lead to inflammation.

Atopy, atopic. Hypersensitivity mediated by IgE (type I) or the tendency to develop this.

Autoantigen. An antigen derived from the same individual; a 'self' antigen.

Autologous. Derived from the same individual.

Avidity. The strength of binding between a multivalent antibody (all antibodies are at least bivalent) and a multideterminant antigen (microbes with repeating antigens). Avidity differs from affinity since it takes into account the valency of the antigen–antibody interaction.

CD. Molecules originally defined by groups of monoclonal antibodies (cluster of differentiation).

CDR. Complementarity determining regions of antibodies and T cell receptors are the most variable regions of the molecules and determine specificity and make contact with the antigen.

Central tolerance. Self tolerance achieved by elimination of self reactive T and B cells in the primary lymphoid organs.

Chemokines. Small chemoattractive cytokines that stimulate the migration and activation of cells particularly lymphocytes and phagocytes; important in inflammation.

Chemotaxis. The movement of cells up a concentration gradient of chemotactic factors such as chemokines.

Class switching. The process mediated through gene rearrangement by which B cells express a new heavy chain isotype without changing the specificity of the antibody produced.

Clonal selection. Antigen selects specific B or T cells to expand into clones.

Complement. A set of serum proteins involved in opsonisation, inflammation and lysis.

Cross-matching. Used to test whether recipients have preformed antibodies to blood group or histocompatibility antigens (HLA) to donor tissues that could interfere with successful transplantation.

CRP. C-reactive protein is an acute phase protein that binds to phosphorylcholine on the surface of many bacteria and acts as an opsonin; serum levels are used as a measure of an ongoing inflammatory response in a variety of autoimmune diseases.

Cytokines. Molecules that affect the behaviour of other cells; if produced by lymphocytes they are called lymphokines, by monocytes, monokines, etc. They can be produced by and act on the same cell, i.e. autocrine.

Cytotoxic. Able to kill cells.

DTH. Type IV or Delayed-type hypersensitivity is mediated by T cells; called delayed since it occurs hours to days after injection of antigen, e.g. the Manteaux test for TB.

Effector cells. Cells mediating immune function such as antibody secretion by plasma cells or cytotoxicity by Tc cells, often used to distinguish from memory cells.

ELISA. Enzyme linked immunoabsorbent assay used to quantitate both antigens and antibodies.

Epitope. an antigenic determinant or small part of an antigen that interacts with an antibody or T-cell receptor.

GALT. Gut associated lymphoid tissue; protects the intestinal tract of the body; see also MALT.

Germ line. The germ cells through which the continuity of the species is maintained; the term used for inherited Ig and TCR genes rather than those generated by gene rearrangement.

Germinal center. Sites of B cell proliferation in secondary follicles in lymphoid tissues. Involved in antibody affinity maturation and the production of memory cells.

Haplotype. A linked set of genes associated with one haploid genome; used mainly for describing inheritance of MHC genes that have infrequent cross-overs and are inherited as one haplotype from each parent.

Hapten. A small molecule that by itself is not immunogenic, but when it is coupled to a larger carrier molecule, can elicit antibodies directed against the hapten, e.g. some drugs.

HLA. Human leukocyte antigens are the major histocompatibility antigens in man that bind peptides and present them to T cells; they are highly polymorphic and act as transplantation antigens.

Humoral. Referring to fluids including the blood plasma and lymph. 'Humoral immunity' is essentially antibody-mediated immunity.

Hybridoma. An 'immortal' hybrid cell line derived by fusion of a B lymphocyte with a tumour cell, a useful technique for making monoclonal antibodies.

Hypervariable regions. Variable amino acid sequences within the variable regions of heavy and light immunoglobulin chains and of the T-cell receptor that contribute most to the antigen-binding site. Synonymous with complementarity determining regions (CDRs).

Hypersensitivity. Heightened immune response directed to innocuous antigens from plants and animals, microbial antigens and autoantigens that often lead to tissue damage; does not occur on first encounter with antigen.

Idiotype. The set of individual antigenic determinants of an immunoglobulin or T-cell receptor variable region, against which other ('anti-idiotypic') B or T cells can react.

Immune-complex. Antibody and antigen bound non-covalently in various proportions. Can cause hypersensitivity reactions.

Immunogen. A substance capable of eliciting an immune response. All immunogens are antigens; but some antigens, such as haptens, are not immunogens. Sometimes also used to describe antigens which induce actual protective immunity, e.g. against infection.

Integrins. One of the 'families' of adhesion molecules.

Interleukins (IL). Generic name for many cytokines/chemokines produced by leukocytes.

Interferons (IFN). Cytokines that inhibit virus replication of which there are three types; IFN-α and β are produced by most nucleated cells while IFN-γ is produced mainly by NK and T cells.

IR genes. Immune response genes are genetic polymporphisms that control immune responses; they include the HLA genes that bind specific peptides and genes controlling cytokines and cytokine receptors.

Isotype. synonymous with antibody class (IgM, IgG, IgA, IgD and IgE). Each isotype is encoded by a separate immunoglobulin constant region gene that is carried by all members of a species (c.f. allotype).

ITAMS. ImmunoTyrosine Activation Motifs; specific tyrosine phosphorylation sites on signalling molecules that are involved in activation of a cell, e.g. on the cytoplasmic tails of CD79 and the ζ chain associated with CD3.

ITIMS. ImmunoTyrosine Inhibitory Motifs; specific tyrosine phosphorylation sites on signalling molecules that are involved in negative signalling of cells, e.g. on the cytoplasmic tails of FcγRII on B cells.

KARs. Killer Activatory Receptors; cell surface receptors on NK cells that activate killing by these cells.

KIRs. Killer Inhibitory Receptors; cell surface molecules on cells of the body that mostly inhibit NK cell activity, e.g. some HLA molecules.

Lectins. Proteins, often derived from plants, that bind specific sugars and oligosaccharides present on animal cell membrane glycoproteins.

Ligand. A molecule that binds to a given receptor (i.e. used in the same sense as in pharmacology).

Lymphatic system. the system of lymphoid organs and vessels that drains the tissues of fluid derived from the blood system.

Membrane attack complex. the terminal complement components C5b, C6, C7, C8, C9 that result in pore formation and membrane damage.

MHC. Major histocompatibility complex; the genetic locus that codes for HLA and, in the mouse, H2 antigens that are involved in peptide binding for presentation to T cells and for graft rejection since the genes are polymorphic.

M cells. specialized epithelial cells in the terminal ileum that transport antigens into the subepithelial Peyers patches.

Mimicry. The mechanism by which microbes, having antigens similar to self-antigens to which the host is tolerant, are able to avoid the immune response.

Monoclonal antibodies. Antibodies produced by a B cell clone and are therefore all identical with regard to specificity. They are used as standard laboratory reagents, e.g. for identification of cell surface markers, bacterial typing, and in immunotherapy.

Necrosis. Death of a cell through chemical or physical injury leading to tissue inflammation; compare apoptosis.

Opportunist. A normally harmless microbe that causes serious infection only when the immune system is compromised (e.g. by HIV or a drug).

Opsonin. A substance (e.g. antibody or C3b) that binds to an antigen and enhances its phagocytosis by a process called opsonization.

Peripheral tolerance. Tolerance to self that develops outside the central lymphoid organs – thymus and bone marrow.

Phagocytosis. The process of internalization of particulate matter by cells, e.g. microbes and dead cells.

Polyclonal. Involvement of many different clones of lymphocytes, or of antibodies secreted by many B cell clones.

Polymorphism. Genetic polymorphism is where a gene has several allelic forms present at a single gene locus (e.g. blood groups, MHC).

Serology. The use of antibodies to detect and measure antigens, e.g. in the typing of infectious agents.

Somatic mutation. A mutation not occurring in the germ-line and therefore not inherited; this form of mutation of the immunoglobulin variable region genes in B cells in the germinal centres is important in maturation of antibody affinity.

Superantigens. Antigens (often bacterial) that stimulate many T cell clones independently of their specificity. This occurs by binding to MHC molecules outside their peptide-binding grooves and to particular T-cell receptor V regions.

Syngeneic. Genetically identical members of the same species, e.g. identical twins or mice from an inbred strain.

Titer. The relative strength of an antiserum. The reciprocal of the last dilution of an antiserum capable of mediating some measurable effect such as precipitation or agglutination.

TLR (Toll-Like Receptors). A group of receptors named after the toll receptor involved in the differentiation of the fruit fly Drosophila. The receptors are used mainly by cells of the innate system to detect microbial components.

Toxoid. A toxin that has been manipulated to eliminate its toxicity while retaining its immunogenicity.

Transgenic. An animal in which a foreign gene has been inserted to study its effect when expressed in a special site or manner.

Transplantation antigens. These are mainly the polymorphic MHC molecules expressed by nucleated cells of the body that are recognised as foreign by recipients not possessing the allelic forms of the donor.

Western blotting. A technique for identification of antigens in a mixture by electrophoresis, blotting onto nitrocellulose and labelling with enzyme or radiolabelled antibodies.

Xenograft. A graft between individuals of different species, e.g. a pig heart in man.

INDEX

Note: Page numbers in **bold** refer to Tables; those in *italics* refer to Figures

accessory molecules 127–8
acid phosphatase 16
acquired immunodeficiency
    disease (AIDS) 6, 165,
    189–90
acquired tolerance 149–51
activation-induced cell death
    (AICD) 145, 147–8, *148*,
    284
  apoptosis and 286, 287–8
acute lymphocytic leukemias
    (ALLs) **257**
acute phase proteins 23, 26–7, **26**
adaptive immune system 5, 6, **6**,
    7
  at birth 59–60
  regulation by 141, 143–4
addressins 57
adenosine deaminase (ADA)
    deficiency 195
adenovirus 182
adhesion molecules 57
  in inflammation and 38–9
adjuvants 177, 178–9, **179**
adrenaline (epinephrine) 157
affinity maturation 77
affinity purification 87, 91–2
African sleeping sickness
    (*Trypanosoma*) 182
agglutination assays 83, 85–6, *86*
aging (immunosenescence)
    283–4
  AICD and apoptosis in 286,
    287–8
  autoimmune disease and 217,
    218
  disease and 294–5
  hemopoiesis and 285
  humoral immunity in 292–3
  immune response genes in
    294, 295
  innate immunity in 288
  monocyte/macrophage
    function in 288, 289, **289**
  morbidity, mortality and
    longevity in 294–6
  nervous and endocrine
    systems in 294, 295–6

  neutrophils and 288, 289
  NK cells and 288, 289
  T cell immunity in 290–1
  T cell phenotypes 290
  T cell receptor usage 290–1
  T cell responses to mitogens
    and antigens 290, 291
  thymic involution in 286, 287
alkaline phosphatase 16
allelic exclusion 72
allergens **203**
allergic rhinitis 201
allografts 240–1
allotypes 78
α-fetoprotein (AFP) 251
α-melanocyte hormone 40
alternative pathway 23, 26
amoebiasis 165
anaphylatoxins 20
anchor residues 121
ankylosing spondylitis 218, 281
antibiotics, antibodies and 192,
    194–5
antibodies to neutrophil
    cytoplasmic antigen
    (ANCA) 23102
antibody/antibodies 3
  affinity 63
  affinity purification of 87, 91–2
  antibody units 61–3
  assays and 87, 88
  chimeric 81
  classes 65–7
  class diversity 73–5, *74*
    antigen-dependent events
    75
    antigen-independent events
    74
  differential splicing and class
    switching 68, 72–3, *74*
  excess 84
  functional diversity 65–6
  functions 93–7
    activation equals
    inactivation 96
    antibody alone 93
    in complement activation
    93–6

    with effector cells 93, 96–7
    major functions of
    complement system 95–6
    regulation 96
    sequence of activation 94–5
  inactivation of 169–70
  molecular components 61
  positive effects 152, 153
  removal of antigen 152, 153
  structure 61–4
  valence and avidity 63, *64*
  see also antibody genes;
    antibody response;
    immunoglobulins
antibody dependent cellular
    cytotoxicity (ADCC) 96,
    97
antibody genes 68, 69–70
  rearrangement 68, 70–2
antibody-mediated protection
    171–2
antibody response
  cellular basis of 108–11
  cross-reactive responses 108,
    111
  in different tissues 112–14
  multiclonal responses 108, 110
  primary and memory
    responses 108, 109–10
  selection and activation of B
    cells 108–9
antigen 7
  affinity purification of 87, 91–2
  dose of, tolerance and 149, 151
  excess 84
  range of 9
  removal by antibody 152, 153
  structure 9–11
  in tolerance 149
  in vaccines 177–8, **178**
antigen processing and
    presenting cells (APCs)
    54, *54*, 134–5
  in vaccination 180
antigenic determinants
    (epitopes) 9, 10, *10*, 11
antigenic drift 169
antigenic mimicry 219

antigenic shifts 169
antigenic variation 167
antinuclear antibodies (ANA)
    231
apoptosis (programmed cell
    death) 15, 16, 93, 287
Arthus reaction 208, *209*
aspirin 202
asthma 67, 202
autoantigens 204, 206, 217, 219,
    220
autoantibodies
    formation of damaging
        immune complexes 227,
        229
    mediation of cell destruction
        227, 228–9
    modulation of cell function
        227
autoimmune disease
    diagnosis 231–2
    factors leading to
        development of 217–21,
        218
    age and gender 217, 218
    autoantigens 204, 206, 217,
        219, **220**
    drugs and autoimmune
        reactions 217, 219
    genetic factors 217, 218–19
    immunodeficiency 217,
        220–1
    infections 217, 219
    mechanisms of development
        222–6
    availability of normally
        sequestered self-antigen
        222, 226
    breakdown of self-tolerance
        222, 223
    defective regulation
        mediated via Th cells 222,
        223–5, *224*
    dysregulation of idiotype
        network 223, 226, *226*
    modification of cell surfaces
        by microbes/drugs 222,
        225–6
    molecular mimicry and T
        cell bypass 222, 223
    polyclonal activation vs
        microbial antigens 222,
        225
    pathogenesis 227–30
    prevalence 215, 216
    replacement therapy 231, 232,
        232
    spectrum 215, 216

suppression of autoimmune
    process 231, 232–3, **232**
tissue damaging reactions in
    227, 228
autoimmune hemolytic anaemia
    (AIHA) 204, 206, 227, 228,
    228
autoimmune thrombocytopenias
    232
autoimmune thyroiditis 232
autoimmunity 215–16
    suppression of 231, 232–3, **232**

B cell anergy 147, *148*
B cell co-receptor 99, 100
    signaling by 99, 101
B cell deficiencies,
    immunodeficiences and
    187, **187**
B cell receptor (BCR) complex
    99, *100*
B cells 5, 7–8, 41, 42, 44–7
    activation 102–7
        biochemical events leading
        to 102, 105–7
        plasma cells 46
        through T cell independent
        antigens *103*, *104*
    bone marrow and B cell
        ontogeny 44–6
    characteristics **42**
    conventional 45
    development and selection
        75–7
    expression of IgM and IgD on
        73
    generation of antigen receptor
        diversity and negative
        selective ion B cells 46
    life history *76*
    surface receptors on **47**
    traffic and recirculation 56
    types 102, *103*
B lymphocytes *see* B cells
B1 cells 102, 103
B2 cells 102, 103
bacteria
    hypersensitivity 210
    immunity to 162, 163
    intracellular 163
    vaccines 181
    *see also under individual
        organisms*; pathogen
        defense strategies
basophils 15, 16, 20–1
Bc cell tolerance 146
bee sting allergy 199
benadryl 202

bird fancier's disease 208
bispecific antibodies (BcAbs) in
    tumors 262, 265
blood, antibody response in 112
blood group antigens 237–8, **237**
bone marrow 48–9
    grafts 242, **242**
    transplants 192, 195
Bordetella pertussis toxin 175
Borrelia burgdorferi 219
breast, lactating 275–6, *276*
breast milk, antibodies in 276–7
bronchus-associated lymphoid
    tissue (BALT) 53, 55
Brucella 163
Bruton's agammaglobulinemia
    105
Bruton's disease 185, 187
Burkitt's lymphoma 249

Candida albicans infection 274
carbohydrate recognition
    domains (CRDs) 34
carcinoembryonic antigen (CEA)
    251
carriers 11
CD3 42, 44
CD8+ 134–5
CD14 35
CD28 290, 291
CD79 42
cecropins 3, 32
cell-mediated immunity 138–9,
    139, 171, 172–3
    deficiencies and 185, 187–8,
    188
central tolerance 145–6, *146*
cervical carcinoma 266
chemokines 7, 24, 27, 30–1, **31**
chemotaxis 15
chemotaxis assays 194
chlortrimaton 202
chronic granulomatous disease
    (CGD) 192, 195
cilia 2
classical pathway 23, 26, 93, 94
clonal deletion 145
clonal expansion 132–3
clonal selection 7, *8*
coeliac disease 217, 228
colicins 4
collectins 24, 31, 32
colony-stimulating factors
    (CSFs) 24
colostrum, antibodies in 276–7
common variable
    immunodeficiency
    (CVID) 185, 187

complement system 7, 23, 25–6, 25, **25**
  activation leading to cell lysis **94**
  C3b 17–18, 25–6, 27
  deficiencies 185, **186**
  immunodeficiency and 185
  inactivation of 170
congenital/primary (inherited) immunodeficiency 183, 184, 185–8
conglutinin 32
contact sensitivity 212, **212**, 213
Coomb's test 85
  indirect 86
cortisol 295–6
co-stimulatory molecules 127, 128–9
C-reactive protein (CRP) 23, 26, 27
Crohn's disease 212, 228, 290
cromolyn 202
cross-reactivity 111
cyclosporin A 232, 242
cytokines 7, 23–4, 26, 27–31, **31**
  immunization and 177, 180
  inhibition of 169
  range of 12, 13
cytolytic T lymphocytes (CTL) 28
cytotoxic T cells 132, 135–7
  mechanisms of cytotoxicity 136–7, 136
  recognition of antigen and activation 135–6

defensins 3, 16, 18, 32
dehydroepiandrosterone (DHEA) 295
dehydroepiandrosterone sulfate (DHEAS) 295
delayed (type IV) hypersensitivity 194, 210–13
dendritic cell vaccines 268
dendritic cells 15, 21–2, 21, **22**
desensitization 199, 202–3, 203
dexamethasone 202
Di George syndrome 185
diabetes 215, 227, 232
dimetane 202
diphtheria, pertussis and tetanus (DPT) vaccine 181
DNA vaccines 177, 179
DNA viruses, oncogenic 142, **143**
dramamine 202
dSR-C1 35

elephantiasis 165
ELISPOT assay 91
endocytosis 35
endogeneous pathway 117, 122
enzyme-linked immunosorbent assays (ELISA) 87, 88, 91, 193, 231
  sandwich 91
eosin 16
eosinophils 15, 16, 22
epinephrine 202
epitopes (antigenic determinants) 9, 10, 10, 11
Epstein–Barr virus 153, 169, 249
equivalence 83, 84
erythrocytes 15, 22
Escherichia coli 1, 35, 181
  toxin 175
estradiol 279
estrogen, effect on immune function 279–80, **280**
exogenous pathway 118, 122
exons 69
experimental allergic encephalomyelitis (EAE) 230

Factor B 94
Factor D 94
Farmer's lung 208
Fas-mediated apoptosis 136, 137
FasL 20
faulty genes in immunodeficiency 195
FcRγRIII 19
FcεR 20
female reproductive tract 271–2, 272
  immunity in 273
  localization of immune cells 271–2
'fetal transplant' 243, 247, 247, 274
filariasis 165
flow cytometry 87, 88–9, 91
fluorescence-activated cell sorter 87, 90
follicular dendritic cells (FDC) 15, 21
fungi, immunity to 162, 165
Fv libraries 81–2, 82

gender
  autoimmune disease and 217, 218
  immune system and 269–70, **269**
gene therapy 192, 195

genetic control of immune responses 155–6
genetic factors, autoimmune disease and 217, 218–19
germinal centers as sites of B cell maturation 112, 113–14
glandular fever 153
gliadin 217
glucocorticoids 40, 157, 202, 232
Goodpasture's syndrome 204, 206, 228, 229
graft rejection
  cross-matching 243, 245–6, 246
  drugs to suppress **246**
  familial grafting 243
  'fetal transplant' 243, 247, 247, 274
  immunosuppression 243, 246–7, **246**
  prevention of 243–7
  tissue typing 243, 244–5, 245
graft versus host reaction 242, **242**
granulocyte-colony stimulating factor (G-CSF) 12, 13, 24, 31
granulocyte-monocyte CSF (GM-CSF) 24, 31
granulomas, production 211–12, 212
granzymes 20
Graves' disease (hyperthyroidism) 204, 207, 207, 215, 217, 218, 227, 229
growth hormone 157
guanine nucleoside exchange factors (GEFS) 131
gut-associated lymphoid tissue (GALT) 53, 54–5

H chains
  genes and translocation 70
  synthesis and assembly 68, 72
Haemophilus 181
  humoral immunity and 187
  vaccines 175
haptens 11
Hashimoto's thyroiditis 228, 231, 269
hayfever 67, 199, 201, 202
heavy chain (HH) 61–3
Helicobacter 181
Helicobacter pylori 159
helper T cells 132, 133–5, 133
  Th1 cells 134–5
    in induction of cytotoxicity by CD8+ CTLs 134–5

helper T cells – *continued*
   in isotype switching and
      affinity maturation 134
   in macrophage recruitment
      and activation 134
   Th2 cells 134
hemolytic anemia 216
hemolytic disease of the
      newborn (HDN) 153, 204,
      205–6
hemopoiesis 12, *13*
   aging and 285
hemopoietic stem cell (HSC) 12,
      13, *13*, 43
hepatitis B
   vaccines 266
   virus 249
herpes simplex virus 175
herpes virus glycoprotein D 180
herpes zoster (shingles) 283, 294
high endothelial venules (HEV)
      56
high zone tolerance 151
histaminase 22
histamine 38
histamine receptor antagonists
      202
hormone replacement therapy
      281
hormones 7
host versus graft reaction 242,
      242
human herpes virus 8 (HHV8)
      249
human immunodeficiency virus
      (HIV) 1, 6, 159, 189–90
   vaccine 182
human leukocyte antigens
      (HLA)
   alleles **238**
   HLA-E 19
human papilloma virus (HPV)
      175
   vaccine 266
human T cell leukemia virus
      (HTLV) 249
humoral immunity 185, 187
   aging and 292–3
5′-hydroxytryptamine (5HT)156
hypergammaglobulinemia 219
hyper-IgM syndrome 185, 192
hypersensitivity
   classification 197–8, **198**
   definition 197
   pathogens **161**
hyperthyroidism (Graves′
      disease) 204, 207, *207*, 215,
      217, 218, 227, 229

idiotype network 152, 154
idiotypes 78–9
IgA 3, 65, 66–7
   in breast milk 276–7
   in female reproductive tract
      273
   maternal 59
   in the newborn 59
   in vaccines 172
Igα 99, 100
Igβ 99, 100
IgD 65, 67
IgE 65, 67
IgE-mediated (type I)
      hypersensitivity 199–203
   common antigens causing
      201–2, **202**
   effector phase 201
   sensitization phase 199, 200
IgG 65, 66
   in female reproductive tract
      273
   maternal 59, *60*
   negative feedback by 152, 153
   in the newborn 59
   structure *62*
   in vaccines 172
IgG-mediated (type II)
      (cytotoxic)
      hypersensitivity 204–7
IgM 59, 65, 67
IgM-mediated (type II)
      (cytotoxic)
      hypersensitivity 204–7
immune-complex-mediated
      (type III) hypersensitivity
      208–9
   associated diseases 208, 209,
      209
   mechanisms 208
immune complexes 83–6
   in vitro 83–4
   in vivo 83, 84
   and tissue damage 83, 84
immune effector mechanisms,
      inactivation of 169–70
immune response genes, aging
      and 294, 295
immune senescence 189, 190–1
immune system 5, 6
   components 183–4
   defects in specific immune
      components 184
   evaluation of different
      components **193**
   evaluation of specific immune
      therapy 192, 193–4
   maturity of 149, 150

immune thrombocytopenic
      purpura (ITP) 227, *228*, 229
immunity
   to bacteria 162, 163, *163*, *164*
   to fungi (mycoses) 162, 165
   to protozoa 162, 165
   to virus 162, 163–4, *164*
   to worms 162, 165–6
immunization 174–6
   active 174, 175
   mucosal 174, 175–6
   passive 174, **175**
   principles of 171
   systemic 174, 175
   see also tumor vaccines
immunoassay 87–92
immunoblotting 87, 90–1
immunodeficiency 6
   autoimmune disease and 217,
      220–1
   classification 183, 184
   diagnosis and treatment 192–5
   family history 192
immunodiagnosis 256–8
   classification 256
   imaging 256, 258
   monitoring 256–7
immunoelectrophoresis 85, 193
immunofluorescence 87, 88–9
   direct 88
   indirect 89
immunogens 9, 11, 150
immunoglobulin 7, 61
   gene superfamily 62
   properties **62**
   see also entries under Ig
immunological synapse 127, 129
immunological tolerance 141
immunosenescence *see* aging
immunotoxins (ITs) in tumors
      262, 265
immuno-tyrosine activation
      motifs (ITAMs) 99, 101,
      131
indirect Coomb′s test 86
indomethicin 202
infections, autoimmune disease
      and 217, 219
infectious mononucleosis 222,
      225
infectious organisms, range of **1**
   see also bacteria
inflammation 36, 37
   acute 37, *37*
   chronic 37
   initiation of 36, 37–8
   termination of response and
      repair 39–40

vascular changes 36, 38–9
inflammatory bowel disease
    216
influenza 159, 291
innate immune system 5, 6, **6**, 7
    aging and 288
    cells of 15–22
    inflammation and 36–40
    molecules of 23–32
innate molecular immune
    defence 23, 24
integrins 30
intercellular adhesion molecules
    (ICAMs) 128
interdigitating cells (IDC) 15, 21,
    22
interferons (IFNs) 23, 27–8, **28**
    IFNα 20, 23, 27, 28
    IFNβ 20, 23, 27, 28
    IFNγ (immune IFN) 15, 20, 23,
        26, 27, 28
interleukin 27
    IL-1 13, 24, 26, 27, 30
    IL-2 20, 23, 29
    IL-3 13, 23, 29
    IL-4 24, 29
        IgE response to 200, *200*
    IL-5 24, 29
    IL-6 24, 26, 27, 30
    IL-8 24, 30
    IL-10 24
    IL-12 24, 30
isohemagglutinins 204, 237, **237**

Jenner, Edward 171
juvenile arthritis 269

Kaposi's sarcoma 190, 249
kidney graft rejection 241, **241**
killer activation receptors
    (KARs) 19
killer inhibitory receptors (KIRs)
    19
Kupffer cells 22

L chains
    genes and translocation *71, 72*
    synthesis and assembly 68, *72*
La Crosse fever 182
lactation, role in immune
    defense 275–7
    localization of immune cells in
        lactating breast 275–6, *276*
lactobacilli 4
Langerhans cells (LH) 15, 21, 22
large granular lymphocytes
    (LGLs) *see* natural killer
    cells

lectins 20
Legionella 159
leishmaniasis 165
leprosy (*Mycobacterium leprae*)
    211
leptin 295
leucine-rich repeat (LRR)
    domain 35
leukemias
    acute lymphocytic (ALLs) **257**
    lymphocytic 249
    subgrouping *257*
leukocyte function antigen (LFA-
    1) 7
light chains (LH) 61–2
lipid rafts 101, 129
Listeria monocytogenes 163
low zone tolerance 151
LOX-1 35
Lyme arthritis 219
Lyme's disease 181
lymph nodes 48, 51–2, *51*
lymphatics, antibody response
    in 112, 113
lymphocyte function-associated
    antigens (LFAs) 128
lymphocyte stem cells (LSC) 44
lymphocytes 7, 41–7, *42*
    in the newborn 59
    specificity and memory 41–2
    traffic and recirculation 56–8,
        57
lymphocytic choriomeningitis
    virus (LCMV) 226
lymphocytic leukemia 249
lymphoid complexes 55, *55*
lymphoid organs 48–52, *49*
    primary and secondary 48
lymphoid stem cell (LSC) *13*
lymphoid tissue, structure of *50*
lymphokine-activated killer
    (LAK) cells 20, 259, 260,
        260
lymphokines 23–4, 27, 29, **29**
lysozyme 2

macrophage-activated killer
    (MAK) cells 261
macrophages 7, 15, 17
    aging and 288, 289, **289**
    surface receptors on **18**
magainins 3, 32
major histocompatibility
    complex (MHC) 155
    antigens 237, 238–9, *238*
    binding peptide 117, 121
    cellular distribution 117, 121–2
    class I genes 117, 120, *120*

class I processing pathways
    117, 122
class II genes 117, 120–1, *120*
class II processing pathways
    118, 122–3
linear amino acid sequences
    10, *10*
structure 117, 120–1
malaria (*Plasmodium*) 165, 182
male reproductive tract 275,
    277–8, *277*
mannose-binding protein (MBP)
    23, 26, 27, 31–2
mannose receptor 34–5
Mantoux test 211
MARCO 35
mast cells 15, 20–1, *20*, 24
    degranulation, IgE-mediated
        201, *201*
    in inflammation 38, *39*
measles 160
    virus 170
membrane attack complex
    (MAC) 26, 94
    components, deficiencies in
        185
memory cells 7
Meningococcus vaccines 175
menstrual cycle, immunological
    changes during 271,
        273–4
mercuric chloride 216
mesothelioma 249
microbes 1
    damage caused by 159, 160–1
    habitat and immune defence
        159, 160
    pathogen protective
        mechanisms 159, 160
    physical barriers to entry 2
    products and competitions 3–4
minor histocompatibility
    antigens 237, 239, 240
mixed lymphocyte reaction
    (response) 244
molecular mimicry 169, 222, 223
monoclonal antibodies 80–2
    fully human 81
    humanization and
        chimerization 80–1
    humanized 81–2, *82*
    preparation 80, *81*
    specificity to tumors 262–3
monocyte chemotactic protein
    (MCP-1) 30
monocyte colony-stimulating
    factor (M-CSF) 12, 13, 24,
        31

monocytes 15, 17, *17*
  aging and 288, 289, **289**
  surface receptors on **18**
monokines 24, 27, 29–30, **29**
mononuclear phagocyte system
    17, **17**
mucin 2
mucociliary escalator 2, *3*
mucosa, antibody response in
    112–13
mucosa-associated lymphoid
    tissues (MALT) 48,53–5
  trafficking in 56–7
mucus 2–3
multideterminant molecules 9
multiple sclerosis (MS) 215, 216,
    227
muramyl dipeptide (MDP) 16
myasthenia gravis (MG) 204,
    206, *206*, 227, 229, 231
Mycobacterium lepri 182
Mycobacterium tuberculosis
    (MTb), immune responses
    to 210
mycoses, immunity to 162, 165
Mylotarg 265

naive cells 56
nasal-associated lymphoid tissue
    (NALT) 53, *54*, 175
nasopharyngeal carcinoma 249
natural killer cells (large
    granular lymphocytes;
    LGLs) 15, 18–20, *19*, 41
  aging and 288, 289
  surface receptors on **19**
necrosis 137
negative selection 145
Neisseria 35, 186
  complement deficiencies and
    185, 186
Neisseria gonorrhoeae 170
neuroendocrine system (HPA
    axis) 155, 157–8
neutrophils 15, 16, *16*
  aging and 288, 289
newborn, antibodies in 59–60
NFAT (nuclear factor of
    activated T cells) 131
nitroblue tetrazolium (NBT) test
    194
nonpathogenic bacteria
    (commensals) 2, 3
noradrenaline (norepinephrine)
    157, 295–6
NSAIDS 202, 232
nuclear factor of activated T
    cells (NFAT) 131

opsonins 17, 31
opsonization 17, 27
origin and host defense against
    tumors 249

passive immunity 172
pathogen defence strategies
    167–70, **168**
  antigen processing 170
  avoidance of recognition 167,
    168–9
    antigenic variation 169
    intracellular habitat 168–9
  inactivation of immune
    effector mechanisms
    169–70
    antibodies 169–70
    complement system 170
    inhibition of cytokines 169
    phagocytosis 169
    T cells 170
  regulatory mechanisms 170
pattern recognition receptors
    33–4, *34*, **34**
penicillin 204
  IgG response to 207
pentraxins 26
peptide antibiotics 3
perforin-induced apoptosis 136
perforins 20
periarteriolar lymphatic sheath
    50
peripheral tolerance 145, 146–8
pernicious anemia 215, 216, 232
peroxidase 16
Peyer's patches 53
phagocytes 6, 15, 16–18, 93
phagocytosis 15, 17, **18**, 169
  assays 194
  defects in 185, 186–7, **186**
plague 159
plasma cell 7
  activated B cells and 46
  ultrastructure *46*
Plasmodium falciparum 165
Plasmodium vivax 165
platelets 15, 22
Pneumococcus 181
  complement deficiencies and
    185
  humoral immunity and 187
  vaccines 175
pneumocystis 190
polio 182
polymorphonuclear cells
    (PMNs) 15, 16, *16*
  in inflammation 36, 38
  surface receptors on **16**

polyvinyl chloride 216
positive selection 145
Prausnitz–Kustner test 200
precipitation assays 83, 84–5
prednisolone 202
pregnancy, immune-associated
    changes during 274–5
primary biliary cirrhosis 269
primary/congenital (inherited)
    immunodeficiency 183,
    184, 185–8
procainamide 216
progesterone, effect on immune
    function 279–80
programmed cell death
    (apoptosis) 15, 16, 93, 287
prolactin 157
prostate-specific antigen (PSA)
    258
protein C 40
proteoglycans 2
protozoa
  immunity to 162, 165
  vaccines to 181, 182
Pseudomonas 170

radial immunodiffusion 85, 193
radioimmunoassay (RIA) 87, 88,
    193
receptor-ligand interactions 99,
    100–1
recombinant vaccines 177, 180
regulatory proteins of
    complement system **96**
rejection, transplant 240–2
  as adaptive immune response
    240
  allografts 240–1
  donor rejection of host tissues
    240, 242
  types of pattern 241, **241**
  xenotransplant 240, 242
reticuloendothelial system 17
rhesus factors 153
rhesus incompatibility 204,
    205–6
Rhesus D antigen (RhD) 205–6,
    205
rheumatic fever, group A
    streptococci and *224*
rheumatoid arthritis (RA) 27,
    215, 216, 231, 269
RNA viruses, oncogenic 142,
    143
rocket immunoelectrophoresis
    85
route of administration,
    tolerance and 149, 150–1

Salmonella 35
Salmonella typhi 163
sandwich ELISA 91
sarcoidosis 212
scavenger receptors (SR) 35
Schistosoma 169
Schistosoma mansoni 165
schistosomiasis 165, 182
scleroderma 216
scrotal cancer 249
secondary (acquired)
    immunodeficiency 189–91
    factors causing 189, **190**
secretions at epithelial surfaces
    2–3, **3**
self-non-self discrimination by
    innate immune system
    141, 142–3
    complement system 142–3
    natural killer cells 142
    phagocytes 142
sequestered antigens 146
serum amyloid protein A (SAA)
    23, 26, 27
serum sickness 208
severe acute respiratory
    syndrome (SARS) virus
    159
severe combined
    immunodeficiency (SCID)
    185, 187, 192, 195
shingles 283, 294
signal transduction 127, 129
single cell suspensions 90
Sjögren's syndrome 281
smallpox 160
sodium dedecyl sulfate
    polyacrylamide gel
    electrophoresis (SDS-
    PAGE) 87, 90
somatostatin 40
spleen 48, 50–1
SR-A I and II 35
SR-CL I and II 35
staphylococcal enterotoxins (SE)
    127, 129
Staphylococcus aureus 35
stem cell factor (SCF) 12, 13
stimulatory and inhibitory
    cytokines 155, 156–7
stimulatory hypersensitivity 204,
    207
streptococcal nephritis 208
Streptococcus
    complement deficiencies and
    185
    humoral immunity and 187
stromal cells 12–13

role in hemopoiesis *13*
substance P 157
switch regions 73
systemic lupus erythematosus
    (SLE) 208, 215, 216, 217,
    218, 230, 231, 269
    kidney failure in 228, 229, 230
systemic vasculitis 216

T cell receptor (TCR) 44, 117,
    118–19
    alpha/beta (αβ) T cells 118
    gamma/delta (γδ) T cells
    118–19
T cell receptor complex 117,
    119–20, *119*
T cells 5, 7–8, 41, 42, 43–4
    activation 127–31
    activation through T cell
    independent antigens *104*
    aging and 290–1
    anergy 146–7, *147*
    bypass 222, 223–5, *224*
    characteristics **42**
    diversity, generation of 124–5
    generation in the thymus 43
    inactivation of 170
    mature T cells and their
    subsets 44
    ontogeny 43
    positive and negative
    selection 43
    recognition of antigen 117–23
    role in immune responses
    115–16
    selection of repertoire 124,
    125–6
    surface receptors on **45**
    thymus function 43
    traffic and recirculation 56
T cytotoxic (Tc) cells 42
T helper (Th) cells 42, 155, 156
T lymphocytes *see* T cells
Tamoxifen 279
testosterone, effect on immune
    function 279, 280, **280**
tetanus toxin 208
theophyline 202
thrombocytopenia 222, 225
thymic involution 286, 287
thymocytes 43
thymosin α1 280
thymus 48, 49–50
thymus-dependent (T-D)
    antigens 102, 104–5
thymus-independent (T-I)
    antigens 8, 102, 103–4
    type 1 103

type 2 103–4
thyroid autoimmune disease 216
thyroid growth-stimulating
    immunoglobulin (TGSI)
    229
thyroid peroxidase antibodies
    231
thyroiditis 215, 216
thyrotropin binding-inhibitory
    immunoglobulin (TBII)
    229
Toll-like receptors (TLRs) 35
Toll proteins 35
toxic shock syndrome toxin
    (TSST) 127, 129
Toxoplasma 165
toxoplasmosis 165
transferrin 2
transforming growth factor β
    (TGFβ) 24
transfusion reactions 204, 206
transglutaminase (tTG) 217, 219
transplantation
    antigens 237–9
    bone marrow 192, 195
    'fetal' 243, 247, *247*, 274
    historical perspective 235
    purging of bone marrow for
    analogous 262, 265
    rejection and 235–6
    rejection mechanisms 240–2
    types of grafts 235–6, **235**
trauma, acquired
    immunodeficiency and
    189, 191
trypanosomiasis 165, 169, 182
tuberculin reaction 210, 211, *211*
tuberculosis 159, 283
    multi-drug resistance 159
    vaccine 181
tumor antigens 250–2
    differentiation 251, **252**
    oncofetal 250, 251, **251**
    virally or chemically induced
    250, **251**
tumor-associated antigens 250
tumor escape 253, 254–5
tumor growth factor β (TgFβ) 31
tumor-infiltrating lymphocytes
    (TILs) 259, 260–1
tumor necrosis factor α (TNFα)
    24, 26, 30
tumor necrosis factor β (TNFβ)
    24
tumor-specific antigens 250
tumor vaccines 181, 182, 266–8
    with APCs loaded with TAA
    266, 267

tumor vaccines – *continued*
  prophylactic vs therapeutic 266
  with transfected tumors 266,
    267
  with tumors and tumor
    antigens 266–7
tumors
  cytokine and cellular
    immunotherapy 259–61
  immunostimulation and
    cytokines 259
  origin and host defense
    against 249
  see also tumors, immune
    responses; tumors,
    immunotherapy with
    antibodies
tumors, immune responses to
  253–5

effector mechanisms 253, 254,
  254
immune surveillance 253
tumor escape 253, 254–5
tumors, immunotherapy with
  antibodies 262–5
with antibodies alone 262,
  263–4
with bispecific antibodies
  (BcAbs) 262, 265
with immunotoxins (ITs) 262,
  265
purging of bone marrow for
  analogous transplants
  262, 265
specificity of mAbs to tumors
  262–3

vaccination *see* immunization

vasoactive intestinal peptide
  (VIP) 40, 157
vasodilation 38
Vibrio 181
viral vaccines 181, 182
virus, immunity to 162, 163–4
vitiligo 215, 216

Wegener's granulomatosis 232
worms, immunity to 162, 165–6
Wuchereria bancrofti 165

xenografts 236
xenotransplant 240, 242,

yellow fever 182